Naturals and Organics in Cosmetics: Trends and Technology

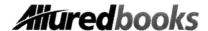

Naturals and Organics in Cosmetics: Trends and Technology

ISBN: 978-1-932633-71-9

Editorial

Book Editor:	Angela C. Kozlowski
Indexer:	Joy Dean Lee
Cover Design:	Bryan Crowe
Interior Design:	Bryan Crowe
Page Layout:	Bryan Crowe

Administration

Publisher:	Marian Raney
Book Sales Executive:	Marie Kuta
Book Coordinator and Web Support:	Anita Singh

Allured books

Allured Business Media
336 Gundersen Drive, Suite A, Carol Stream, IL 60188 USA
Tel: 630-653-2155 Fax: 630-653-2192
www.AlluredBooks.com
E-mail: books@allured.com

Table of Contents

Introduction

Over the last thirty years, the personal care market has undergone many trends, embraced many fads and responded to many consumer demands. Some trends were a flash in the pan; others have come and gone many times without becoming firmly established. After all, our business is in many ways the convergence of technology and fashion. The consumer has the final say as to the direction of our market.

Some market trends become so entrenched that they become a permanent part of our industry. In past times these trends have been established by regulations and product safety. Products have ceased to be used in particular applications or have been banned in one or more applications based upon safety. A good example of this type of change in our industry is preservatives. In the 1970s, formaldehyde was an accepted, commonly used preservative. Today it is absolutely forbidden. David Steinberg; long-time expert in cosmetic preservation has often stated, "Booze and formaldehyde are the only two preservatives that nature produces!" This change in our industry is a permanent one. There is no chance that we will revert to formaldehyde as a preservative.

The move toward green, sustainable, natural products is a trend that has been growing over the years. The permanence of a particular idea or concept can only be established over a long period of time, but it is fair to say this movement will be with us for a long time.

Malcolm Gladwell, in his now classic book *The Tipping Point: How Little Things Can Make a Big Difference* describes tipping points as points in time when "the levels at which the momentum for change becomes unstoppable."[1] I believe we are at a tipping point relative to green chemistry. This does not mean that the concept will not evolve.

As one looks at this compilation, several things become apparent:

The concept is evolving. The older articles in this compilation show that the concepts of what is green was both new and not terribly clear. Even the newer articles do not show uniformity of concept.

The definitions are developing. Many competing terms have been used to describe the products of interest. They include the terms "green", "sustainable", "renewable", "natural", "non-petro" and many others. What they mean, how they are used, what products can be classified in that way and by whom are topics that continue to be debated and defined.

The target is changing. Is green a process or a place? In other words, do we treat green as a process of continual rethinking and re-formulation to make our product with the best green profile consistent with consumer expectations, or is there one final target that makes the product acceptable, independent of the consumer? What about cost, how much is a consumer willing to pay for the added benefit of improved greenness? How does one measure green? Will research and development actively search out and develop green products?

The consumer will ultimately determine what is successful. All these questions will be determined by the consumer and what sells in the market. Will the woman at the fashion show in Paris or New York wash her hair with soap, even if it is natural? Clearly, the product needs to meets the consumer demand, not merely be green.

Finally, it is suggested that you keep an open but skeptical mind. By that I mean question the most basic assumption. Everything needs to pass the reality test of "does it make sense?" And "will the consumer buy it?"

In a speech in Cape Town, South Africa, on June, 7 1966, Robert F. Kennedy said, "There is a Chinese curse which says, 'May we live in interesting times'. Like it or not, we live in interesting times..." There has been some debate as to where this saying originated, but there is no debate of its accuracy. The corollary of this is "embrace interesting times, become part of them."

Tony O'Lenick
February 25, 2010

References

1. Malcolm Gladwell, *The Tipping Point: How Little Things Can Make a Big Difference*, Little Brown (2000)

CHAPTER 1

Current Status

Tim Kapsner

Aveda Corp., Blaine, Minn., USA

As Kermit so famously said, it's not easy being green. But it certainly is increasingly popular, for consumers as well as marketers. Environmental awareness has seeped into and permeated most aspects of society, culture and trade. It has become a big part of the advertising and marketing scene as consumers' increased interest in health and wellness, as well as this increased concern for the environment, has fueled the move to buy products that make environmental, natural, or organic claims.

While the overall market for cosmetics in the United States is very mature and experiencing slow growth in the range of 1 to 3%, the sector of cosmetics making environmental, natural or organic claims ("green claims", "green products" or the "green cosmetics market") is projected to experience double digit growth for the foreseeable future[1]. Although representing only a small segment of the market (3 to 10% in most product categories), the fast growth of the green cosmetics market is both a cause and an effect of increasing attention by marketers. The green product trend has moved into the mainstream in most consumer product categories. In the cosmetics markets, the large multinationals are either buying smaller green product brands or launching their own green product lines, or both. Green claims are increasingly popular in all marketing channels, from prestige to drug stores.

Imaginative researchers in progressive companies are pushing the envelope in the use of plant-based ingredients. Topics as diverse as natural insect repellants, carotenoids for skin brightening and anti-inflammatory effects of magnolia are explored in the articles contained herein. New cosmetic products in the marketplace are using many food ingredients, such as acai and papain, and other ingredients derived from plants, such as USP salicylic acid made from oil of wintergreen. Glucosides and polyglyceryl esters are replacing ethoxylates and propoxylates in emulsions. Ingredients derived from plants, marine biology, algae, yeasts, enzymes and bacteria are found in many cosmetic products. The opportunities are limited only by the reach of the imagination.

The use of plant ingredients is not new to the current generation of formulators. The protein/fatty acid condensate surfactants were developed shortly after World War II. Their mildness helped inspire Madge the manicurist to soak several generations of clients' fingertips in that famous green dish soap. These types of ingredients, however, have been improved dramatically since those early days. The breakthrough of making amino acids by fermentation instead of hydrolyzing proteins has allowed these dark brown smelly ingredients (remember Potassium Coco-Hydrolyzed Animal Protein?) to evolve into much more elegant, albeit still relatively expensive, surfactants whose use has blossomed in foaming cosmetic cleansers. A mind-boggling array of cosmetic esters has been used by several generations of formulators to produce many elegant effects. One of the articles in this volume, "Bio-based Esters for a Smaller Footprint", shows that a new green frontier exists even for this relatively mature technology.

The growth in the green product category has included the development of various natural and organic standards by governments and private organizations. Some think that it is taking the cosmetics industry forever to develop a system for standardization. It's easy to forget, however, looking over from our industry's paroxysms of passion and strife in this area that it took the food industry decades to achieve their current state of relative peace and harmony. It's also easy to miss the fact that words and concepts like "synthetic" and "nonagricultural", so central to the natural and organic claims of both the food and cosmetic industries, are still adding "spice" to the food industry and creating conflict after almost a decade of government regulation

The organic food industry started from a vision to improve the environmental sustainability of food production and also as a way to increase the value and profit margins of food products. The origins of the movement can be glimpsed as early as the 1920's, when farmers were still selling directly to consumers[2]. As the organic market grew and became more complex, the desire to standardize organic claims led to the development of many private certification standards for food throughout the world. Eventually, government regulation resulted after key principles and practices resulted from these private standards. In the three major markets, the United States, Europe and Japan, organic food claims have been regulated by government standards for about a decade.

The development of cosmetic standards has also been pioneered by the private sector. One of the most widely recognized natural cosmetic standards in Europe was created by BDIH, the Association of German Industries and Trading Firms (*www.kontrollierte-naturkosmetik.de/e/index_e.htm*), which works in the pharmaceutical, health care, food supplement and cosmetics industries. Ecocert, one of the EU's largest organic food certifiers, also certifies products to a private cosmetic standard (www.ecocert.com/-Cosmetics-.html), created by Cosmebio, another cosmetics industry trade organization. After many years of certifying to this standard, Ecocert led a group of European certifiers in the creation of a new organization called the European Cosmetics Standards Working Group. Their standard, called COSMOS (www.cosmos-standard.org), is in development. NaTrue (www.natrue.org) is the other major player in the European cosmetic standards arena. Originally created to help influence the government in its eventual move to regulate these claims, NaTrue formed an alliance with IKW, the German Cosmetics, Toiletry, Perfumery and Detergent Association. Soon after this, the new group (which retained the NaTrue name) announced that it was developing its own standard for organic and natural cosmetics. These two groups, NaTrue and COSMOS, have emerged as the major European forces in the future of natural and organic cosmetic certification.

The US has also seen a great deal of activity in this area. A task force with representation across the industry was adopted by the

Organic Trade Association early in the new millennium to create a standard for certified organic cosmetics. The baton was eventually passed on to NSF (*www.nsf.org*), which recently finalized a standard. Another trade organization, OASIS (Organic and Sustainable Industry Standards, *www.oasisseal.org*) was created to foster education, communication and collaboration among green cosmetic companies. It launched that effort by drafting an organic cosmetic standard. The Natural Products Association (*www.naturalproductsassoc.org*) also has a standard, this one for cosmetic marketers that want to make "natural" claims for their products. The USDA's National Organic Program (NOP, *www.ams.usda.gov/nop*), which sets the US standard for organic claims for agricultural products, may also be used to certify qualifying cosmetic products. This highlights two interesting differences in the way this process has evolved in Europe compared to the US. Most of the major cosmetic standards in Europe have provisions addressing both "organic" and "natural" claims within the same standard. In the US, by contrast, separate standards (and organizations administering them) have developed for "natural" and "organic" claims. In the US, the government regulated organic food standard (the NOP, run by the USDA) can be used to certify a cosmetic product that meets its organic standard. In the EU and Japan, the government regulated food standard cannot be used to certify cosmetics. These differences have had a significant effect on how the marketplace has developed for these products.

In addition to the standards discussed above, all cosmetic product claims, including their natural and organic status, are regulated by the Federal Trade Commission (FTC) through the Fair Package and Labeling Act. This act requires any claim on the packaging and labeling of any retail product to be truthful and not misleading. In addition, the Lanham Act requires advertising to be truthful and not misleading. This fundamental requirement is enforced not only by FTC but by the National Advertising Division of the Better Business Bureau (the NAD) through both competitive challenges and challenges brought directly by the NAD as part of its routine monitoring of the marketplace.

So where are the frontiers of green cosmetic products? The most widely recognized and consumer friendly claims may still be "natural" and "organic"; some of the newer ones on the horizon are "green" (from the Twelve Principles of Green Chemistry[3]), "sustainable" and "Cradle to Cradle"[4]. Responsibly drawing from cultures around the world can by done by sourcing ingredients from traditional/native/ indigenous communities, as well as by adapting the vast knowledge of traditional Chinese medicinal practices and Ayurveda. Words and phrases recently added to the discussion are "biomimetics", "carbon footprint", and "life cycle analysis". These concepts and technologies will lead us in new and exciting directions for many years to come, as all of these approaches are used to move our industry further down the path to products that are simultaneously more environmentally responsible and highly functional.

Of course we can't ignore the question of whether "green" in its many guises, is a trend or a new reality. One of the answers to that question is a single word: authenticity. Consumers are pretty smart and can often distinguish between the pioneers and the pretenders. There will always be products and marketers in any category that jump on any new trend, play with it for a time and then move on to the next hot trend. Consumers will still vote with their pocketbook, and the authentic companies will still survive and flourish.

References

1. Kline & Company, May 2009 presentation to Estee Lauder.
2. Lockeretz, William, *Organic Farming: An International History*, CABI Publishing Series, 2007.
3. Anastas, Paul T. and Warner, John C., *Green Chemistry: Theory and Practice*, Oxford University Press, Oxford UK, 1998.
4. Donough, William and Braungart, Michael, *Cradle To Cradle, Remaking the Way We Make Things*, North Point Press, 2002. See also *www.epea.com*.

CHAPTER 2

Organic Cosmetic Standards: A New Formulation Challenge

Tim Kapsner

Aveda Corp., Blaine, Minn., USA

KEY WORDS: *NSF standards, Ecocert, COPA, organic calculation, allowable chemical processes*

ABSTRACT: *The popularity of the Ecocert cosmetic standards and the publication of the NSF standards have increased the complexity of the organic cosmetic landscape. This chapter reviews organic standards in cosmetics and contrasts how to formulate products based on Ecocert vs. NSF standards*

A vast array of US cosmetic products is being labeled "organic"—from certified organic massage oils to shampoos containing synthetic surfactants and preservatives. The resulting confusion in the marketplace indicates that the organic food and cosmetics industry do not know what to think of, or do with, each other. The major organic food markets in the United States, the European Union (EU) and Japan have all struggled with whether—and how to—embrace the emerging cosmetic "stepchild" of organic foods. Regulators in each of these three markets have referred to cosmetics in their organic food programs, but these references have not always helped to clarify the situation. The regulatory answer to the question of using the food standards to certify cosmetics could be paraphrased in each of these markets as follows:

- United States: "Yes you can. No you can't. OK, I suppose you can."

- European Union: "Not now, not ever."
- Japan: "Go ahead—just do not translate it into Japanese."

To a company entering the organic cosmetics market, the worldwide picture will be overwhelmingly confusing. To an experienced marketer, the worldwide picture also is overwhelmingly confusing.

Standards Background

A recent article[1] provides a history of the organic cosmetic standards process in the United States and a brief summary of the worldwide organic cosmetics landscape. As the present article hits press, that process should have resulted in the publication of a US organic cosmetics standard by NSF International (*www.nsf.org*), a world-renowned standards organization. NSF is accredited by the American National Standards Institute (ANSI), to create ANSI standards. ANSI is the US representative in the International Standards Organization (ISO).

The public comment portion of the NSF process (see **NSF Process**) will hopefully result in broad feedback to this standard from the cosmetics and food industries. The NSF standard, when finalized, could be used on a voluntary basis for certifying cosmetic products in the US market.

Ecocert, a private food certifier in the European Union, has developed a private organic cosmetic standard that has been in use in Europe for several years. The Ecocert standard was registered with the French government in 2002 as the official organic cosmetic standard in France. Products certified to this standard are beginning to appear in the United States, which has increased the awareness of the many different standards in use and in development.

Ecocert vs. NSF

Organic foods can be certified at three different levels to make three different claims—"100% organic;" "certified organic" requiring 95% organic content; and "made with organic ingredients," which requires 70% organic content. The decision was made by the NSF standard committee to default to the United States Department of Agriculture's (USDA's) National Organic Program (NOP) food standard for the two higher levels of certification, "100% organic" and "certified organic."

According to the NOP,[2] a food can make a front label claim of "certified organic" if the organic content is at least 95%. The NSF standard redefines the category of "made with organic ingredients" to allow for the use of cosmetic ingredients prohibited by the NOP food standard. Examples of these ingredients are fatty alcohols and surfactants such as sodium coco-sulfate. The organic content requirement of this category, 70% minimum, mirrors the standard.

The state of California also has passed its own organic food law, the California Organic Products Act (COPA).[3] COPA requires that any cosmetic product sold in California contain at least 70% ingredients that are certified to the NOP food standard, for either a "certified organic" claim or a "made with organic ingredients" claim. This law is mandatory, not voluntary, for California. The provisions in COPA for cosmetics do not restrict the content of the 30% nonorganic portion of the product. This portion may contain any ingredients acceptable for use in cosmetics.

The European Ecocert standard has two levels of certification: "organic" and "ecological." The "ecological" level is a lower level of certification, akin to the NSF/NOP standard of "made with organic ingredients." The organic content requirement is lower for the Ecocert "ecological" certification than for its "organic" certification.

The content requirements for Ecocert are much more complicated than for NSF. There are three content requirements to meet the Ecocert standard. First, the natural and naturally derived content (including water) must be at least 95% of the formula.

The second and third calculations for Ecocert certification concern organic content. The second requirement is that 95% of the plant ingredients must be certified organic. The third is that at least 10% of the finished product ingredients, not counting water, must be certified organic. At the lower "ecological" level of Ecocert certification, the natural requirement is the same as the organic level—95% of the finished product. The organic content requirements are lower—50% of the plant ingredients and 5% of the finished product. These requirements are summarized in **Table 1.**

Table 1. Organic Content Requirements

Standard	Organic Claim	Lesser Claim (Made with/Ecological)
NSF	95% organic food ingredients	70% organic content from allowed processes
COPA	70% NOP food ingredients	70% NOP food ingredients
Ecocert	95% natural/95% organic/	95% natural/50% organic/ 10% organic 5% organic

It is important to note that the NSF standard is built on the USDA's NOP organic food standard, so the organic content in the NSF standard must be NOP organic. The Ecocert standard starts from the EU's organic food program, so it is written to require organic ingredients certified to the European Union's EC2092/91 organic program.[4]

Allowed Ingredient Processing

The NOP food standard, which defines the organic category of the NSF standard, is not concerned with the chemical reactions that produce the ingredients or food products. Any cosmetic ingredient produced by an NOP-allowed process such as heating, mixing or steaming is allowed. Some chemical conversions can be accomplished by the use of NOP-allowed processes and the use of sodium hydroxide, which is an "allowed synthetic" in the NOP food standard. Three of these chemical conversions are hydrolysis, esterification and saponification. Any ingredients that can be made by these reactions such as soap (e.g., sodium cocoate) can be used in a cosmetic product that is labeled "certified organic" by the NOP food standard.

The Ecocert cosmetic standard does recognize the chemistry used to produce cosmetic ingredients. This standard includes a list of the chemical reactions that can be used to make ingredients for products to be certified by Ecocert. This list is much longer than the NSF/NOP organic list, as can be seen in **Table 2**.

The NSF standard also recognizes and allows a list of chemical processes at the "made with organic ingredients" level of certification. The main difference in allowed chemical processes between the NSF "made with organic ingredients" standard and the Ecocert organic standard is the allowance of amphoteric surfactants by Ecocert. **Table 2** summarizes the chemical processes that can be performed under each standard and gives examples of ingredients that can be made by each process. Imaginative ingredient manufacturers will come up with many more ingredients that fit into each category.

Table 2. Allowable Chemical Processes

Standard	Allowed Processes	Ingredients
NOP Organic	Hydrolysis	Wheat amino acids
	Esterification	
	Glyceryl stearate	
NSF "Made With"	Everything above plus:	
	Protein condensation	Sodium cocoyl glutamate
	Etherification	Lauryl glucoside
	Hydrogenation	Hydrogenated castor oil
	Hydrogenolysis	Coconut alcohol
	Sulfation	Sodium coco-sulfate
Ecocert	Everything above plus:	
	Amphoterics	Cocamidopropyl betaine
		Sodium cocoamphoacetate

Example Formulas

The Ecocert standards and the NSF "made with" category allow a much broader range of cosmetic ingredients than the NSF/NOP organic category, so it follows that more functional, elegant formulas can be made in the first two categories than in the NSF/NOP organic category. With the exception of amphoteric surfactants, the NSF standards will allow the same formulation chemistry to be used in products labeled "made with organic ingredients" as the Ecocert standards allow for products labeled "certified organic." Example formulas for a lotion and a shampoo/body wash formulated to the two standards will show the differences.

Formula 1 shows a lotion formulated to the NOP food standard. There are a few emulsifiers that could be made to the NOP food standard. Glyceryl stearate, made from vegetable-derived glycerin and stearic acid, and sodium stearoyl lactylate, made from vegetable-derived lactic acid and stearic acid, would comply. Natural lactic acid, like natural acetic acid—the acid in vinegar—is produced by fermentation of sugar.

Formula 1. NOP organic lotion

Organic aloe	62.00%
Organic sunflower oil	8.00
Organic shea butter	10.00
Glyceryl stearate	2.50
Sodium stearoyl lactylate	2.00
Xanthan gum	0.50
Organic ethanol	15.00
	100.00

Organic Calculation:
95% Organic Ingredients

Organic oils and butters would comprise the oil phase. Preservation would be the major issue, with ethanol being one of the few antimicrobial ingredients allowed.

The Ecocert standard allows the use of fatty alcohols and their derivatives. This gives a great deal of formulation flexibility in the use of the fatty alcohols themselves and in the form of sugar ethers (polyglucosides) and fatty alcohol/fatty acid esters. Preservation would be much easier with the use of benzoic and sorbic acids. Formula 2 shows a typical lotion made to the Ecocert standard.

If the hydrogenated vegetable oil is produced in a certified facility, it counts toward the organic content under the two standards.

The organic content of the Ecocert organic lotion is 24.8%. In order to increase the organic content up to the 70% requirement for the NSF "made with organic ingredients" category, the batch water and the floral water would have to be replaced by an organic plant liquid such as aloe gel. If the synthetic preservatives also were replaced by NSF-allowed preservatives, such as organic acids, the Ecocert organic lotion could be labeled by the NSF standards as "made with organic ingredients."

Soaps made from sodium hydroxide and organic oils such as coconut would be the main candidate for foaming ingredients under the NSF/NOP organic category. A very simple organic body wash, shown in Formula 3, could be made using soap.

Formula 2. Ecocert organic cream (from standards)

Sucrose cocoate	2.00%
Cetyl alcohol	3.70
Organic hydrogenated castor oil	1.50
Isostearyl behenate	5.00
Ethyl palmitate	5.00
Organic plant extract (in organic ethanol)	8.00
Plant active substance	1.00
Vegetable-derived glycerin	3.00
Water (*aqua*)	55.00
Organic floral water	15.00
Preservatives (synthetic)	0.50
Organic fragrance	0.30
	100.00

Note: All of the fatty alcohols and fatty acids are of natural origin.

Ecocert Organic Calculations:

1. Percent natural–only synthetic is 0.5%   99.50%
2. Percent organic of total plant ingredients:
   $(1.5 + 8 + 15 + 0.3)/(1.5 + 8 + 15 + 0.3 + 1) =$ 96.12%
3. Percent organic of total formula:
   $1.5 + 8 + 15 + 0.3 =$ 24.80%

Formula 3. NOP organic body wash

Organic aloe	69.00%
Organic coconut oil	12.00
Sodium hydroxide	3.00
Organic olive oil	0.50
Xanthan gum	0.50
Organic ethanol	15.00
	100.00

Organic Calculation:
96.5% Organic Ingredients

Preservation is again the major issue, with ethanol being a practical choice. An organic shampoo similar to the example used in the Ecocert standards (**Formula 4**) shows the use of a sugar/fatty alcohol ether (polyglucoside) and an amphoteric surfactant (betaine) to give a very acceptable foam.

Using this formula as a starting point, it could be modified to make it acceptable in the NSF/NOP "made with organic ingredients" category by replacing the batch water and floral water with organic aloe, using an acceptable preservative system such as ethanol and organic acids, and replacing the amphoteric surfactant with an acceptable surfactant, such as sodium coco-sulfate.

Formula 4. Ecocert organic shampoo

Lauryl polyglucose citrate	12.00%w/w
Cocamidopropyl betaine (65% fatty acid of natural origin, 15% synthetic acetate, 20% synthetic amine)	13.00
Hydrolyzed vegetable protein containing 40% organic vegetable protein, 59.8% water and 0.2% preservatives)	6.00
Water (*aqua*)	53.70
15% Organic floral water	15.00
Preservatives (synthetic)	0.30
	100.00

Ecocert Organic Calculations:
1. Percent natural:
   12 + (13 X 65%) + (6 X 99.8%) + 53.7 + 15 =   95.40%
2. Percent organic of total plant ingredients:
   15 / 15 =   100%
3. Percent organic of total formula:
   15 =   15%

Beyond the differences in finished product organic content calculations, there are also differences between the NSF and Ecocert standards in organic content calculations in the ingredients themselves. The organic content of a floral water such as rosewater in the NSF standard is only the amount of water that was contained in the fresh plant material. The Ecocert standard allows the entire floral water to count as organic content if the distillation used at least 20% fresh plant material or 5% dried plant material. The NSF standard allows a standard portion of processed ingredients such as fatty alcohols (98%) or sulfates such as sodium coco-sulfate (60%) to count toward the finished product organic content. Readers interested in these complex details are referred to the standards and appendices.

It is important to note that the overall organic content of the Ecocert example formulas are 24.8% and 15%. This organic content would also be EU organic, not NOP organic. Thus, neither of these formulas would comply with COPA, so neither could be sold as an organic product in California.

NSF Process

NSF International has created a comprehensive standards development process that requires broad representation from the industry. Food certification inspectors, cosmetic manufacturers, certifiers, cosmetic chemists, consumer groups and government regulators are all taking part in the creation of the cosmetic standard. Once published to the industry, all feedback on the standards will be considered by the committee in order to produce a final document that is presented to the NSF board for more modification or final NSF approval. The standard can then be used on a voluntary basis to certify cosmetic products. NSF is also well-versed in the process of taking a standard from development through government regulation.

Conclusion

The popularity of the Ecocert cosmetic standard and the development of the NSF standard have certainly increased the complexity of the organic cosmetic landscape. Marketers of organic cosmetic products will have to choose their organic certification program based on what they feel best fits their company's marketing goals. They will need to spend time and effort to educate the consumer about what makes their product "organic."

Consumers may be increasingly overwhelmed and confused by the complexity of the organic options. Sorting through this mass of confusion, in addition to new marketing opportunities and consumer education, will mark the progress of the industry as it strives to figure out what "organic" means to personal care. Stay tuned.

Published July 2007 *Cosmetics and Toiletries* magazine

References

1. TR Kapsner, Personal care standards go public, *Organic Processing Magazine* 4(2) (Apr–Jun 2007)

2. USDA Web site, *NOP Organic Food Standards*; Available at: *www.ams.usda.gov/nop* (Accessed May 24, 2007)
3. California Department of Food and Agriculture Web site, *California Organic Products Act*, Available at: *www.cdfa.ca.gov/is/fveqc/organic.htm*; (Accessed May 24, 2007)
4. European Union Law Web site, *EU's EC 2092/91 food standards*; Available at: *http://eur-lex. europa.eu*; (Accessed May 24, 2007)

CHAPTER 3

Greening Personal Care Chemistry

James H. Clark and Louise Summerton
Green Chemistry Centre of Excellence

KEY WORDS: *green chemistry, sustainable development, clean synthesis, renewable resources, greener products, substitution*

ABSTRACT: *Multiple economic, legislative and customer pressures are forcing an unprecedented level of change in chemical manufacturing and the design of chemical products. The authors examine the drivers for change and opportunities across the product lifecycle for green and sustainable chemistry including the use of renewable resources, cleaner synthesis methods and greener products.*

The challenges for chemical-intensive industries, including the producers of personal care products, in the 21st century are as great as those faced by almost any industry.[1] The chemical industry, which has been effective in supplying a diverse range of intermediates and formulation components largely based on low-cost petroleum feedstock, is now under pressure to change the way it operates. The drivers for change affect all aspects of production, notably feedstock, manufacturing processes and the choice and key design features of products (**Figure 1**).

While the impact of increasing oil prices on the cost of transportation and heating fuels is frequently and often dramatically publicized, the effects on other oil-dependent industries and their downstream users receive less attention. Some 20% of the petroleum used in the European Union (EU) goes into chemical manufacturing such as feedstock and energy, and more than 90% of the organic chemicals used today are oil-derived.

To add to the problem of increasing costs, the industry also faces concerns over reliability of supply due to the demand from rapidly growing chemical industries in areas such as China. When the price of phenol, a major building block petrochemical, tripled in 2005, the price hike could be attributed to both oil price increases and demand from the growing industries of the East.

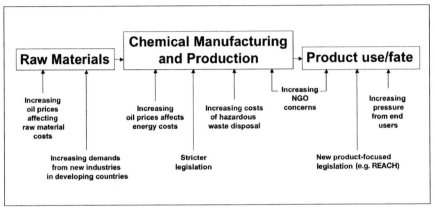

Figure 1. Drivers for change in chemical production

Chemical manufacturing has also had to face a climate of heightened legislation for the last 10 years and many companies have significantly "cleaned up their act" by reducing levels of pollution and improving workplace health and safety records. Pressures continue to mount, however, with rapidly increasing energy costs and restrictions over the storage of chemicals and disposal of hazardous waste, making competitiveness with the new industries in the East more difficult. While the 1990s can be seen as a period of improvement in "good housekeeping," it is now apparent that step-change improvements such as the introduction of new, clean technologies are needed.

The early years of the 21st century have seen an unprecedented level of attention on the human and environmental safety of products. Perhaps inevitably, chemicals have come under the microscope from new legislation, notably REACH, but also from more sector-specific regulations such as Restriction of Hazardous Substances (RoHS), reflecting public concerns.[2,3] One outcome of this is the increasing awareness by retailers of the range of chemicals they effectively sell that are disguised in the form of food, medicines, clothing, electronic goods, cleaning products and, of course, personal care products.

In the rush to be seen as "green," retailers are competing over their green credentials, encouraged by frequently published reports from nongovernmental organizations (NGOs). Currently retailers are only aware of chemicals that can attract negative publicity; hence, the focus is almost entirely on avoidance of headline-grabbing substances such as phthalates and brominated flame-retardants. With a newly found inquisitiveness over supply chains using "green-tinted" spectacles, retailers and their customers are likely to ask more difficult questions relating to overall environmental footprints.

Personal care product producers are subject to these changing attitudes and need to respond early through their own lifecycle awareness. Future products need to be verifiably green and sustainable with well-understood and controlled supply chains.

Green Chemistry

Research for finding more environmentally friendly replacements for hazardous chemical processes dates back more than 20 years but the term *green chemistry* was suggested in the mid 1990s by the US Environmental Protection Agency (EPA). The term has become widely accepted—if sometimes interchanged with *sustainable chemistry*, which strictly speaking, is different—and has helped to provide focus to the movement towards more environmentally compatible chemical processes and products. The US EPA led the charge with grants to support green chemistry R&D, as well as an awards program.

Green chemistry centers, institutes and networks have been established in numerous countries including the United States, United Kingdom, Japan, Greece and Spain. A dedicated and high-impact factor journal, *Green Chemistry*, has been in business for almost 10 years and each year sees numerous national and international green chemistry conferences and other events.

Green chemistry can basically be considered a series of reductions (**Figure 2**). Greater resource efficiency and less waste will obviously benefit a company's bottom line. Energy and water will be increasingly important resources in manufacturing, especially in many developing countries where numerous Western companies have outsourced all or part of their manufacturing. Reducing the number of process auxiliaries and, in particular, process steps, is also likely to provide financial savings as well as improved environmental performance—green chemistry is simple chemistry.

While most of the green chemistry research in the 1990s was process-focused, the last two years have seen growing interest in the other stages of the product lifecycle, notably raw materials and, with increasing user awareness, the product itself including its fate, once released into the environment. Personal care chemists need to take measures to improve the green credentials of their products, to ensure the sustainability of their raw materials, and to minimize manufacturing costs through green chemistry reductions. By looking at the use of renewable resources as feedstock, cleaner synthesis methods in manufacturing, and greener products based on "benign by design" ideology, practical measures can be considered to achieve these goals.

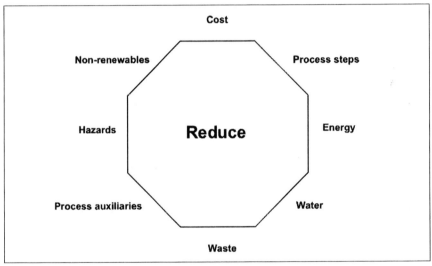

Figure 2. Green chemistry reductions

Renewable Resources[4-6]

There is a false assumption by many individuals that green equals natural, and that when the industry refers to green(er) chemicals, it means natural or plant extracts. The first stage of developing a truly green and sustainable chemical product should be based on a renewable resource; in the case of an organic chemical, this means biological materials including trees, grasses and agricultural residues.

However, it is likely that the majority of these future products will require green chemical modification of that resource to give it the necessary properties for effective use. The best examples of this are the so-called bio platform molecules—relatively simple compounds that can be obtained in simple one or two-stage processes from biomass (see **Figure 3**).[7]

Some of the key platform molecules that are expected to become widely available from bioresources via the fermentation route are shown in **Figure 4**.

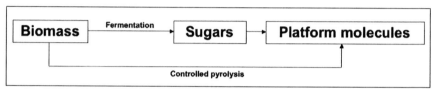

Figure 3. Biomass-derived platform molecules

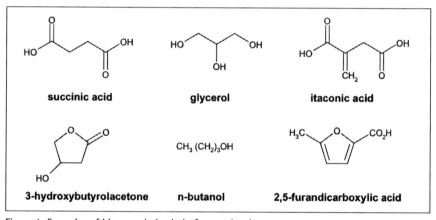

Figure 4. Examples of biomass-derived platform molecules

These are all oxygenated and hydrophilic. Nonetheless, their high degree of functionality makes them good candidates for chemical transformations as shown, for example, by succinic acid (see **Figure 5**).[8]

It is important to note that these molecules are produced in fermentation broths—aqueous, high dilution (< 10% w/w) and mixed with other products plus nutrients, enzymes, etc. Energy-demanding and wasteful separation and purification processes will massively reduce the economic and environmental credibility of such chemicals, and green chemistry needs to be chemistry that is effective under such conditions.

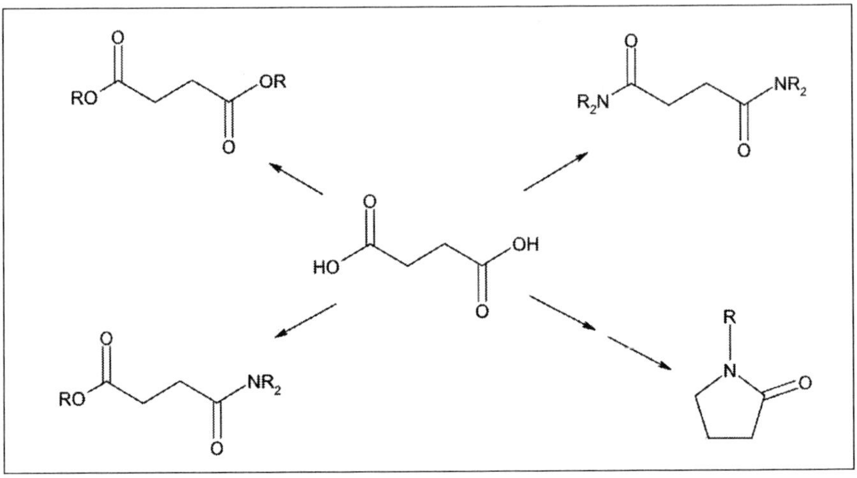

Figure 5. Products that are easily accessible from succinic acid

Some heterogeneous catalysts including those based on carbonized polysaccharides can achieve this, and when combined with membrane technology, provide future routes to the continuous conversion of dilute aqueous feedstock to nonaqueous chemical products.[9] Other renewable molecules to be considered for future feedstock in green and sustainable supply chains include vanillin, a rare aromatic example, and fatty acids and esters that are now produced in ever larger quantities from biodiesel manufacture.

Clean Synthesis

Clean synthesis and clean chemical production are where the green chemistry movement began and remain in the heart of the area. The starting point for developing a clean synthesis strategy is to set metrics to measure reaction efficiency by means other than the traditional value of yield alone.[10] Atom economy, or the percentage of atoms in the substrates that go into the desired product, and the E factor or the ratio of waste to product weights, are the best established of these, although both have limitations. Atom economy ignores any reagents, catalysts and solvent, whereas with an E factor, one has to decide on the system boundaries and whether to include the process auxiliaries, such as the solvent and quench or wash water. In a typical documented synthetic procedure for an organic reaction, apart from the substrates, the reaction mixture contains solvent and frequently other auxiliaries such as acid, base or catalyst, and the work up can involve large amounts of water and organic solvent.

In a way it does not, within reason, matter what one includes— e.g., it is often prudent to ignore solvents that are clearly and practically recyclable—as long as like-for-like comparisons can be made with alternative procedures. One increasingly serious omission from all of the major green chemistry metrics that currently exists is energy; given the increasing cost of energy it would be foolish to ignore this in route selection.

The major and most widely applicable solutions to inefficient, wasteful or otherwise dangerous synthetic routes are:

1. Alternative routes, carefully evaluated by green chemistry metrics and other critical parameters, including energy and the use of hazardous chemicals;

2. Catalysis and especially heterogeneous catalysis such as supported $AlCl_3$ and other solid acids and bases;

3. Solvent avoidance or substitution with a nonvolatile solvent such as an ionic liquid or an easily recyclable and benign solvent such as supercritical CO_2. Given the immaturity or limitations of alternative solvents, the industry can also use a series of parameters to thoroughly compare the credentials of different VOC solvents such as solvent power, toxicity, safety, recoverability and even a mini-life-cycle assessment to allow the inclusion of sustainability as a factor.

4. Avoiding auxiliaries—including protecting and deprotecting agents but also extending to avoiding solvents altogether wherever possible.

It should also be remembered that the bulk of process chemistry waste tends to come after the actual reaction. Separations or reaction quenches are often achieved by drowning the reaction in a large volume of water; organic solvents can be used to wash out products; and other process auxiliaries can be used to clean up and purify the product.

Through the use of the right reagents and catalysts, as in heterogenized forms or permanently separated by a membrane reaction, much of this can be avoided. It may also be possible through the use of a membrane or other flow reactor such as a spinning disc reactor to continually remove product from the reaction zone. Even in a static reactor the use of supercritical CO_2 as a reaction solvent or simply as an extraction medium has the advantage of easy separation simply through a reduction in pressure.[11]

Greener Products

There will be an increasing number of occasions where substitution of a process reagent or more significantly of a final product will become important. This may be driven by availability and cost issues, difficulty in manufacture, legislation, expedient application of greener product guidelines, as in assessing the probable need for substitution on the basis of known or extrapolated persistence, bioaccumulation and toxicity data, or customer or NGO and media pressure. A good strategy for substitution is to consider both existing "green" chemicals and biomass-derived products likely to emerge in the near future (see **Figure 6**). The acceptability criteria may set limits to change, such as "no more than 20% greater cost;" or "no more than two process steps from the raw material;" or "commercially available feedstock."

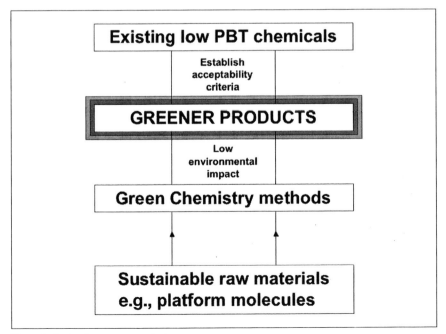

Figure 6. Routes to greener products

Some examples of classes of compounds and substances where either substitution is becoming important and/or where renewable, i.e., biomass-derived, sources are becoming available, are briefly discussed in the following.

Future sources of aromatic compounds are particularly uncertain. Among the most promising bio-platform molecules for future chemical manufacturing, the only aromatic compound is vanillin, which can be obtained from lignin in low, 2–3% yields. Some other natural materials also contain aromatic compounds, although their yields by extraction or even reactive (e.g., oxidation) extraction are similarly low. One different approach is to start from glucose, which is widely and easily available from numerous biomass materials, and to use a combined biochemical process to produce simple benzenoid aromatics (see **Figure 7**).

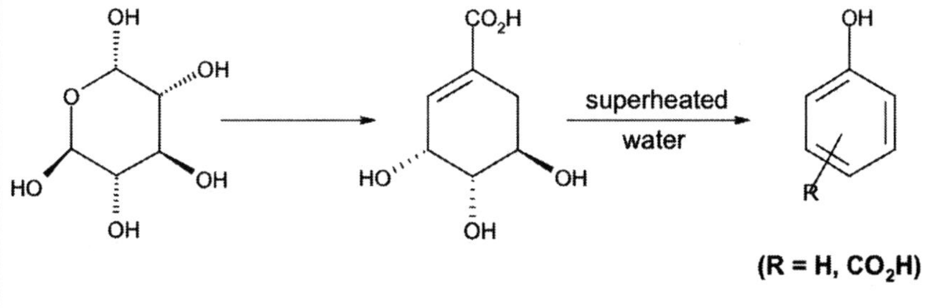

Figure 7. Production of simple benzenoid aromatics

The para-substitution pattern of one of these products is consistent with that used in some sunscreen agents in personal care products. Some emollients contain ortho-substitution patterns, commonly ortho-substitutional phenols, that may be accessible from vanillin.

There is concern over the apparent poor biodegradability of some chelants including EDTA, although this has been contested. Nonetheless, there has been a great effort directed towards more environmentally friendly substitutes for EDTA. One example of this is EDDS (see **Figure 8**).

Unfortunately the activity of EDDS is not as effective as EDTA. Phosphonates have also been proposed but its biodegradability may not be much better than that of EDTA.[12]

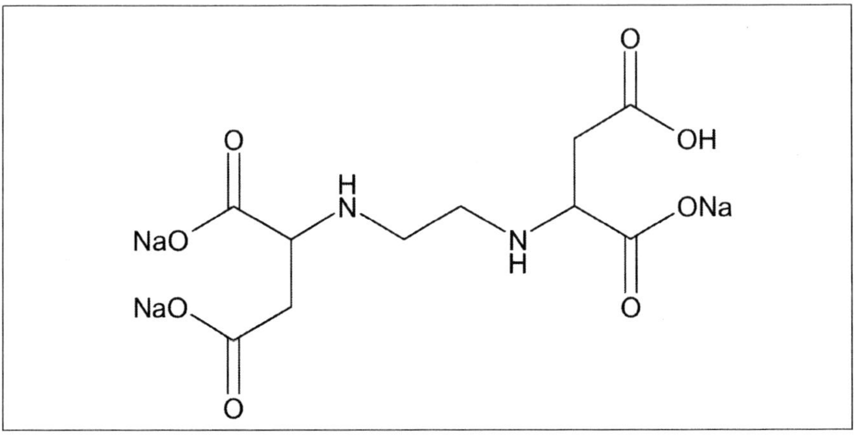

Figure 8. A more environmentally friendly substitute for EDTA, EDDS

Plant waxes can be extracted using environmentally benign supercritical carbon dioxide. One of the most interesting sources is wheat straw, which is abundant, widely available in Europe and of low value.[13] The benign extraction technology has the additional advantage of being tunable so that different fractions of the complex mixture of chemicals called waxes can be collected. These have different properties and different application values including cosmetics as well as nutraceuticals and insect semiochemicals. All UK waxes are imported. Furthermore, there is a growing desire to avoid animal-derived waxes in products such as cosmetics.

In other current research at the Green Chemistry Centre at York, natural polysaccharides such as starches are being used to stabilize nanoparticles. This could have value in applications such as sunscreens where titanium dioxide nanoparticles are known to be more efficient UV light reflectors than larger particle aggregates, but where there are concerns over the particles' ability to trigger damaging electron-transfer processes if they can migrate through the skin.

By using "neutral" materials such as starch in more imaginative ways, and by building up new products using bio-derived platform molecules, new formulations of sustainable chemical products can be created. And by using clean synthesis methods and green chemical technologies to carry out the chemical conversions en route, the industry can ensure green and sustainable chemical products.

Published March 2008 *Cosmetics and Toiletries* magazine

References

1 JH Clark, Green chemistry today (and tomorrow), *Green Chem*, 8 17 (2006)

2 DJ Knight, Regulation of Chemicals, *RAPRA Review Report*, 16 181 (2006)

3 J Garrod, The current regulation of environmental chemicals, RE Harrison and RE Hester, eds, in *Chemicals in the Environment*, RSC: Cambridge 1–20 (2006)

4 JH Clark, Green Chemistry for the second generation biorefinery, *J Chem Technol Biotechnol* 82 803 (2007)

5 L E Manzer, Biomass derivatives: A sustainable source of chemicals, J Bozell and K Patel, eds, in *Feedstock for the Future*, ACS: New York 40–51 (2006)

6 AJ Ragouskas et al, The path forward for biofuels and biomaterials, *Science* 311 484 (2006)

7 T Werpy and G Petersen, Top Value Added Chemicals from Biomass, technical report No. DOE/GO-102004-1992, National Renewable Energy Lab, Golden, CO USA (2004) available at: *www.osti.gov/bridge*

8 V Budarin, JH Clark, R Luque and DJ Macquarrie, Versatile mesoporous carbonaceous materials as acid catalysts, *Chem Commun* 634 (2007)

9 V Budarin, R Luque, D J Macquarrie and J H Clark, *Chem European J*, 13 6914 (2007)

10 DJ Constable et al, Green chemistry measures for process research and development, *Green Chem*, 3 7 (2001)

11 N Tanchaix and W Leitner, Supercritical carbon dioxide as an environmentally benign reaction medium for chemical synthesis, JH Clark and DJ Macquarrie, eds, in *Handbook of Green Chemistry & Technology*, Blackwell: Oxford 482-501 (2002)

12 B Nowack, Environmental chemistry of phosphonates, *Water Research* 37 2533 (2003)

13 FEI Deswarte, JH Clark, JJE Hardy and PM Rae, The fractionation of valuable wax products from wheatstraw using CO_2, *Green Chem* 8 39 (2006)

CHAPTER 4

Building Natural Products

Eric S. Abrutyn
TPC2 Advisors Ltd., Inc.

KEY WORDS: *beeswax, lip balm, lemongrass, deodorant, hand cream, green tea, sunscreen, styling gel, natural*

ABSTRACT: *Are consumers actually interested in products that contain natural materials, or are they really interested in products that are safer and have a minimal impact on the planet (i.e., they are renewable)? The key to meeting consumer demand is to understand what natural means in order to produce formulations that meet expectations.*

It appears that consumer interest in natural and organic products is growing. The question is: What does this mean? Are consumers actually interested in products that contain natural materials, or are they really interested in products that are safer and have a minimal impact on the planet (i.e., they are renewable)? The key to meeting consumer demand is to understand what natural means in order to produce formulations that meet expectations.

Since the cosmetics and personal care industry is not regulated, various organizations have offered conflicting positions on standardized guidelines for natural and organic claims. To improve communication on this topic, it will therefore become important to dissociate claims regarding the naturalness of ingredients from the perception of safety.

Safety is inherent in the raw materials used for formulating, regardless of their origin and in the synergies among ingredients— for more than 50 years, the industry has worked hard to monitor the safety of products on the market, supported by the US Food and Drug Administration (FDA). And recently, more governmental agencies such as the FDA, the US Department of Agriculture (USDA) and the Council of Europe's Committee of Experts on

Cosmetic Products have taken a proactive role in sorting out the meanings of natural and organic for the cosmetics and personal care industry. Such organizations act as a clearer scientific focal point in deciding what ingredients are safe for use in cosmetic products. In addition, several organizations currently are monitoring the safety of cosmetics and personal care ingredients, such as the Cosmetic Ingredient Review (CIR) panel.

General Formula Standards

As noted, an ever-growing list of organizations with standardized guidelines exists that measures the naturalness of a product formula. The definition for *natural* in chemicals legislation was introduced in 1981, and in 2000, the Council of Europe's Committee of Experts on Cosmetic Products issued guidelines for natural cosmetic products. Only as recently as 2008, however, did the USDA and the European Cosmetic Standards Working Group (COSMOS)[1] provide additional guidance for formulating to meet natural claims. Nongovernmental, for-profit organizations offering organic and/or natural certification for cosmetic products include: Quality Assurance International,[2] the National Science Foundation,[3] ECOCERT,[4] OASIS,[5] Nature,[6] the Soil Association, Guaranteed Organic Certification Agency,[7] BDIH,[8] the Natural Products

Formula 1. Burt's Bees beeswax lip balm

Beeswax	qs
Coconut oil	2.05–5.0%
Sunflower oil	2.5–5.0
Tocopheryl acetate	0.5–1.0
Tocopherol (vitamin E)	0.5–1.0
Lanolin	0.5–1.0
Peppermint oil	< 0.25
Comfrey root extract	< 0.1
Rosemary extract	< 0.1

Formula 2. Tom's of Maine lemongrass natural deodorant body bar

Soaps of coconut and palm	qs
Sage extract	< 0.1%
Rosemary extract	< 0.1%
Ascorbyl palmitate	< 0.1%
Lemongrass oil	<0.25%

Note: These vegetable-based soaps include a blend of rosemary and vitamin C for preservation, and of sage and lemongrass for their reported natural odor-fighting properties.

Association,[9] and Certech[10]—to name a few. However, organic and natural certifications for cosmetics are not backed by specific legislation, such as in the foods industry.

Formulas 1–5 are examples of natural products on the market, taken from sources of public domain and including estimates of the ingredient percentages used and/or their function in the formula, to provide readers with a starting point for their own formulation work. It is suggested that readers perform a patent

Formula 3. Green By Nature mint green tea hand cream

Water (*aqua*)	Carrier
Butyrospermum parkii (shea butter)	Emollient/moisturizer
Sesamum indicum (sesame) seed oil	Emollient
Beeswax	Structurant
Prunus persica (peach) kernel extract	Emollient
Pistacia vera seed oil (pistachio oil)	Emollient
Glycine soja (soybean) seed extract	Emollient
Chamomilla recutita (matricaria) flower extract	Emollient
Stearic acid	Emulsifier
Aloe barbadensis leaf extract	Skin calming
Camellia oleifera leaf extract (green tea extract)	Claim support
Yogurt powder	Co-emulsifier
Rosa moschata seed oil (rose hip oil)	Claim support
Sorbitan olivate	Emulsifier
Tocopherol (vitamin E)	Antioxidant
Citrus grandis (grapefruit) seed extract	Skin calming
Mentha piperita (peppermint) oil	Skin calming
DMDM hydantoin	Preservative
Iodopropynyl butylcarbamate	Preservative
Citrus aurantium amara (bitter orange) fruit extract	Skin calming/aroma
Ascorbic acid (vitamin C)	Antioxidant
Citric acid	pH Adjuster
Malic acid	pH Adjuster
Glycerin	Humectant

search to ensure they are not infringing on any existing and protected technologies. In addition, two supplier-submitted examples of natural formulas are provided, for reader consideration.

Most natural products launched consist of at least 90% naturally derived materials and they omit certain ingredients construed as being unsafe, such as parabens. Cosmetic products meeting organic standards tend to follow USDA food standards, where no chemical fertilizers, herbicides, pesticides or other toxins were used to grow the non-hybridized plant sources from which the raw materials are derived. The most common denominators among formulas that meet claims for natural standards include:

- Ingredients based on environmentally conscious and ecologically sound practices that are socially responsible with regard to the use of resources, and that impart minimum human impact on the environment;

Formula 4. All natural styling gel*

A.	Dehydroxanthan gum (AMAZE XT polymer, Azko Nobel)	0.85% w/w
B.	Deionized water (aqua)	50.00
C.	Tapioca starch (Naviance Tapioca certified organic biopolymer, Azko Nobel)	2.50
D.	Deionized water (aqua)	44.95
	Glycerin (vegetable grade)	0.25
E.	Sodium benzoate	1.00
	Benzyl alcohol	0.25
	Hydrolyzed wheat protein (and) hydrolyzed wheat starch (and) water (aqua)	0.20
		100.00

Procedure: Without heat, slowly sift A into B with good agitation (700 rpm), until completely dispersed. Reduce mixing speed to 400 rpm and mix for 15 min to completely hydrate. In a separate mixing vessel, sift C into D with good agitation (~ 400 rpm) and mix until completely dispersed. Slowly add CD to AB. Continue mixing at ~ 400 rpm and heat to 80°C. Hold for 25 min. Cool to 45°C before adding E in order. Mix until homogenous. Fill containers. Viscosity: 15,000–20,000 cps; Brkfld Heliopath Spindle #T-C /10 rpm; pH 5.0–7.0

Note: Formula provided courtesy of Akzo Nobel; naturally derived ingredients in this styling gel provide moderate stiffness with humidity resistance and a pleasant aesthetic feel. Tapioca starch offers texture and hold with excellent aesthetics while dehydroxanthan gum polymer yields rheology and high humidity hold.

- Water is considered a basic ingredient; therefore, it is not included in the calculation for total percentage of natural or organic ingredients;
- At least 90% of the formula composition, sans water, is based on renewable feedstock and ingredients with neutral carbon footprints;
- Incidental ingredients such as preservatives, chelating agents and antioxidants do not have to be included in the calculation so long as they represent less than 1% of the non-water portion of the composition, and there are no renewable resource alternatives; and
- All raw materials used should represent the best approach to safe exposure to humans; safety measurements are based on scientific studies demonstrating their long-term safety to humans.

In general, the key to formulating natural products is to choose safe and effective raw materials of as natural an origin as possible.

Formula 5. All natural sunscreen lotion*

A. Deionized water (*aqua*)	qs
Zinc oxide	10.00% w/w
B. Glycerin	2.50
Xantham gum	0.50
C. Cetearyl alcohol (and) coco glucoside	3.00
Sorbitan sesquioleate	0.75
White beeswax	1.50
Butyrospermum parkii (shea butter)	1.50
Simmondsia chinensis (jojoba) seed oil)	1.00
Prunus amygdalus dulcis (sweet almond) oil	0.50
Sesamum indicum (sesame) oil	0.50
Tocopheryl acetate (vitamin E acetate)	0.50
Bisabolol nat.	0.20

Procedure: Combine A, mix well and heat to 75–80°C. Premix B and add to A at 75°C while homogenizing. Separately combine C, heat to 75°C and add C to AB at 75°C, homogenizing until batch is uniform. Transfer batch to sweep mixing and cool to 40°C. Add D in order and mix until room temperature. Homogenize at slow to medium speed till batch uniform, then stop.

Note: Formula provided courtesy of BASF.

Their renewability also should be incorporated into the product development process, to result in the smallest possible negative footprint on the environment. However, for product developers to meet the specific requirements of a given standard, it is important to fully understand the requirements since they can vary as to how the percentage of natural ingredients is calculated, or the degree of modification allowed to a natural source material. This is important because some natural ingredients are either not functionally suitable to create good aesthetics, are not stable, or are not sufficiently pure—odorless and colorless.

Conclusions

The continued market demand for natural products is growing, and while the definition of *natural* remains an ongoing discussion, there is a definite push toward eliminating classical, "chemical-sounding" ingredients, even if they are proven safe and have little or no impact on the planet. Since the concept of *natural* and how it is positioned in the marketplace is still a moving target with minimal legal standardization, it will take some time to provide formulators with a clear idea of how to find and utilize the right materials that support this market claim.

Current standards are dependent upon the marketing division within individual companies and their legal department. For now, it is best for formulators to work with their company's legal, regulatory and marketing groups to agree on how *natural* will be defined and stay true to the course. Then it will be easier to work with raw material suppliers to document and match to these specification requirements.

Various organizations including those previously listed, whose Web sites may be found in the concluding references to this chapter, have developed a list of acceptable and unacceptable renewable ingredients that would meet their standards for natural and organic claims. Also, a number of raw material suppliers have published prototype formulations for use as starting points for natural product formulations.

The development of personal care products for this market requires clear communication regarding whether said products will be positioned as *natural*—meaning either containing natural ingredients or being safer for the environment; *organic* and thus meeting a set of specified standards; or *renewable*, referencing low impact on resources in the environment. In addition, such products should outline the source of feedstock from which their ingredients derived, as well as the renewability and greenness of the source; and safety assurance based on reliable, peer-reviewed science and scientific organizations.

The personal care industry must take a leadership role, as it has for the past 50 years with other issues, to control the misleading association of terms such as *natural* and *organic* with the consumer's expectation of implied safety; the industry must continue in its defense of ingredients with established safety.

Published October 2009 *Cosmetics and Toiletries* magazine

References

1. *www.cosmos-standard.org*
2. *www.qai-inc.com*
3. *www.nsf.gov*
4. *www.ecocert.com*
5. *www.oasisseal.org*
6. *www.natrue.org*
7. *www.goca.ws/organic-certification*
8. *www.kontrollierte-naturkosmetik.de/e/bdih.htm*
9. *www.naturalproductsassoc.org*
10. *www.certechregistration.com/1_organic_certification.htm*

CHAPTER 5

Green Star Rating for Cosmetic Compounds and Formulations

Anthony J. O'Lenick, Jr
Siltech LLC

KEY WORDS: *green star rating, renewable, nonrenewable, natural, green*

ABSTRACT: *The following is taken from U.S. Patent Application 20090259409, which directed toward "a process that can be used in the formulation of more environmentally friendly, greener formulations for consumer applications. The process includes evaluating the components in a formulation, then determining the percentage of the molecule that is green, establishing a green star rating and determining the effect of that component on the overall green star rating of a formulation."*

Background

Today's consumer and formulator have become increasingly aware of the consumption of resources that are not renewable. Products derived from fossil fuels are nonrenewable. This includes products like gasoline, coal, natural gas, diesel and other commodities. Green resources are defined as renewable resources, replenished by natural processes. Green products are renewable resources and include oxygen, fresh water, timber and biomass (renewable energy source—biological material derived from living organisms). Green products also include commodities such as wood, paper and leather.

Furthermore, alcohol, oils from plants and seeds are considered green products.

Green raw materials are preferred in the preparation of cosmetic products, as they are both renewable and biodegradable. However, these basic green products cannot be combined in a way that provides consumer products that meet the demands of the consumer. For example, soap can be a green detergent, but it does not possess all the desirable properties that give the consumer a laundry detergent. In order to make high-performance formulations, some materials that are not green are required.

While the concept of a green product is straightforward, the ability for the formulator and the consumer to quantify the greenness of a given shampoo or other consumer product is more difficult. Given a proper understanding, the consumer and formulator can make informed, educated decisions about creating products with the best combination of green properties and formulation attributes. In other words, the need of the consumer and the need of the environment can be intelligently determined.

All too often in the past, the determination of the greenness of a raw material or formulation was more emotional than scientific and required either an all or nothing approach to environmental stewardship. Simply put, materials are green or they are not. Unfortunately, the formulations of consumer products that are commercially acceptable require a trade-off in optimizing the performance and greenness. Consumers demand many formulation benefits that cannot be achieved with only green ingredients. Some non-green products are required. To educate the consumer, a systematic approach to measure the level of greenness in a formulation was needed. This quest resulted in the development of the "Green Star Rating" system or simply "GSR".

The Green Star Rating provides a process by which a formulator can easily ascertain the "greenness" of a raw material and a consumer can determine and compare the "greenness" of a formulation to similar types of products. This process allows the formulation chemist a way to break a molecule down into green portion and a non-renewable resource portion. The evaluation of this data allows for the generation of a Green Star Value, which is the percentage of the molecule that is based upon green chemistry divided by 10. Once this number is known, the effect of replacing one ingredient in a formulation with a "greener" compound can be ascertained. Specifically, if a raw material used in a formulation at 20% by weight with a Green Star Rating of 1 is replaced with a product with a Green Star Rating of 7, the impact on the formulation is (7-1) times 0.20 or 1.2. This means that much more renewable resources are being used in the formulation and its consumption will have less of a negative impact on the environment. This approach allows the formulator to make greener products and the consumer to choose greener products.

The Green Star Rating is determined using the following steps:

Step 1   Determine the empirical formula for chemical compounds used to make formulated products;

Step 2   Determine which portions of the molecule are green;

Step 3   Determine the percentage by weight of the green portion of the molecule;

Step 4   Determine the green star value and, optionally;

Step 5   Optimizing the formulation by selecting components with the greatest green star value.

Raw Materials

There are two areas in which the Green Star Rating process can be applied: 1) to raw materials to allow for the prudent selection of products for inclusion into formulations, and to formulations themselves allowing for the generation of a Green Star Rating, a method for the consumer to understand the relative degree of greenness in a finished product.

Example 1—Sodium Coco Alcohol Derived from Natural Alcohol

Step 1—Determine the empirical formula for chemical compounds used to make formulated product.

Sodium Coco Sulfate   C12H23SO4Na

Step 2—Determine which portions of the molecule are green.

Sodium coco sulfate

Renewable Material   Natural Alcohol   C12H23

Non-Renewable   Synthetic Sulfation SO_4Na

Step 3—Determine the percentage by weight of the green portion of the molecule. This is done by multiplying the weight of each atom by the number of atoms in each portion.

Renewable Material   Natural Alcohol $C_{12}H_{23}$

Carbon has a molecular weight of 12, there are 12 present in the renewable portion, so the molecular weight contribution of the carbon is 12 times 12 or 144. Hydrogen has a molecular weight of 1, there are 23 hydrogen atoms present in the renewable portion, so the molecular weight contribution of the hydrogen is 1 times 23 or 23. The sum of all the elements in the renewable portion is 144+23 or 167.

Non-Renewable   Synthetic Sulfation SO_4Na

Sulfur has a molecular weight of 32, there is 1 sulfur atom present in the non-renewable portion, so the molecular weight contribution of the sulfur is 1 times 32 or 32. Oxygen has a molecular weight of 16, there are 4 oxygen atoms present in the non-renewable portion, so the molecular weight contribution of the hydrogen is 4 times 16 or 64. Sodium has a molecular weight of 23, there is 1 sodium atom present in the non-renewable portion, so the molecular weight contribution of the sulfur is 1 times 23 or 23. The sum of all the elements in the non-renewable portion is 32+64+23= 119

Total Molecular Weight = Renewable Portion + Non-Renewable portion
Total Molecular Weight = 167+ 119= 289
Renewable Portion/Total = 167/289 = 57.7%

Step 4—Determine the Green Star Value.
Green Star Value (GSV) = % Renewable rounded to unit = 58

Example 2—Sodium Laureth 3 Sulfate,
$$C_{12}H_{23}O(CH_2CH_2O)_3SO_3Na$$

Step 1—Determine the empirical formula for chemical compounds used to make formulated product.

Empirical Formula: $C_{18}H_{35}O_7SNa$

Step 2—Determine which portions of the molecule are green.

| Renewable | $C_{12}H_{23}$ (Natural Alcohol) |
| Non-renewable | $-(CH_2CH_2O)_3SO_4Na$ (EO-Sulfate) |

Step 3—Determine the percentage by weight of the green portion of the molecule. This is done by multiplying the weight of each atom by the number of atoms in each portion.

Calculations

Renewable Portion

	C	H	N	O	P	S	Na	K
Number	12	23	0	0	0	0	0	0
MW	144	23	0	0	0	0	0	0
Total	167							

Non- Renewable

	C	H	N	O	P	S	Na	K
Number	6	12	0	7	0	0	1	0
MW	72	12	0	112	0	0	23	0
Total	219							

Total	386
% Renewable	43
Green Star Rating	43

Example 3—Sodium Lauryl Sulfate (Ziegler Alcohol derived)

Step 1—Determine the empirical formula for chemical compounds used to make formulated product.

Sodium lauryl sulfate $C_{12}H_{23}SO_4Na$

Step 2—Determine which parts of the molecule are natural (derived from green natural raw materials) and which are synthetic.

Non-renewable (Synthetic) $C_{12}H_{23}SO_4Na$

Step 3—Determine the percentage by weight of the green portion of the molecule. This is done by multiplying the weight of each atom by the number of atoms in each portion.

Calculations

Renewable Portion

	C	H	N	O	P	S	Na	K
Number	0	0	0	0	0	0	0	0
MW	0	0	0	0	0	0	0	0
Total	0							

Non- Renewable

	C	H	N	O	P	S	Na
Number	12	23	0	4	0	1	1
MW	144	23	0	64	0	31	23
Total	285						

Total	285
% Renewable	0
Green Star Rating	0

Example 4—Cocamidopropyl Betaine

Step 1—Determine the empirical formula for chemical compounds used to make formulated product.

$$\begin{array}{c} CH_3 \\ | \\ C_{11}H_{23}C(O)\text{-}N(H)\text{-}(CH_2)_3\text{-}N^+\text{-}CH_2C(O)\text{-}O^- \\ | \\ CH_3 \end{array}$$

Formula $C_{18}H_{38}O_3N_2$

Step 2—Determine which parts of the molecule are natural (derived from green natural raw materials) and which are synthetic.

Renewable $C_{12}H_{23}O$

Nonrenewable $C_6H_{14}O_2N_2$

Step 3—Determine the percentage by weight of the green
portion of the molecule. This is done by multiplying
the weight of each atom by the number of atoms in
each portion.

Calculations

Renewable Portion

	C	H	N	O	P	S	Na	K
Number	12	23	0	1	0	0	0	0
MW	144	23	0	16	0	0	0	0
Total	183							

Non- Renewable

	C	H	N	O	P	S	Na	K
Number	6	14	2	2	0	0	0	0
MW	72	14	28	32	0	0	0	0
Total	146							

Total	329
% Renewable	55.6
Green Star Rating	56

Example 5—Cocamid DEA

Step 1—Determine the empirical formula for chemical
compounds used to make formulated product.

$$C_{11}H_{23}\text{-C(O)-N-(CH}_2\text{CH}_2\text{OH)}_2$$

$$C_{16}H_{30}O_3N$$

Step 2—Determine which parts of the molecule are natural (derived from green natural raw materials) and which are synthetic.

$$C_{11}H_{23}\text{-}C(O)\text{-}N\text{-}(CH_2CH_2OH)_2$$

Renewable $C_{12}H_{23}O$

Non-renewable $C_4H_{10}O_2N$

Step 3—Determine the percentage by weight of the green portion of the molecule. This is done by multiplying the weight of each atom by the number of atoms in each portion.

Calculations

	C	H	N	O	P	S	Na	K
Number	12	23	0	1	0	0	0	0
MW	144	23	0	16	0	0	0	0
Total	183							

Synthetic

	C	H	N	O	P	S	Na	K
Number	4	10	1	2	0	0	0	0
MW	48	10	14	32	0	0	0	0
Total	104							

Total	287
% Renewable	63
Green Star Rating	63

Example 6—Cocamid MEA

Step 1—Determine the empirical formula for chemical compounds used to make formulated product.

$$C_{11}H_{23}\text{-}C(O)\text{-}NH\text{-}CH_2CH_2OH$$

$$C_{14}H_{29}O_2N$$

Step 2—Determine which parts of the molecule are natural (derived from green natural raw materials) and which are synthetic.

$$C_{11}H_{23}\text{-}C(O)\text{-}NHCH_2CH_2OH$$

Renewable $C_{12}H_{23}O$

Non-renewable C_2H_6ON

Step 3—Determine the percentage by weight of the green portion of the molecule. This is done by multiplying the weight of each atom by the number of atoms in each portion.

Calculations

Renewable Portion								
	C	H	N	O	P	S	Na	K
Number	12	23	0	1	0	0	0	0
MW	144	23	0	16	0	0	0	0
Total	183							

Non- Renewable								
	C	H	N	O	P	S	Na	K
Number	2	6	1	2	0	0	0	0
MW	24	6	14	32	0	0	0	0
Total	76							

Total	259
% Renewable	70.6
Green Star Rating	71

Formulations

The Green Star Rating System can also be used on any formulation. All of the individual components in the formulation are rated and the overall Green Star rating is established.

Conditioning Shampoo

	% weight
Water	55.0
Sodium Lauryl Sulfate	18.0
Sodium Laureth 3 Sulfate	16.0
Cocamidopropyl Betaine	8.0
Cocamid DEA	3.0

Example 1 Conditioning Shampoo

This product is based on sodium lauryl sulfate (synthetic alcohol)

Ingredient	%weight	% Solids	Example	GRS	Contribution
Water	55.0	-	-	-	-
Sodium Lauryl Sulfate	34.0	9.5	3	0	0 (.095 times 0)
Cocamidopropyl Betaine	8.0	2.8	4	56	1.6 (.028 times 56)
Cocamid MEA	3.0	3.0	6	71	2.1 (.03 times 71)

Total   3.7

Example 2 Conditioning Shampoo (Version 1)

This product is based on sodium lauryl sulfate (synthetic alcohol) and SLES-3

Ingredient	%weight	% Solids	Example	GRS	Contribution
Water	55.0	-	-	-	-
Sodium Lauryl Sulfate	17.0	4.5	3	0	0 (.045 times 0)

Sodium Laureth 3 Sulfate	17.0	4.5	2	43	2.0 (.045 times 43)
Cocamidopropyl Betaine	8.0	2.8	4	56	1.6 (.028 times 56)
Cocamid DEA	3.0	3.0	5	63	1.9 (.03 times 63)

Total   5.5

Example 3 Conditioning Shampoo

This product is based on sodium coco sulfate (renewable alcohol)

Ingredient	%weight	% Solids	Example	GRS	Contribution
Water	55.0	-	-	-	-
Sodium Coco Sulfate	17.0	4.5	1	58	2.6 (.045 times 58)
Sodium Laureth 3 Sulfate	17.0	4.5	2	43	1.9 (.045 times 43)
Cocamidopropyl Betaine	8.0	2.8	4	56	1.6 (.028 times 56)
Cocamid DEA	3.0	3.0	5	63	1.9 (.03 times 63)

Total   8.0

Example 4 Conditioning Shampoo

This product is based on sodium coco sulfate (renewable alcohol)

Ingredient	%weight	% Solids	Example	GRS	Contribution
Water	55.0	-	-	-	-
Sodium Coco Sulfate	17.0	4.5	1	58	2.6 (.045 times 58)
Sodium Laureth 3 Sulfate	17.0	4.5	2	43	1.9 (.045 times 43)
Cocamidopropyl Betaine	8.0	2.8	4	56	1.6 (.028 times 56)
Cocamid MEA	3.0	3.0	6	71	2.1 (.03 times 71)

Total   8.2

These simple formulations show the power of the new system. Minor changes in the formulation made by properly selecting raw materials result in a 2.2 times improvement in the green star rating. This process allows the formulator to fine-tune formulations to maximize greenness and to inform the consumer about the amount of a given formulation that is renewable. The same approach works not only on shampoos but all formulations.

Conclusion

The Green Star Rating System provides the formulator and consumer with a metric by which both formulations and raw materials can be evaluated. The determination allows for the consumer to pick the product with the *highest Green Star Rating that provides the attributes consumers demand.* Inherent in this system is the belief that consumers can make educated selections of cosmetic formulations that balance the desire for green products and at the same time answer all the consumer's demands about performance.

CHAPTER 6

Green Formulations: Not All Components Are Equal

A. Cristoni, G. Maramaldi and C. Artaria
Indena SpA, Milan, Italy

KEY WORDS: *natural cosmetics, skin health, safety, efficacy, quality*

ABSTRACT: *In the consumer's mind, a natural or green cosmetic is automatically safe; however, the safety, quality and efficacy of botanical ingredients used in formulations need to be carefully assessed. Stability is also an important issue. Current research is directing analyses of final formulations to evaluate not only their cosmetic raw materials, but also their active materials.*

Nature has always been a generous source of wellness for mankind. Since ancient times, the healing properties of various plants have represented the first medicines and cosmetics. The study of tribal and native traditions has many times laid the foundation to successfully isolate new and effective cosmetic active ingredients.

Modern functional cosmetics represent valid alternatives to dermatological treatments for preventing the signs of aging, and the plant kingdom can provide many active compounds to counteract those signs, including: skin tone and elasticity loss,[1] wrinkle formation,[2,3] capillary fragility,[4] and increased skin sensitivity.[5]

However, natural ingredients require specific expertise not only in their research, but also in their analysis and formulation. The quality of botanical extracts, which needs to be standardized, is a crucial point for the quality of the final formulation, among others.

Standardized Extracts

To demonstrate the efficacy and reproducibility of a botanical active's variables in a cosmetic formulation, the consistency of the natural extract is a key factor. Reproducibility is also important when considering regulatory aspects aimed to assess the toxicity and tolerability of a cosmetic ingredient.

The consistency of a botanical extract is relatively achievable when dealing with a pure product such as escin or esculin from *Aesculus hippocastanum*; glycyrrhetinic acid from *Glycyrrhiza glabra*; or with a dry extract highly purified up to the isolation of a unique class of molecules such as triterpenes from *Centella asiatica*, flavolignans from *Silybum marianum*, polyphenols from *Vitis vinifera* and anthocyanins from *Vaccinum myrtillus*.

In some cases it is convenient to purify a unique active principle up to 80–90%, whereas in other cases a complete extract of numerous different compounds may be more active than the single isolated molecules. Research in this field is complex and involves not only the identification of the active principle, it also aims to investigate the interactions between the active ingredients and other molecules present in the phytocomplex.[6]

Different technologies or manufacturing methods may be necessary for different types of extracts but the main parameters include: composition constancy, stability, microbe counting and the limitation of residual solvents and pesticides. These parameters should be carefully monitored as required by health authorities.

The crucial stages of the process include, as a rule of thumb, choosing the raw material first, followed by extraction and purification. While the choice of extraction solvents in the preparation of standardized extracts is an important factor for the finished product quality, the choice of the raw material is pivotal.

From a practical point of view, the botanical source must be thoroughly checked before extraction, as far as botanical and chemical aspects are concerned (see **Table 1**).

The next phase is the preparation of the extract in standardized conditions, which requires the steps described in **Table 2**.

Extracts prepared according to the criteria in **Tables 1** and **2** can be classified as standardized. Although some of these parameters appear obvious, they can be difficult to achieve. For instance, all the botanical materials must be gathered within in a short, specific time period then stored after analysis to avoid the degradation of the active ingredients. In some cases, crops from homogeneous, genetically selected strains of plantules or seeds are grown in controlled agrochemical conditions. Cultivation can be a solution for plants whose harvesting in the wild could endanger the species' survival.

Table 1. Raw material characteristics and preliminary analysis

Parameter	Action to control the parameter
Part of plant	Botzanical identification, macro and microscopic analysis, control of sophisticant and contaminant presence
Harvesting	Careful selection and control of the region, area and harvesting period
Storage	Control of harvesting, drying and storage conditions
Active principle content	Chemical analysis in order to adequately mix different batches
Heavy metals and pesticides	Chemical analysis in order to discard the polluted batches

Table 2. Standardization and analysis

Parameter	Action to control the parameter
Extraction	Follow a defined method, with specified grinding, solvent, temperature, pressure
Concentration (if necessary)	Follow defined procedures, with analysis at the key steps of production
Chemical analysis	Control of the content in active principles, and of their reciprocal ratio; control of the presence of impurities, heavy metal, pesticides and residue solvents
Microbiologic analysis	Control of the microbial presence and of pathogen absence
Stability	Periodical analysis, in order to confirm the extract quality

Safety Issues

From a safety standpoint, the quality of a botanical extract needs to be carefully evaluated both on the raw material itself and within the final formulation—whether it is intended as a topical or oral cosmetic.

Recent evaluations[6] have in fact demonstrated that, besides labelling claims, only a small percentage of commercial products had chemical profiles that complied with their declared content. This research focused on the commercial preparation of bilberry extract purchased from different countries.

The HPLC method developed and validated in Indena research laboratories was optimized to analyze the content of anthocyanins, the polyphenols that bestow beneficial properties to bilberry extracts. (see **Figure 1**).

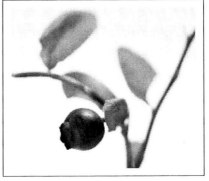

Figure 1. Case study: Bilberry

Bilberry: A Case Study

Chemical and pharmacological studies of bilberry extract have identified anthocyanosides, also known as anthocyanins, as the major components responsible for the biological properties of bilberry. They have been demonstrated to possess a broad range of activities, including: antioxidant activity,[7,8] antiplatelet aggregation,[9] phosphodiesterase inhibition,[10] interaction with collagen, phospholipids and proteoglycans,[11] a relaxing effect on vascular smooth muscle,[12] and arteriolar vasomotion stimulation.[13]

Bilberry is exploited for its capacity of reinforcing the blood vessel wall: it strengthens capillary walls by linking with the endothelial cell membranes, thus increasing their resistance and reducing capillary permeability by stimulating the synthesis of perivascular tissue constituents. In topical applications, these properties are particularly useful in case of heavy legs or couperose, where microcirculation improvement and capillary tone are crucial to the relief of disorders.

According to Indena research,[6] 40 different preparations containing bilberry, marketed under 24 different brands, were collected in four different countries for analysis. The samples came from the United States, Italy, Japan and Malaysia. The labels indicated three different types of preparations:

- bilberry extracts with a 36% anthocyanin content;
- bilberry extracts with a 25% anthocyandin content; and
- bilberry extract without content indication.

The analytical work based on HPLC revealed that 25% of the tested products had a different profile from a typical bilberry profile of either an anthocyanins content at 36%, or anthocyanidin at 25%. In fact, 10% did not even contain the active anthocyanins molecules and only 15% were found to possess a sufficient quantity of anthocyanins to be effective, as proven by clinical trials.

The fact also emerged that only 65% of the tested commercial products sold in the United States contained a quantity of ingredients matching the label claim.

Regarding the issue of appropriate labelling, a recent review[14] of the described analytical work highlighted some of the confusing information provided to the final consumer. For instance, the identity of the botanical species *Vaccinium myrtillus*, the only species with a sound tradition of medicinal use and well-documented by the scientific literature, is reported in 60% of labels, whereas the genus *Vaccinium* comprises over 450 species and the part of the plant is indicated on 70% of labels.

It needs to be taken into consideration that different parts of the same plant may have different biological properties. Bilberry leaves, for instance, have been traditionally used as a remedy for diabetes. This is not surprising since bilberry leaves, although they contain few anthocyanosides, are rich in tannins. The active ingredients are not defined on the labels, making it difficult for the consumer to understand the differences between the products. The quantity it contains in either milligrams or as a percentage concentration also is not listed.

Conclusions

Callaghan observed[15] that when the cosmetic industry wants to demonstrate how supplements can benefit the skin, it needs to be innovative and address questions relating to safety, toxicity, bioavailability, molecule interactions that control biological function, and age-related physiology.

The commercial preparations that have been analyzed recently highlight differences in content and variations between labelling and actual concentration, revealing a scenario of the herbal preparations that require the development of reliable analytical methods to analyze finished formulations.

It is important for formulators to be aware of the different qualities of natural extracts that may, by all means, affect the quality of the final formulations.

Published March 2008 *Cosmetics and Toiletries* magazine

References

1. FR Maffei, M Carini, R Stefani, G Aldini and L Saibene, Anti-elastase and anti-hyaluronidase activities of saponins and Sapogenins form *Hedera helix, Aesculus hippocastanum* and *Ruscus* aculeatus: Factors contributing to their efficacy in the treatment of venous insufficiency, *Arch Pharm 328* 720–724 (1995)
2. RF Maffei, M Carini, G Aldini, R Stefani, E Bombardelli and P Morazzoni, Free radical scavenging action and anti-enzyme activity of proanthocyanidine A2, a new polyphenol from *Aesculus hippocastanum* L., 18th IFSCC Congress, Venezia, Italy (Oct 3–6, 1994)
3. E Bombardelli, M Spelta, LR Della, S Sosa and A Tubaro, Aging skin: Protective effect of silymarin phytosome, *Fitoterapia* vol LXII 2 115–122 (1991)
4. E Bombardelli, P Morazzoni and A Griffini, *Aesculus hyppocastanum* L., *Fitoterapia* vol. LXVII 6 483–511 (1996)
5. A Cristoni, F Di Pierro, G Guglielmini, A Giori and P Morazzoni, Soothing activity of terpenoid fraction of *Ginkgo biloba* and of its phospholipidic complex, proceedings of 22nd IFSCC Congress, Edinburgh (2002)
6. C Cassanese, E De Combarieu, M Falzoni, N Fuzzati and R Pace R, New liquid chromatography method with UV detection for analysis in anthocyanins and anthocyanidins in *Vaccinum myrtillus* fruit dry extracts and commercial preparations, *J AOAC Int 90* 4 911–919 (2007)
7. R Salvare, P Braquet, Th Perruchot and L Douste-blazy, in *Flavonoids and Bioflavonoids 1981*, L Farkas, M Gabòr, F Kàllay and H Wagner, eds, Elsevier: Amsterdam, Oxford, New York (1982) pp 437–442
8. P Morazzoni and S Malandrino, Anthocyanosides and their aglycons as scavengers of free radicals and antilipoperoxidant agents, *Pharmacol Res Comm 20* suppl 2 254 (1988)
9. P Morazzoni and MJ Magistretti, Activity of myrtocyan, an anthocyanoside complex from *Vaccinum myrtillus* (VMA) on platelet aggregation and adhesivness, *Fitoterapia* 61 13 (1990)
10. C Ferretti, M Blengio, S Malandrino and G Pifferi, Effect of *Vaccinum myrtillus* on some phosphodiesterase isoforms, XI Internat Symp on Medicinal Chem, Jerusalem, Israel (Sep 2–7, 1990)
11. E Bombardelli and SB Curri, Antocianosidi, sostanza fondamentale del connettivo e correlazioni istangiche, *Terapia angiologia* 32 117 (1976)
12. V Bettini, F Mayellaro, E Patron, P Ton and V Terribile Wiel Marin, *Fitoterapia 55,* 323 (1984)
13. A Colantuoni, S Bertuglia, MJ Magistretti and L Donato, Effects on *Vaccinum myrtillus* anthocyanosides on arteriolar vasomotion, *Arzneim Forsch* 41 905 (1991)
14. C Artaria, R Pace, G Maramaldi and G Appendino, Different brands of bilberry extract—A comparison of selected components, *Nutrafoods* (2007) 6 (4), pp 5–10
15. T Callaghan, Challenges, opportunities in clinical evaluations of oral beauty supplements, *Cosm & Toil* 120 9 (Sep 2005)

CHAPTER 7

Keeping Cosmeceuticals Cosmetic

Wen Schroeder
SEKI Cosmeticals LLC, Appleton, Wisc., USA

KEY WORDS: *Antiaging, cosmeceuticals, drugs, cosmetics, claims substantiation, regulation*

ABSTRACT: *Global demand for cosmeceuticals continues at an explosive rate and the discovery of antiaging medical interventions, coupled with new functional active ingredients, provides a fertile innovation ground for product developers. This paper discusses current scientific and regulatory affairs to take into consideration for the successful commercialization of cosmeceutical products.*

According to market research, baby boomers' unprecedented purchasing power, coupled with a youth-dominated cultural shift and modern technological advancements, have fueled a rapidly growing US antiaging industry that exceeded US$45.5 billion in 2004, $7.7 billion of which was spent on appearance products alone.[1] Another report anticipated sales of cosmeceuticals in the United States to grow to more than $16 billion by 2010.

Oftentimes, cosmeceutical products incorporate such age-reversing and appearance-rejuvenating claims as: "aging is reversible and optional"; "regenerates damaged skin"; "penetrates deeply into the layers of the skin"; "erases wrinkles and boosts collagen synthesis within 10 days"; "stimulates cellular metabolism within days"; and so on. An Australian survey conducted by CoreData and *www.news.com. au* reported that 55% of the respondents did not trust the accuracy of the scientific claims made by cosmetic companies, and many were cynical about those claims.[2]

It is therefore unclear whether cosmeceutical products should be considered a new regulatory subcategory of cosmetics, or if they should be regarded as medicinal products. So what are the rules regulating product claims for this category, and what are the substantiation standards?

Legal Distinction Between Drugs and Cosmetics in the United States

In the United States, regulatory requirements for cosmetics and drugs are established by the Federal Food, Drug and Cosmetic Act (FD&C Act) of 1938 and enforced by the US Food and Drug Administration (FDA).

The act defines cosmetics as:

"Articles intended to be rubbed, poured, sprinkled or sprayed on, introduced into, or otherwise applied to the human body … for cleansing, beautifying, promoting attractiveness or altering the appearance."[3]

Drugs are defined by this act as:

"(A) Articles intended for use in the diagnosis, cure, mitigation, treatment or prevention of disease …; and

(B) Articles (other than food) intended to affect the structure or any function of the body of man or other animals."[4]

Currently, products are classified by this legislation based on their intended use. A product's intended use may be established through its direct advertising or product claims. However, the FDA advises that consumer perception and expectation of the product also constitute the basis for determining the intended use, be it through direct advertisement or indirectly implied promotional messages.[5, 6]

The FDA sets specific requirements governing cosmetic product labeling, including details such as the product identity display, placement of the name and business location, appropriate ingredient listing, accurate statement of the net quantity of contents, appropriate directions for safe use and appropriate warning statements when deemed necessary. Labeling is defined as including all written, printed or graphic material that appears on the products, containers, packaging inserts and any material accompanying the product.

Therefore, any promotional material or statement, including those that appear on the Internet, in product catalogs and in flyers, are considered cosmetic product labeling. These requirements are regulated under two main regulations: the FD&C Act, and the Fair Packaging and Labeling Act (FPLA).

The primary enforcement focus of the FDA on cosmetic products is in regards to misbranding. To qualify as a cosmetic product, the labeling must not imply any physiological effect, must not suggest an impact on structure or function, must not contain ingredients that are commonly regarded as drugs, and must not contain unapproved color additives. If an ingredient is known by the public to have certain therapeutic effects, its use in a cosmetic product without drug claims would in fact violate the FDA misbranding rule. For instance, incorporating acetaminophen[a] into a cosmetic product would instantly classify it as a drug by FDA standards, even if no drug claims are made. Therefore, incorporating drug claims on a cosmetic label deems the product to be misbranded, leading to FDA enforcement action.

In general, a cosmetic product is not allowed to contain ingredients that are commonly regarded as drugs, such as active ingredients recognized for therapeutic benefits. In addition, International Nomenclature of Cosmetic Ingredients (INCI) names should be listed on cosmetic labels instead of the chemicals names associated with therapeutic benefits.

For example, alpha-tocopherol should not be listed as *vitamin E* in the declaration of ingredients because listing it as such would imply a therapeutic effect. Other examples of ingredients well-known for therapeutic effects include hormones and hydrocortisone.

The Global Situation: Cosmetics vs. Drugs

The definition of a therapeutic drug is quite similar around the world. Most countries agree that a drug is intended for the diagnosis, cure, mitigation, treatment or prevention of diseases via some means of physiological action. When it comes to cosmetics, however, differences exist in major world markets including Australia, the United States, Europe, Canada and Japan.

---

[a] Acetaminophen is the active ingredient in Tylenol, a product of McNeil PPC, Inc.

Australia: In Australia, a cosmetic is defined by the Therapeutic Goods Association (TGA) as:

A substance or preparation intended for placement in contact with any external part of the human body, including the mucous membrane of the oral cavity, and the teeth, with a view to altering the odors of the body; or changing its appearance; or cleansing it; or maintaining it in good condition; or perfuming it; or protecting it.

Similar to the classification standard practiced in the United States, a cosmetic product will be considered therapeutic if it is intended to treat, alleviate or prevent disease; if it claims to affect the structure or function of the human body or have therapeutic effects; or if it contains ingredients possessing therapeutic effects.[7] The two major factors used to differentiate cosmetics from therapeutic products are the composition and the proposed use and claims. According to the third edition of *Guidelines for Cosmetic Claims* by the TGA, cosmetics may not make therapeutic claims unless they are listed in the Australian Register of Therapeutic Goods.[8]

Sunscreen products in Australia must comply with a different set of mandatory product labeling requirements. Sunscreens are divided into two subcategories—primary and secondary. Although both are regulated by the TGA Department of Health and Aging as therapeutic goods under the Therapeutic Goods Act, their category determines the appropriate labeling requirements. In general, if the main purpose of the product is to protect the skin from UV radiation, then it is usually considered a primary sunscreen. If the product serves a major cosmetic function, such as a color cosmetic or a moisturizer, but contains additional UV protection claims, then it is considered a secondary sunscreen. Primary sunscreens must have the SPF listed clearly on the main label, whereas the SPF in a secondary sunscreen must appear on the package but not necessarily on the main label.

Canada: The Canadian Food and Drugs Act defines a cosmetic as:

Any substance or mixture of substances manufactured, sold or represented for use in cleansing, improving or altering the complexion, skin, hair or teeth; and includes deodorants and perfumes.

Similar to the FDA, Health Canada further stipulates that claims of physiological effect are not allowed in cosmetics. A cosmetic product making a therapeutic claim, for example to "prevent or treat disease," would be classified as a drug under the Food and Drugs Act and therefore a drug identification number (DIN) would be required.[9]

Personal care products sold in Canada may be regulated under one of the three regulatory schemes: natural health product (NHP) regulations, food and drug regulations, or cosmetic regulations. The determining factors are the ingredients used, the intended uses and product claims. Health Canada estimated that most personal care products sold in Canada are cosmetics.

NHPs in Canada are defined based on their function and ingredients. They must be used for: the diagnosis, treatment, mitigation or prevention of a disease, disorder or abnormal physical state; restoring or correcting organic functions in humans; and modifying organic functions in humans, such as modifying those functions in a manner as to maintain or promote health.

To qualify as an NHP, the product must not contain ingredients prohibited in NHPs and must contain medicinal ingredients approved for use in NHPs. In general, NHPs include vitamins and minerals, herbal remedies, homeopathic medicines, traditional medicines such as traditional Chinese medicines, probiotics and other products such as amino acids and essential fatty acids. Sunscreen, as an example, is regulated as a nonprescription OTC drug product in Canada but depending on the types of actives used, those actives could be grouped as either NHPs or drugs.

A sunscreen that is considered an NHP contains inorganic UV filters such as titanium dioxide and zinc oxide, with a 25% maximum level allowed. Products containing organic UV filters such as avobenzone, oxybenzone, cinoxate and so on, are regulated as drug products. Again, these products are further divided into either primary or secondary sunscreens, depending on their intended primary UV protection claims.

Japan: The Japanese Pharmaceutical Affairs Law regulates all pharmaceuticals, quasi-drugs, cosmetics and medical devices in

Japan. Its definition of a cosmetic is stated as:

A substance with mild effect on the human body that is intended to be put on the human body for the purpose of cleansing, beautifying, enhancing attraction, changing appearance or maintaining skin or hair health.

This definition differs from the others in that it allows cosmetics to have a mild effect on the human body.[10]

Europe: In the European Union, the Seventh Amendment to the Cosmetic Directive (original Directive 76/768/EEC) defines a cosmetic as:

Any substance or preparation intended to be placed in contact with the various external parts of the human body (epidermis, hair system, nails, lips and external genital organs) or with the teeth and the mucous membranes of the oral cavity with a view exclusively or mainly to cleaning them, perfuming them, changing their appearance and/or correcting body odors and/or protecting them or keeping them in good condition.[11]

The directive further instructs in Article 7a,1(g) that proof of the effect claimed for the cosmetic product be kept readily accessible to competent authorities of the member state. Based on this definition, one could expect cosmetic products to show some "effect."

Although product classification standards may differ between continents, regulatory requirements for cosmetics are quite similar in these major markets, in terms of: demanding the manufacturer to carry the full responsibility for product safety; not requiring pre-market product approval or registration; establishing cosmetic-specific Good Manufacturing Practice (GMP) guidelines; and imposing no restrictions on sales distribution channels.

Cosmeceutical Product Labeling

The term *cosmeceutical* has been used by the cosmetic industry to refer to cosmetics that possess drug-like effects. Antiaging products are among this fast-growing segment of the skin care market, and many of these products are being deemed cosmeceuticals since they claim to deliver rejuvenation benefits far beyond skin moisturization or merely camouflaging wrinkles.

However, the FDA does not recognize cosmeceuticals as a valid product class and does not plan to include it as a subcategory of cosmetics. In addition, the FDA plans to apply the same structure and function standard to cosmeceutical and antiaging products. If a product is intended for cosmetic use but its claims suggest physiological or drug-like properties, the product will be subjected to both drug and cosmetic regulations.[12] By doing this, the FDA is simply reinforcing the fact that a personal care product can be either a drug or a cosmetic but it cannot be both while only adhering to one set of regulations. If a company chooses to claim a product as both, it must be prepared to provide the claims substantiation required for both product types— and not just the easier of the two. A cosmetic provides a superficial effect, is temporary and does not affect the structure or function of the body; therefore, it is not regulated. The FDA will not permit manufacturers to "hide" under this cosmetic product category while still claiming drug effects without complying with drug regulations.

Cosmeceutical claims using language such as "enhanced cellular turnover rate"; "DNA repair"; "molecular energy renewal at the mitochondria level"; and "collagen synthesis stimulation," suggest affecting the structure and function of the user. Therefore, the FDA considers these products as drugs and will regulate them as such.

Health Canada takes a similar stance as the FDA on cosmeceuticals. It does not recognize them as a legitimate product category; they are regulated either as a cosmetic or a drug depending on the claims that are made and/or the composition of the product. Acceptable cosmetic claims that are provided in the *Guidelines for Cosmetic Manufacturers, Distributors and Importers*[13] include: "softens skin"; "reduces the look of cellulite"; "removes oil"; "helps to eliminate odor-causing bacteria"; "soothes"; or "helps to prevent the look of aging." Using phrases such as: "heals," "slims/slimming," "stops acne," "kills germs," or "eliminates wrinkles," may lead the Canadian authority to consider a product as mislabeled.

The Australian National Coordinating Committee on Therapeutic Goods allows antiaging cosmetic product claims such as: "covers up" or "hides age spots, blemishes or dark pigmented areas"; makes the consumer "feel younger" or "look younger"; "helps to prevent, reduce or slow the signs or appearance of aging"; "moisturizes aging skin"; or "smoothes wrinkles."[14] It, however, does not allow claims such as "antiaging" and "temporarily reduces the depth of wrinkles by moisturization" without substantiation. Unacceptable wording for a cosmetic, but not necessarily acceptable for a drug, includes anything claiming to "eliminate, prevent, stop, reduce, slow or reverse aging, wrinkles, premature aging, or the aging process." It also includes products claiming to rejuvenate cells or any references to fading age spots, de-pigmenting, skin bleaching and so on.

In the EU, antiaging products were among the 32 "borderline cosmetics" listed by the Council of Europe Publishing in 2000.[15] These products are not adequately covered by the EU Cosmetic Directive and can be regulated differently by each member state as consumer products, cosmetics or even drugs, depending on the claims and ingredients used, essentially creating a regulatory and marketing complication for the industry.

FDA Enforcement—Drugs or Cosmetics

The FDA cosmetic regulatory branch has been seriously weakened in recent years due to significant budget constraints, limited resources and the need to allocate resources to handle more pressing and life-threatening public health issues. Cosmetics generally are not likely to cause serious adverse effects and historically have been relatively safer than food, drugs and medical devices. As a result, the cosmetic industry has not experienced major FDA enforcement actions against extravagant antiaging product claims.

However, recent warning letters[16-17] may indicate a trend in future FDA enforcement actions. In both cases, the FDA stated that the claims being made were considered to be "structure/function" claims and that the cited products were not generally recognized as safe and effective for the intended use. Those products were thus considered as unapproved new drugs. New drugs may not be marketed without prior FDA New Drug Application approval. The FDA has specified some of the "structure/function" drug claims that are inappropriate for cosmetic products (see **Inappropriate Cosmetic Product Claims**).

Inappropriate Cosmetic Product Claims Based on FDA Regulations

"Clinically proven to dramatically reduce the appearance of existing stretch mark length, depth, texture, and discoloration ..."

"A stretch mark-reducing emulsion ... to diminish fine lines, wrinkles and crow's-feet"

"[S]uperior wrinkle-reducing properties of a patented oligo-peptide (called Pal-KTTKS)...on 'photo-aged skin'... [A] key ingredient in the ..."

"[S]ignificant improvement' in wrinkle depth, length, wrinkle volume ..."

"... actually increases the synthesis of new collagen"

"is proven to reduce deep wrinkles up to ... 70%"

"Stimulates your skin's own collagen-building network"

"Reduces deep wrinkles from within the skin's surface ..."

"Visible results that won't fade away ..."

"Vitamin C helps reduce the effects of aging ... by helping to strengthen collagen and elastin fibers"

"Clinical studies proved a 50% reduction in wrinkles ..."

FTC Enforcement: Claims Substantiation

The Federal Trade Commission (FTC) was first established in 1914 to prevent unfair business competition in the market place. From a regulatory standpoint, product claims and advertisements should be truthful and not mislead consumers; claims substantiation must pass the "reasonable basis of support" requirement for both the expressed and implied claims.[18] Deception is defined by the FTC as:[19]

- A representation, omission or practice likely to mislead the consumer.
- Being judged based on the standpoint of "reasonable consumers."
- Being determined to provide an overall impression as such by considering the net direct impression, expressed claims, and those that are implied via the context.
- Claims that are "material" and that lead to a consumer's purchasing decision.

The FTC's policy stipulates that, in order to be deemed as competent and reliable scientific evidence, "tests, analyses, research, studies or other evidence must be based on the expertise of professionals in their relevant area, and that the tests have been conducted and evaluated in an objective manner by persons qualified to do so, using procedures generally accepted in the profession to yield accurate and reliable results."[20]

The FTC Act assigns liability broadly. Advertisers, ad agencies and endorsers all carry various degrees of responsibility. There are many legal remedies and penalties available for FTC enforcement actions, including warnings, injunctions, refunds, profits disgorgement, corrective advertising, and surveillance. The FTC also has been known to use litigation via both the administrative and federal courts to make its case.

In general, the FTC tends to pay more attention to nationwide advertising campaigns that have a far-reaching impact, advertisements raising health and safety concerns, blatantly false or extreme claims, and serious disease claims. In recent years, its main focus has been on dietary supplements and weight-loss programs or products.

Being Global WithoutGlobal Regulation

Global regulatory definitions and requirements can lead to confusion for personal care product companies. To launch a global product, personal care companies face the daunting task of navigating through a vast sea of uncertainties including conflicting regulatory product definitions, borderline product categorization, varying allowances for product claims and different product labeling requirements. In this highly regulated and inter-related modern world, a company cannot measure its success simply by its ability to develop the most scientifically advanced formula with measurable and effective skin care benefits. The biggest challenge currently facing the cosmetic industry is how to walk the fine line when considering the following:

- What the cosmetic industry would like to claim for marketing advantages;
- What the industry can truthfully say from the scientific point of view;

- What the consumers will perceive as believable;
- What cosmetic competitors are claiming for their products; and
- What can be said about a product under the regulations.

Today's consumer product companies face a tremendous task of bringing newer, more value-added products into the market within a much shorter time frame. Aging baby boomers' desire to remain forever young will continue to add fuel to the already feverish global growth of the antiaging skin care product segment. Complex marketing strategies, global supply chain distribution and product positioning often collide with last minute, unexpected regulatory restraints, causing costly delays in product launches.

In extreme cases, unforeseen and/or unresolved regulatory road-blocks can sink a profitable product line, which is unfortunate but avoidable. Incorporating a comprehensive and well-orchestrated regulatory strategy and analysis during the early conceptualization phase is essential to overall product development success.

It is imperative that the successful implementation of any global marketing plan take into consideration different regional regulatory requirements for ingredient selection, product claims, and advertising and promotional materials. To avoid financially disastrous last-minute hurdles for any product launch, the best operational rule for success is to scope out the marketing scheme during the early product development cycle and to develop potential claims through careful examination of regulatory allowances and scientific support evidence, taking into consideration current consumer perception and awareness; and finally, following up with a well-designed product safety review and testing, both pre- and post-market.

Published September 2008 *Cosmetics and Toiletries* magazine

References

1. J Dvorko, Antiaging Products and Services, BCC Research, Report ID: PHM041A, Feb 2005
2. L. Bjorksten, Ad claims 'bogus,' but we still pay, Apr 23, 2007, *www.coredata.com.au/pdf/2007042301.pdf* (Jul 11, 2008)
3. FD&C Act, sec. 201(i)
4. FD&C Act, sec. 201(g)(1)

5. Senate Report No. 361, 74th Congress, 1st session. 4, 1935.
6. PB Hutt, The Legal Distinction in the United States Between a Cosmetic and a Drug. *J Toxicol Cut Ocular Toxicol* 20(2–3) 203–210 (2001)
7. Australian Therapeutic Goods Act (1989)
8. Cosmetic Claims Guidelines, 3rd edition, National Coordinating Committee on Therapeutic Goods, May 9, 1997, *www.tga.gov.au/docs/pdf/cosclaim.pdf* (Jul 11, 2008)
9. The Canadian Food & Drugs Act F-27, 1985, *laws.justice.gc.ca/en/showtdm/cs/F-27* (Jul 11, 2008)
10. Pharmaceutical Administration & Regulations in Japan. Mar 2006, published by the Pharmaceutical Manufacturers Association, *www.jpma.or.jp/english/parj/pdf/2006.pdf* (Jul 11, 2008)
11. Council Directive on the approximation of the laws of the Member States relating to cosmetic products (76/768/EEC) Jul, 27, 1976 (OJ L 262, 27.9.1976, p. 169). *eur-lex. europa.eu/LexUriServ/LexUriServ.do?uri=CONSLEG:1976L0768:20070508:EN:PDF* (Jul 11, 2008)
12. C Rados, Science Meets Beauty: Using Medicine to Improve Appearances *FDA Consumer Magazine* Mar–Apr (2004)
13. Guidelines for Cosmetics Manufacturers, Importers and Distributors, *hc-sc.gc.ca/cps-spc/pubs/indust/cosmet_guide/act-loi_e.html* (Jul 11, 2008)
14. Cosmetic Claims Guidelines, National Coordinating Committee on Therapeutic Goods. 3rd Edition. May 9, 2007 *www.tga.gov.au/docs/html/cosclaim.htm* (Jul 11, 2008)
15. Cosmetic Products—Borderline Situations. Strasbourg, France: Council of Europe Publishing; 2001:200.
16. FDA-amended Warning Letter from the Director of the Denver District to Basic Research LLC, Jan 20, 2005 *www.fda.gov/foi/warning_letters/archive/g5195d.htm* (Jul 11, 2008)
17. FDA Warning Letter from Director of the Los Angeles District to University Medical Products USA, Inc, Jan 22, 2004 *www.fda.gov/foi/warning_letters/archive/g4511d.htm* (Jul 11, 2008)
18. FTC Policy Statement Regarding Advertising Substantiation Mar 11, 1983.
19. FTC Policy Statement on Deception, appended to Cliffdale Associates Inc, 103 FTC 110, 174 (1984)
20. FTC vs. Prolong Super Lubricants Inc. Decision and Order, Docket No. C-3906 Nov 22, 1999

CHAPTER 8

Organic and Natural: Caveat Emptor

David C. Steinberg
Steinberg & Associates

KEY WORDS: *USDA organic Seal, Natural Products Association Seal, OASIS Organic Seal*

ABSTRACT: *COSMOS is the European Union's (EU) newest effort to outline organic and natural standards, with draft guidelines published in November 2008. But how is it different than other standards?*

Every once in a while, readers ask how topics are selected for this column. This time, the idea came from an e-mail inquiring what COSMOS standards are. Previous columns have discussed Canadian Natural Health Products regulations but have steered clear of the natural and organic debate, although this author previously published an article[1] that debates animal versus vegetable ingredients, in which he explains that a chemical is a chemical regardless of its origin; a molecule of glycerin is just that, whether from natural sources like animal or vegetable fat, or from petroleum or biodiesel sources.

COSMOS is the European Union's (EU) newest effort to outline organic and natural standards, with draft guidelines published in November 2008. But how is it different than other standards? This calls for a review of the various natural and organic standards for the personal care industry and how they have evolved.

What is Natural?

According to the author, when he first began to learn during the Dark Ages, the elements of earth, air, fire and water were understood to be natural; thus everything made from them was considered natural. Later, industry expert Ken Klein stated that anything made from the first 92 elements of the periodic table are natural, and that no man-made elements should be used in products claiming to be natural; however, this philosophy did not seem a sufficient answer for what marketers where claiming.

An Internet investigation retrieved several meanings for the term *natural*, among which were: being present in or produced by nature; i.e., *a natural pearl*; being inherent or not acquired; not being produced or changed artificially; and not being altered, treated or disguised.

The US Food and Drug Administration (FDA) does not define natural in the Food, Drug and Cosmetic Act or any other FDA regulation; the closest definition[2] for natural personal care products was established in Canada as a regulated category called Natural Health Products. This regulation, which went into effect on Jan. 1, 2004, defines natural health products (NHPs) as: vitamins and minerals, herbal remedies, homeopathic medicines, traditional medicine such as traditional Chinese medicine, probiotics, and other products like amino acids and essential fatty acids.

While these materials are found in nature, Canada took it a step further to describe acceptable substances as being synthetic duplicates of those materials listed above. Synthetic duplicates are substances that share identical chemical structures and pharmacological properties with their natural counterparts; an example of such is vitamin E anddl alpha-tocopherol.

A semi-synthetic substance may also be acceptable as an NHP, provided that it shares identical chemical structures and pharmacological properties with its natural counterpart. Semi-synthetic substances are produced by processes that chemically change a related starting material that has been extracted or isolated from a plant or a plant material, an alga, a fungus or a non-human animal material. An example of such is ginsenosides, which are produced from the starting compound betulafolienetriol.

In the end, whatever marketing deems natural is natural; the critical inference is that consumers believe products marketed as natural are safer than products that are not marketed as natural. This has given rise to an increase in use of the word *organic* within the cosmetic industry.

Organic

Recalling studies from his youth, the author notes that the term *organic* originally referred to the chemistry of the carbon atom. Then in 1973, an organization called the California Certified Organic Farmer was formed to promote organic farming in California, instilling in the public a new sense of the word *organic*. This group became one of the first to certify products with an organic seal of approval on the label. In 1979, the state made the organic labeling of foods a law subject to their controls.

In 1980, the US Department of Agriculture (USDA) published its "Report and Recommendations on Organic Farming,"[3] in which organic farming was described as a "production system that avoids or largely excludes the use of synthetically compounded fertilizers, pesticides, growth regulators and livestock feed additives. To the maximum extent feasible, organic farming systems rely upon crop rotations, crop residues, animal manures, legumes, green manures, off-farm organic wastes, mechanical cultivation, mineral-bearing rocks and aspects of biological pest control to maintain soil productivity and tilth, to supply plant nutrients and to control insects, weeds and other pests."[4]

Reasons for interest in this system included:
- Increased cost and uncertain availability of energy and chemicals;
- Increased resistance of weeds and insects to pesticides;
- Decline in soil productivity from erosion and accompanying loss of organic matter and plant nutrients;
- Pollution of surface waters with agricultural chemicals and sediment;
- Destruction of wildlife, bees and beneficial insects by pesticides;
- Hazards to human and animal health from pesticides and feed additives;
- Detrimental effects of agricultural chemicals on food quality;
- Depletion of finite reserves of concentrated plant nutrients (e.g., phosphate rock); and

- Decrease in numbers of farms, particularly family-type farms, and disappearance of localized and direct marketing systems.[5]

By the late 1980s, a number of private and state-run certifying bodies were operating in the United States. Standards varied among these entities, causing trouble in commerce. Certifiers often refused to recognize products certified as organic by other agents, which was a problem particularly for organic livestock producers seeking feed, and for processors trying to source ingredients. In addition, a number of well-publicized incidents of fraud began to undermine the credibility of the organic industry.

In an effort to curb these problems, the organic community pursued federal legislation. The result was the Organic Foods Production Act of 1990, which mandated the creation of the National Organic Program (NOP) and the passage of uniform organic standards. These standards were incorporated into NOP regulations.[6] Implementation of the regulations began on April 21, 2001, and all organic certifiers, producers, processors and handlers were required to be in full compliance by Oct. 21, 2002.[7]

Beyond federal legislation, the California Organic Products Act (COPA) was signed into law in 2003, and beginning Jan. 1, 2003, all products sold in California containing a total of less than 70% organic ingredients were no longer allowed to use the word *organic* on the front labeling panel. Later in 2003, the State Assembly repealed the non-food provision of the COPA but in the end, cosmetics remained a part of the Act.

With the growth of nationwide food stores based on certified organic foods, interest in the organic market has spread to cosmetics and other personal care products. From this interest, several groups have emerged with varying standards for organic certification; most use a seal that appears on product labels to indicate organic certification. Following are some of the major bodies, as well as their requirements. This is not a comprehensive list but it will provide an overview.

National Organic Program (NOP, United States): Within this program are four levels of organic claims for foods. The NOP defines the claims that can be used for agricultural products by their content, excluding water and salt.

- *100% Organic:* For this claim, 100% of the ingredients in the product must be certified organic products and in this case, the USDA Organic seal may be used (see **Figure 1**).
- *Organic:* To make this claim, 95% of the materials in the product must be certified organic products; the same USDA Organic seal may be used in this instance.
- *Made with organic ingredients:* For this label claim, 70% to 94.99% of the product's ingredients must be certified organic; in this case, use of the USDA Organic seal is not permitted.
- *Contains organic:* This label claim requires less than 70% of certified organic ingredients in a product and also cannot bear the USDA Organic seal.

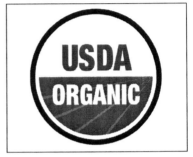

Figure 1. USDA Organic seal

Natural Products Association (NPA, United States): This organization was founded in 1936 and was principally concerned with dietary supplements. The group represents more than 10,000 retailers, manufacturers, wholesalers and distributors of natural products, including foods, dietary supplements, and health and beauty aids. On May 1, 2008, the group issued its certification program for personal care products. In order to display the NPA seal (see **Figure 2**), a product must meet the following requirements:

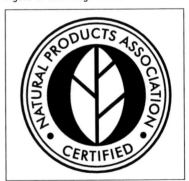

Figure 2. NPA seal

- Contain at least 95% truly natural ingredients or ingredients that are derived from natural sources;
- Contain no ingredients linked with potentially suspected human health risks;
- Not be processed in ways that significantly or adversely alter the purity of its natural ingredients;
- Include ingredients derived from a purposeful, renewable/plentiful source found in nature (flora, fauna, mineral);

- Be minimally processed and avoid the use of synthetic or harsh chemicals so as not to dilute the material's purity; and
- Should contain non-natural ingredients only where viable natural alternative ingredients are unavailable, and only when they pose absolutely no potentially suspected human health risks.

The Natural Products Association also has published[8] a list including 839 ingredients that it considers meets these requirements.

Cosmetics Organic and Natural Standard (COSMOS, EU): As noted above, COSMOS is one of the EU's newest efforts, with its draft published in November 2008. This standard was developed from collaborations between working groups including: the Instituto per la Certificazione Etica e Ambientale (ICEA in Italy); the Federation of German Industries and Trading Firms for Pharmaceuticals, Health Care Goods, Dietary Supplements and Personal Hygiene products (BDIH in Germany); Bioforum in Belgium; the French Professional Association of the Ecological and Organic Cosmetics, and a French certification organization (Cosmebio/Ecocert in France); and an environmental charity promoting sustainable, organic farming and championing human health (The Soil Association in the UK). The COSMOS draft is available at *www.cosmos-standard.org.*

These standards describe five categories of ingredients: water, minerals, physically processed agro-ingredients, chemically processed agro-ingredients and synthetic materials. The draft details what materials are and are not allowed. It is interesting to note the chemical reactions that are and are not allowed (see **COSMOS Chemical Reactions**).

Under Appendix II of the COSMOS standard, the following synthetic ingredients are allowed: benzoic acid, benzyl alcohol, dehydroacetic acid, denatonium benzoate, heliotropine, salicylic acid, sorbic acid and tetrasodium glutamate diacetate. The second part of Appendix II lists the mineral origin products allowed—which contradicts the initial five categories of organic ingredients listed since "mineral" is included one of the organic ingredient categories.

COSMOS Chemical Reactions

Allowed physical processes:

- Extractions must use natural materials with any form of water or with a third solvent of plant origin such as ethyl alcohol, glycerin, vegetable oils and CO_2 absorption (on an inert support that conforms to these standards);
- Bleaching or deodorization (on an inert support conforming to these standards);
- Grinding, centrifuging (solid/liquid separation, spin-drying);
- Settling, decanting, desiccation or drying (progressive or not by evaporation/natural under sun);
- Deterpenation (if fractionated distillation with steam);
- Distillation, expression or extraction (steam);
- Filtration and purification (ultra filtration, dialysis, crystallization and ion exchange);
- Lyophilization, blending, percolation, cold pressure and hot pressure (depending on the fluidity of the fatty acids to be extracted);
- Sterilization with thermal treatments (according to a temperature respectful of the active substances); and
- Sifting, maceration and ultrasound

Allowed chemical processes:

- Alkylation, amidation, calcination of plant residues and carbonization (resins, fatty organic oils);
- Condensation/addition, esterification, etherification and fermentation (natural/biotechnological);
- Hydration, hydrogenation, hydrolysis and neutralization (to obtain Na, Ca, Mg and K salts);
- Oxidation/reduction processes for the manufacture of amphoterics; and
- Saponification, sulphation and roasting

Unallowed processes:

Any other processes that are not listed above are not allowed, including but not limited to:

- Bleaching or deodorization (on a support of animal origin);
- Use of enzymes derived from GMOs;
- Deterpenation (other than with beam);
- Ethoxylation, irradiation and sulphonation (as the main reaction);
- Techniques employing genetic engineering;
- Treatments with ethylene oxide or using mercury (mercurial soda);
- Use of petrochemical solvents (hexane, toluene, benzene, etc.); or
- Propoxylation.[9]

California Organic Program (United States): Products sold in California must comply with the 2003 COPA Act[10] to be labeled organic. These products also must be at least 70% organic, not including water and salt content. Like the USDA program, this program attempts to apply a food law to cosmetics. All organic ingredients used in organic products must be certified by one of the organizations listed by the USDA. There are additional registration fees and other labeling requirements.

Organic and Sustainable Industry Standards (OASIS, United States): OASIS was developed and is observed by major cosmetic companies in the United States such as L'Oréal and Estée Lauder. This standard certifies products at two levels—*organic* or *made with organic.* The *made with organic* designation requires 70% minimum organic content with additional criteria for the remaining 30% of ingredients. The *organic* label claim will require a minimum of 85% organic content until January 2010, at which time it will increase to a requirement of 90% minimum organic content; the minimum requirement will increase a third time to 95% by 2012. Products that cannot achieve a 95% organic level, such as soap, must use the *made with organic* claim.

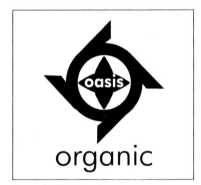

Figure 3. OASIS seal

This interval approach takes into consideration the fact that at least two years are necessary for surfactant and emulsifier manufacturers to put enough products into the commercial stream to supply the industry with organic versions of functional ingredients. Since one of the goals of OASIS is to promote the development of more raw materials developed from organic starting materials, this approach works with chemical manufacturers to achieve these goals.[11]

Whole Foods—Premium Body Care Seal (United States): One of the major retail outlets for organic products is the Whole Foods supermarket chain. This group has established its own rules and symbol. As of press time, the author has not been able to obtain the rules or the symbol. The group lists more than 250 ingredients that are not allowed, and also does not allow animal testing or organic UV filters. The group is aligned with the Environmental Working Group (EWG).

Organic Consumers Association (United States): This final group was established in 1998 in opposition to the USDA's NOP program, and deals primarily with the food area. It has been involved in litigation with other standards.[12]

Comments

What chaos. Why are there so many different organizations, standards, symbols—and now, lawsuits? There is only one answer: marketing. One may question whether the companies selling cosmetics stamped with these symbols care about anything more than selling products. The underlying message is that consumers have been misled to believe that these products are safer than non-natural or non-organic cosmetics.

These organizations' definitions are contradictory and in some ways, amusing. One set of rules states that water found in the *Aloe barbadensis* leaf is organic while water from the faucet is not. Water is water is water. Also, natural minerals are allowed as colorants but they cannot be processed; as a minor point, this means that with the exception of mica, none of these natural minerals would be permitted in cosmetics. Natural iron oxides, for example, would be in violation of FDA, EU and Japanese standards since ground iron oxide ores have enough lead, mercury, arsenic, cadmium, etc., in them to keep Proposition 65 lawyers in California busy filing lawsuits forever.

Natural does not mean safe. In fact, the NPA's list of permitted "safe ingredients" includes 15 of the EU's 26 listed fragrance allergens. Perhaps natural allergens are better, then? And while one firm stands behind the EWG and proclaims that synthetic UV filters are dangerous, only permitting ZnO and TiO_2, the International Agency for Research on Cancer has in the meantime declared TiO_2 to be a known human carcinogen; plus, synthetic ZnO is the only ZnO used since its natural ore only exists with lead.

How far can this go?[13] Do natural or organic cosmetics impart real benefits or are they just another marketing fad? As the economy in the United States declines, it appears that consumers are still spending money for organic foods but are foregoing higher priced organic personal care products.

This column is titled "Caveat Emptor," which means "let the buyer beware." This column also calls to mind a quote by David Hannum, among others, that states: "There's a sucker born every minute." In this author's opinion, that is what keeps these products on the store shelf.

Published April 2009 *Cosmetics and Toiletries* magazine

References

1. DC Steinberg, Ingredient Review: Animal vs. Vegetable, A Continuing Controversy, *Skin Inc.* 11(3) 58–62 (Apr 1999)
2. Natural Health Products Regulations, Health Canada Web site, available at *www.hc-sc.gc.ca/dhp-mps/prodnatur/legislation/acts-lois/prodnatur/index-eng.php* (Accessed Feb 4, 2009)
3. Report and Recommendations on Organic Farming, USDA Web site, available at *http://nal.usda.gov/afsic/pubs/USDAOrgFarmRpt.pdf* (Accessed Feb 4, 2009)
4. *Ibid Ref 3*, pp 13
5. *Ibid Ref 3*, pp 16–17
6. National Organic Program, USDA Web site, available at *www.ams.usda.gov/nop* (Accessed Feb 4, 2009)
7. ATTRA Web site, National Sustainable Agriculture Information Service, available at *www.attra.org* (Accessed Feb 4, 2009)
8. Illustrative "Positive List" of Ingredients, Natural Products Association Web site, available at *www.naturalproductsassoc.org/site/DocServer/Natural_Ingredients_List.pdf?docID=7341* (Accessed Feb 4, 2009)
9. OASIS draft document, available at: *www.oasisseal.org* (Accessed Feb 4, 2009)
10. California Organic Products Act of 2003, California Department of Food and Agriculture Web site, available at *www.cdfa.ca.gov/is/docs/copa2003.pdf* (Accessed Feb 4, 2009)
11. *Ibid Ref 9*
12. Round One Legal Victory for Organic Consumers and Dr. Bronner's against "Organic Cheater" Personal Care Brands and Certifiers, Organic Consumers Association Web site, available at *www.organicconsumers.org/articles/article_15126.cfm* (Accessed Feb 4, 2009)
13. 100 Percent Pure Web Site, available at *www.100percentpure.com/fruitpigmentedintro.html* (Accessed Feb 4, 2009)

CHAPTER 9

DNA: Hard Evidence of Cosmeceutical Claims

Katie Schaefer

Cosmetics and Toiletries Magazine, Carol Stream, IL, USA

KEY WORDS: *FDA, Better Business Bureau, cosmeceutical, nutricosmetic, RNA, DNA, genome*

ABSTRACT: *Regulatory bodies such as the Better Business Bureau and the US Food and Drug Administration are cracking down on manufacturers for the messages they convey, requiring they be backed by solid science.*

Products have evolved to serve multiple functions, treading the line between industries and stirring the emergence of such terms as *cosmeceutical* and *nutricosmetic*. While some dismiss this as mere marketing, the associated claims cannot be ignored; and as an over-abundance of claims becomes more indecipherable for the consumer, regulatory bodies such as the Better Business Bureau and the US Food and Drug Administration are cracking down on manufacturers for the messages they convey, requiring they be backed by solid science.

To support finished product or raw material claims, Anna Langerveld, PhD, of Genemarkers LLC, has developed two in vitro methods—the Affymetrix microarray and the Taqman Real Time Polymerase Chain Reaction (PCR)—to measure the up-regulation or down-regulation of genes.

Testing Preparations

Before tests are performed, RNA solutions are prepared and converted into complementary DNA (cDNA) using the reverse transcriptase enzyme. For the Affymetrix microarray, the cDNA samples are converted back into fluorescently labeled cRNA. This cRNA is fragmented into small pieces and loaded onto a gene chip.

"The labeled cRNA binds to its complementary DNA sequence on the gene chip and the fluorescence is measured," said Langerveld.

For the Real Time PCR method, cDNA is mixed with small pieces of DNA called *primers* and *probes*. These pieces contain DNA sequences and bind only to specific genes of interest. The enzyme taq polymcrase is added to the reaction and the mixture is placed in a PCR device to create millions of copies of the specific cDNA, determined by the primer or probe. Fluorescence is used in both methods.

Scanning the Genome

In the Affymetrix mircroarray, samples with more cRNA for a given gene generate a larger fluorescent signal. "Fluorescent signals for each gene are compared across all the samples," said Langerveld. This method differs only slightly from the PCR method, where the probe has a fluorescent tag and is measured by the device. Again, the greater amounts of cDNA for a specific gene will generate a larger fluorescent signal, which is compared across all samples.

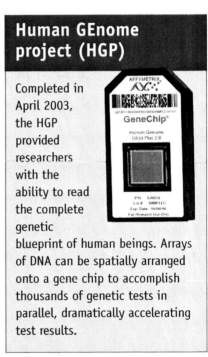

Human GEnome project (HGP)

Completed in April 2003, the HGP provided researchers with the ability to read the complete genetic blueprint of human beings. Arrays of DNA can be spatially arranged onto a gene chip to accomplish thousands of genetic tests in parallel, dramatically accelerating test results.

Nearly 25,000 genes can be analyzed at once with the Affymetrix microarray, says Langerveld, who explained that this method typically is used first to examine a formula's activities across the entire genome. The formula is then further refined to up-regulate or down-regulate specific genes, and those mechanisms are verified via the Real Time PCR method, which scans appriximately 180 genes. In one example, Langerveld tested a finished product manufacturer's antiaging formula via the PCR method to validate its activity on collagen 1A1 and sirtuin, among 89 other genes, to support anti-aging label claims.

Langerveld stressed the importance of choosing genes carefully for the Real Time PCR so as not to omit potentially affected genes. "You have to know what genes you are looking for. For example, if you choose 15 different collagens, you might miss a collagen that was changed by the ingredient or product," said Langerveld.

Beyond Cosmeceuticals

Langerveld's work thus far has focused on substantiating claims for cosmeceuticals and antiaging products. However, these methods could extend to new areas such as safety and toxicity. "It is very easy to generate a panel of toxicity-related genes or genes that trigger inflammation, [although] you would not want to turn on those genes."

In addition to safety, the methods could aid in formulation work. "Formulators could use these methods to determine how much of a particular ingredient is needed to turn on a certain gene," said Langerveld. "For example, some antioxidants are more powerful at lower concentrations. Formulators could look at several doses to turn on a particular gene and find the most effective dose," said Langerveld.

Besides dosage amounts, combinations of ingredients could be tested to determine whether they act synergistically on genetic markers. The absorption of certain molecule sizes into the skin could also be substantiated via genetic mechanisms.

The future of gene expression testing extends to a number of industries. Beyond testing hormones for anti-acne products or sirtuins for antiaging products, Langerveld's team is currently using the method to identify biomarkers in the blood that identify Multiple System Atrophy, a degenerative and deadly disease.

Published May 2009 *Cosmetics and Toiletries* magazine

CHAPTER 10

Natural and Organic: The Emerging Revolution

John William Corley
Royal Aromatics, Neptune, NJ, USA

KEY WORDS: *certification, statistics, definitions, regulations, supply chain, fragrance*

ABSTRACT: *In light of consumer demand for natural and organic products, companies and suppliers are responding with products and ingredients.*

Imagine a world in which the price of gasoline is 25 cents a gallon, where Starbucks Frappuccinos are nutritious and contain no calories, and where you actually like your mother-in-law. Unrealistic, perhaps, but for those involved in the organic world, and organic personal care specifically, the announcement in August 2005 that the United States Department of Agriculture (USDA) will allow for USDA certification of personal care products was received with equal disbelief. Why? Because, just four months earlier, the organization declared that it would have nothing to do with certification of personal care products.

Fast-forward to 2006, and we see the emergence of an flavor and fragrance industry that views the organic movement as much more than a short-term market aberration. This is indicative of nothing less than a social and lifestyle evolution among consumers and the flavor and fragrance industry.

Consider the Facts (and Nonfacts)

The interest in organic and natural products in personal care continues to expand and grow. Market researcher Packaged Facts projects that the US natural and organic skin care, hair care and cosmetics market will grow from 2004's $5 billion to $7.9 billion by 2009. (Organic oral care and cosmetics, to cite just two market segments, totaled $589 million and $336 million, respectively.) These numbers may seem modest, considering that the global personal care sector is about $150 billion in manufacturer sales (2004). However, if you consider the fact that natural and organic personal care is a segment growing at a 25 percent rate, it takes on an entirely different meaning.

The increasing movement of consumers to healthier lifestyles coupled with a growing fearful perception of the possible carcinogenic effects of certain chemicals has encouraged the market to look for alternative products containing natural ingredients. In the United States, for example, consumer interest in natural and organic products has risen in conjunction with the demand for cosmeceuticals, aromatherapy and spa-type products.

Growth has been attributed to baby boomers and Generation X consumers who increasingly crave safer nonchemical-based fragrances, shampoos, lotions, deodorants, tooth-pastes, etc. It is important to state here that the average consumer likely associates the adjectives "synthetic" or "harmful" with the term "chemical," as opposed to the true definition offered, for example, in J.W. Hill et al.'s *General Chemistry*: "A chemical substance is any material with a definite chemical composition, no matter where it comes from." Consumers, after all, are not, generally speaking, chemists. It is important to keep in mind that buyers' opinions often are shaped by misperceptions—a true challenge for all personal care industries.

The Money Trail

Consumers perceive the term "organic" to represent a superior level of purity, wellness, and overall health and well-being. This can translate into big money for the flavor and fragrance industry and personal care overall. A number of recent acquisitions lend credence to this trend. Colgate's major stake purchase in Tom's of Maine, for example, is just the most recent. According to Tom Chappell, CEO of Tom's of Maine, "More and more people are looking for safe and effective natural products from plants and minerals from a company that shares their values…we realized that we cannot meet this growing demand alone. We decided to seek a partner to help us."

Scott Van Winkle, managing director of equity research for international investment firm Canaccord Adams and an analyst in the natural products arena, said he expects Colgate to honor those promises, although it probably will impose "more of a corporate culture" on Tom's.

"Colgate has to keep [Tom's] the same for its brand integrity to remain," he said. "I can't imagine seeing the Colgate label on Tom's products anytime soon."

So, although customers' corporate structure might be changing, their focus on being perceived as natural/organic remains paramount.

Van Winkle said that the fact that an $11 billion company such as Colgate is willing to pay a valuation of $119 million for Tom's gives "a lot more validation for the natural personal care category." (L'Oréal's recent 652-mm euro offer for The Body Shop further reinforces the premise that natural is good business.)

Reuters recently reported that "the rising tide, it seems, does lift all boats—including even the largest ship, Wal-Mart Stores Inc. At the Reuters Food Summit in March, Wal-Mart announced plans to double its organic SKUs [stock keeping units] and become the 'mass-market provider of organic food.'"

Elaine Lipson, organic program director for New Hope Natural Media, parent company of *The Natural Foods Merchandiser*, was cautiously optimistic: "Wal-Mart has tremendous economic power, and I hope that within the organic realm it will use that power to uphold the integrity of the organic standards, and to help educate consumers about the meaning and benefits of organic farming.

"In the long run," Lipson continued, "I hope that Wal-Mart's decision means that many more consumers will learn more about how their food is grown and produced, and will make choices accordingly, and that more farmers will be able to find the funding, research and market support to make the transition to organic."

"Mass" market is an understatement for retailing's 800 pound gorilla. With $314 billion in sales in 2006, Wal-Mart is the world's largest retailer. It employs 6 million worldwide, operates more than

3,800 stores in the United States and nearly 2,400 more around the globe, and serves more than 138 million customers per week.

The implications of Wal-Mart's decision are far-reaching. It means that natural/organic products have broken out from the traditional health food/health and beauty care channel, and are exploding in mass-retail supermarkets, chain drugstores and now mass merchandisers.

The cover story in the April 2006 issue of GCI (*Global Cosmetic Industry*) ("Sustaining Natural Growth," *www.gcimagazine.com/articles*) makes an excellent point in explaining that consumers' interest in natural and organic foods appears to extend to personal care products, as well. According to Jason Naturals' director of marketing, Laura Setzfand, "Most consumers are introduced to natural personal care through their interest in food. Enhanced packaging and marketing also are encouraging nonusers to try natural (and organic) for the first time, and formula improvements are changing the perception that natural products are less effective."

Another perspective on the emerging natural and personal care market comes from the financial community. "It's the same progress we saw in natural foods—the success of the naturals companies attracted the mainstream brands," says Canaccord Adams' Van Winkle. So how soon might we see L'Oréal lavender essential oil shampoo or Suave 70 percent organic lotion? One to three years, he predicts. "The natural personal care market is growing like a weed. The market is probably bigger than we think."

Consumers are responding to the proliferation of new natural and organic personal care products throughout the world, which is coinciding with a whole slew of new natural and organic personal care marketing and advertising. Increased competition has resulted in targeted ads and communication support at the retail level, and companies are doing a good job of differentiating their product history, formulation, quality, brand and philosophy. Coty recently entered the field with its own organic personal care line under its Healing Gardens brand, which includes *Jasmine Therapy* cologne spray and *Green Tea* body mist. Similarly, Aubrey Organics has debuted its new line of natural and organic fragrances.

Challenges

The flavor and fragrance industry faces several daunting challenges in the organic and natural arena—particularly in the supply chain area. Finding a reliable supply chain that can support all aspects of product development according to natural or organic requirements is the most serious hurdle. The supply chain for natural and organic ingredients used in personal care is evolving constantly. Specialists are emerging in all areas, from packaging to preservative systems. The challenge is balancing supply and demand. Customers are afraid to commit to projects because they view suppliers as evolving, with the availability of ingredients limited and prices too high. Suppliers are afraid to commit to farmers and ingredient processors unless *they* have a commitment from the customer. As more and more flavor and fragrance/personal care companies step forward to meet consumer demand, the supply chain will evolve, and the issues concerning availability, quality and price will improve.

As we look into the crystal ball at the future, we see some interesting and challenging supply shifts occurring in the natural and organic area—particularly for essential oils. Wal-Mart's decision to expand its offerings in the organic agriculture area certainly will push the envelope in third-world countries to develop and cultivate more organic agriculture. And it should come as no surprise that India, China, Thailand, Vietnam, Indonesia and other countries are lining up to take advantage of this newfound market. The shift in supply of agricultural products to lower-cost labor markets is not new; we've seen this development unfold throughout the past 15 years in the essential oil market. What *is* new is the natural and organic flavor and fragrance/personal care movement, which is challenging companies to come up with products that contain safe ingredients. The biggest selling point of essential oils is that they can offer consumers both olfactive and therapeutic benefits.

India and China stand at the forefront of the emerging supply chain. According to a recent article in the *Financial Times*, the value of essential oils as ingredients (natural extracts from herbs, flowers and wood used in fragrances and flavors, and as aromachemical feedstock) is more than $11 billion and growing at 8 percent per annum. India remains the largest producer at 17 percent of the world market, followed by China (15 percent) and the rest of the Pacific Rim (8 percent), Latin America, North Africa, Eastern Europe, Europe and the United States.

India and China are not only the largest producers of essentials—they are also the *fastest-growing* producers. In addition, these countries are conducting more and more value-added research and development into the properties of essential oils to satisfy company and consumer demand, as well as to protect and retain their positions in the market.

India and China also are seizing the opportunity to become leaders in the certified organic arena. A number of well-known international certification associations have set up shop in both countries in reaction to the increased demand for organic certification for a whole host of agricultural products. Although still in an embryonic stage, the need for organic certification in light of Wal-Mart's strategy could be staggering in the next couple of years.

Regulatory, Definitions and Labeling

Manufacturing and marketing natural and organic personal care products presents many challenges for those companies that wish to comply with USDA regulatory standards in accordance with the National Organic Program (NOP).

As previously mentioned, the USDA reversed its original position (from 2005) and agreed to regulate organic personal care products with this statement:

"There are agricultural products, including personal care products, that, by virtue of their organic agricultural product content, may meet NOP standards and be labeled as '100 percent organic,' 'organic' or 'made with organic,' pursuant to NOP regulations. Businesses that manufacture and distribute such products may be certified under the NOP, and such products may be labeled as '100 percent organic,' 'organic' or 'made with organic,' as long as they meet NOP requirements."

This now allows companies that manufacture personal care products in accordance with NOP requirements to make reference to this in their product labeling, if they so desire.

As mentioned earlier, "organic" is no longer a foreign term to consumers, but there is still confusion about its exact meaning.

(Consumer fuzziness on definitions of key industry terms such as "organic," "natural" and "chemical" continues to plague the industry.) Simply put, "organic" is a method of growing and processing natural ingredients under controlled conditions that must meet stringent purity standards. It is a system of crop cultivation employing biological methods of fertilization and pest control as substitutes for chemical fertilizers and pesticides. In general, these regulations prohibit the use of genetic engineering (GE), ionizing radiation and sewage sludge. However, contrary to popular perception, organic is not a formal health claim, although perhaps this will change in the future.

Although most organic producers may see personal care as marginally related to their organic endeavors, the expansion of organic standards to cover the sector continues to have profound conceptual and regulatory implications for the entire organic industry.

Fervent organic supporters consider personal care products to be notoriously underregulated. Any number of chemical and synthetic additives can be used in their processing.

It is widely accepted in the industry that consumers buy organic fragrance/personal care products under the illusion that the items are held to organic food standards. Despite this awareness, the word "organic" is used on the labels of products that often contain toxic materials that do not comply with NOP guidelines.

The NOP regulations are fairly clear on what is and what is not organic. Aside from the general categories previously mentioned, the National List of Allowed Synthetic and Prohibited Non-Synthetic Substances details exceptions to organic standards (*www.ams.usda. gov/nop*). New standards for organic personal care products are currently under review and likely will be published before the end of this year. The goal of the improved standards is to promote sustainable agriculture, elevate integrity in organic personal care products and impose penalties on violators.

Interestingly enough, all organic products are natural, but not all natural products are organic. Although the number of companies engaged in organic agriculture and processing is increasing, there are far greater numbers of companies participating in "natural" product manufacturing and marketing.

And there is far greater abuse and misuse of the term "natural" in marketing, labeling and packaging due to the fact that it is completely unregulated. There are, of course, advocacy organizations that are trying to promote natural via a whole host of eco-labeling mechanisms, but consumers need to be wary, as the word "natural" often is just that…only a word.

Fragrance

Next to finding an organic preservative system that really works, the fragrance area represents the greatest challenge for personal care companies. Studies indicate that only around 2–3 percent of all personal care products contain natural or organic fragrance. This is amazing when you consider that fragrance is one of the main criteria in consumer choice of a personal care product.

There are many reasons for this low percentage. Natural and organic personal care is an "emerging" product category, and the need for good fragrance and perfumery, until recently, has not been a requirement. Substantivity and complexity are common attributes of traditional perfumery, where perfumers can work with thousands of aroma chemicals and molecules.

The building blocks for these aroma chemicals are either crude sulfate turpentine or petrochemicals that generally do not meet the definition of natural and almost never of organic, as I just reviewed.

In order for perfumers to create natural or organic fragrances (with organic being even more limiting, due to more structured certification and licensing requirements), they must work with essential oils, botanical extracts, tinctures, resinoids or vegetable oils. Generally, among this group, only essential oils, tinctures and resinoids have olfactive value.

Unfortunately, most perfumers today have limited experience in working with these ingredients and have been trained to create fragrance using a proliferation of aroma chemicals. If essential oils are used, it is often done more for marketing reasons than for olfactive reasons. Why? Many perfumers favor the use of synthetics in fragrance creation to achieve interesting/novel effects. In some cases, synthetics provide flexibility and cost savings that cannot be found in naturals/organics. Further complicating matters is the fact that concretes and absolutes are almost always produced via petrochemical solvent (i.e., hexane) extraction from flowers, and thus cannot meet organic standards.

The desire to have more substantive and complex fragrance notes is now becoming more prevalent in natural and organic personal care briefs—a tall order, but a necessary one. It simply makes little sense to produce a skin cream, body lotion or shower gel that is 100 percent natural or organic, only to add a synthetic fragrance to the product.

One trend in naturals/organics is that companies' desire to maximize the natural or organic content in personal care product development—either for therapeutic reasons or simply for marketing appeal—results in a strict adherence to single-theme olfactive notes (i.e., lemon, bergamot, lavender, rosemary, peppermint and eucalyptus). There are a few reasons for this. First and foremost, labeling is unforgiving. If you use a synthetic fragrance in your product, you likely will need to declare it. So, a number of natural and organic personal care companies have elected to obtain odor from natural or organic essential oils—particularly those that are more prevalent, such as lavender, lavandin, peppermint, orange, lemon, etc. This has been the extent of their perfumery. But, as I mentioned a bit earlier, companies need to challenge themselves. Fragrance is one of the key purchasing criteria used by consumers in selecting a personal care product. As this category matures, companies are going to have to work harder to distinguish themselves.

Another reason for the persistence of single-theme olfactive fragrances in naturals/organics is that naturals tend to be expensive. Even if a company could source an organic fragrance, it would be concerned about the cost impact on the finished product. Ironically, there is a fallacy that I would like to try and dispel. Yes, fragrances—particularly those made with organic essential oils—can be expensive. But companies in the personal care business need to focus more carefully on what that fragrance "expense" really represents in terms of the overall product cost. Generally, fragrance load levels in lotions and creams are low, ranging from 0.5 percent to perhaps as high as 2 percent, depending upon the application. The impact on product cost is far less than the cost of surfactants or new nonparaben-based preservative systems. And let's not forget the expense of the bottle, label and, yes, all that marketing. It is important to remember that the economic paradigm is the same, whether you are creating a traditional skin care product or an organic one.

My point is that product developers of organic and natural personal care products should consider fragrance to be a key criterion when creating their personal care products. They need not shy away from organic fragrance due to cost or availability any longer. The availability of organic essential oils, vegetable oils, botanical extracts, tinctures and resinoids is far better today then it was just a couple of years ago. For example, it would have been next to impossible five years ago to find lavender, lavandin, orange, peppermint and many other essential oils as "certified organic." If you did, you might find just a few kilos at an extremely exorbitant price. Today, production of certified organic lavandin oil produced in France is big business, resulting in 30,000–40,000 kg or more per year. And two years from now there will be far greater choices and quantities available as the demand for natural and organic personal care continues to grow and evolve. The good news is that organic fragrances can and do exist. We'll discuss more about that in a minute.

I have found semantics to be a big problem in promoting organic "scents." Many health and beauty care companies presume that the word "fragrance" means synthetic. It does not, as history tells us. About 4,000 years ago, Egyptians were busy concocting fragrances containing myrrh, cinnamon, rose, galbanum and olive oil, referring to incense as "the fragrance of the gods."

In 1792, Jean Marie Farina created the famous *Eau de Cologne*, based on Italian citrus oils of neroli, lemon and bergamot combined with French lavender and rosemary. This natural perfume became known as the first popular "bouquet" and was the genesis for the custom fragrance manufacturing industry. Farina's bouquet led to the creation of the fragrance *4711*, named after the address of the building in which it was invented, 4711 Glockengasse, Cologne, Germany. There was nothing remotely synthetic about *4711*. Back in those days, there were no pesticides, aroma chemicals or other products that could violate an organic claim!

Back to substantivity and efficacy. Perfumers today are "limited" to working with essential oils, tinctures, resinoids and botanical extracts in creating organic fragrances. Anthony Caputo and his creative staff at Royal Aromatics have spent the past three years creating blends using these organic ingredients to give customers what they want: more substantive and complex fragrance notes. When asked about the challenges he has faced throughout the years, Caputo summarizes it like this: "My experience and training always have focused on creating fragrances using aroma chemicals. When first faced with creating without products such as Galaxolide (IFF), Hedione (Firmenich), Cedramber (IFF) and many other aroma chemicals, and working ostensibly with essential oils, I struggled. I really had to go back to my roots to understand the synergies, chemotypes and complementary nature of these essential oils. The more oils I could get my hands on, the more creative I became. The learning curve of our creative team has grown as more and more organic essential oils become commercially available. Initially, I did not think it could be done, but you can create wonderful complex bouquets with patience and perseverance. I would, however, like to see more in the way of organic and natural floral and musk notes."

Beyond Essential Oils

Caputo and others involved in natural fragrance creativity still desire more substantive, unique and complex notes with which to create. These likely will come to perfumers from flavor and fragrance companies that are focused on value-added products and technology. These include natural isolates, or fractions, processed without petrochemical solvents, chemical catalysts or mediums. The technology is not new. Fractionation is a method of isolating certain naturally occurring volatile active components in botanicals and plants using simple steam distillation or more sophisticated molecular and super-critical carbon dioxide distillation methods. These volatile active components can produce extremely concentrated notes or flavors that add value to a fragrance or flavor compound.

The great appeal is that these isolates are produced via methods that not only qualify them as natural, but organic under the NOP, as well. For example, analysis of the chemotypes (isolates) in a sample of ylang-ylang oil reflects key natural components, including natural germacrene, natural β-caryophyllene and natural benzyl acetate. 1,8-Cineole occurs naturally in Spanish and Tunisian rosemary oil, and can be isolated and used as a concentrated note in fragrances. The same can be said of natural linalool and natural linalyl acetate, which are key chemotypes in French lavender oils.

As demand increases for organic flavor and fragrance ingredients, the greater the availability will be. Companies such as Citrus and Allied Essences Ltd., a flavor and fragrance ingredient manufacturer based in the United States, have made a significant investment in natural and organic chemotype fractionation. Stephan Pisano, a vice president in the organization, believes that the investment is timely and necessary in order to support the demands of its customers. Other manufacturers will follow. I expect India to become an important player in the natural and organic fractionation area, as well.

New isolates that qualify as organic will provide perfumers, flavorists and other formulators with the ability to create better-quality products that meet organic standards and add value to their finished products. However, some ingredient manufacturers are taking a "wait-and-see" attitude before committing resources, because the organic personal care market is just beginning to emerge, and there is some reservation about "applying" for and participating in the organic certification process. Frankly, it is not a complicated process. It is rigorous, but not complicated.

In summary, an increasing number of consumers want organic products. Recent company acquisitions and new product introductions reflect how the markets are reacting to this consumer demand for healthier personal care products. There is a need for new, functional and olfactively pleasing fragrance ingredients to support consumer preference in natural and organic fragrances.

Published September 2006 *Perfumer & Flavorist* magazine

CHAPTER 11

The Blossoming of Naturals I: The Buying Public

Jeb Gleason-Allured

Perfumer & Flavorist Magazine, Carol Stream, IL, USA

KEY WORDS: *definitions, teens, flavors, marketing trends*

ABSTRACT: *Discussion of 13 truths about natural/organic/wellness consumers and how the industry can reach them*

Who are your customer's customers, the 'naturals consumer'? What do they want? What are their values? How do they interact with the world?

Today, products touting natural/organic/wellness aspects have become ubiquitous—reflecting a changing consumer public that is ostensibly better educated and, thus, more product- and service-conscious.

There are 13 truths of natural/organic/wellness consumers—what drives them, what they think matters, and how the industry can communicate and deliver the promise of naturals to them.

Truth 1: 'Natural' can mean anything and thus means nothing. While most consumers likely conceive of 'natural' as synonymous with 'organic', nothing could be further from the truth. The lack of regulation or coherent industry initiatives to settle on definitions means that it is up to finished product companies to set benchmarks, fluid as they may be. Intuiscent's Helen Feygin points out, "Burt's Bees, for example, labels all of its products with a bar that depicts the amount of natural materials in a product. Of course, natural certification is based on producers'/vendors' certification of natural ingredients that go into the manufacture of a finished product. How accurate this standard is depends entirely on the integrity of the producer."[1]

Truth 2: Every day, naturals consumers are inundated with medical and nutritional information on television, in print and online, the result being a wary but naturals-hungry buying public. These consumers seek a more sophisticated connection to their purchases—education is key—and expect natural-touting products to be safe and effective.

Truth 3: Although naturals of every variety really have come into their own on the market, organic launches suffer from higher costs. Wal-Mart has recently tried to remedy this, using its vast network and purchasing power to bring organics to the mainstream consumer. However, the limitations of the category continue. Unilever global food group vice president, Alan Jope, told *The Boston Globe*, "At the end of the day consumers buy benefits, and it's not exactly clear what the benefits are from organic. They [organic products] might end up being niche propositions."[2] In addition, because world governments have yet to unify behind natural and organic standards, consumers are left to wonder what exactly they are getting. The lack of transparency may ultimately limit the market's growth.

Truth 4: The key to naturals is consumers' growing association of beauty with health and wellness. Notions of longevity and mortality now are commonly linked with personal care and spa offerings. Considering the wide acceptance of organic shopping, as well as the existence of an aging baby boomer population, all things natural have a promising future. As *Drug Store News* reported, "One person well on the way to seniority turns 50 every 7.5 seconds in [the United States]. And according to ACNielsen, those people 50 years and older control 80 percent of the nation's financial assets and 50 percent of the discretionary income."[3]

Truth 5: Unfortunately, the corollary between health/wellness and beauty has not yet reached the majority of teens. The sad fact is that many adolescents are willing to do almost anything for the sake of beauty. This presents a huge opportunity for the spa and beauty industries, which are grooming this demographic for growth. If they can help teens make the health-beauty connection, the opportunities will be vast.

Truth 6: One of the key factors in naturals is the "trading-up" principle, in which consumers pay a bit more for an indulgence—opting for Starbucks in lieu of the corner coffee shop, for example. We also are beginning to see the rise of guiltless indulgence, such as food-scented candles—sensory pleasure without the health consequences.

Notions of guilt manifest in other ways as well. Naturals are the arena in which social responsibility and personal well-being/ health meet. By embracing natural products, consumers are making a choice not just about the items, but about how they want to live their lives. Most importantly, companies serving these consumers need to reflect and telegraph these beliefs in no uncertain terms. As Tom's of Maine co-founder, Tom Chappell, emphasizes, "I believed it was possible to combine environmental concerns and capitalism in a for-profit company."[4]

Truth 7: I'm sure many of you know someone who buys or doesn't buy products based on political or personal values. In naturals, this sense of responsibility sends a strong message of fair trading relationships, coupled with the perception of a greater benefit from naturals. Just as a vanilla-scented candle offers sensory pleasure without the caloric guilt, natural/organic products provide sensory benefits without the attendant social guilt. Natural products declare that you can indulge yourself with a clear conscience, because you are what you buy!

Truth 8: The way to consumers' hearts is through their bellies. Kitchens are a major gateway into the naturals market, with the increasing presence of all natural and ethnic foodstuff creating familiarity and acceptance. The lesson here: If consumers are willing to eat it, they will be willing to slather it on their skin. Some examples of this phenomenon include products containing chocolate, vanilla and a variety of fruit flavors.

Truth 9: As naturals break into mass-market channels, a split reveals itself between natural newbies and old-school enthusiasts. The latter are label scrutinizers who cannot be fooled by greenwashing—the process of simply slapping the word "natural" on a jar. They know what to look for, and they know when they are being lied to. Old-school naturals consumers also could be called cultural creatives.

CulturalCreatives.org describes this group as: "50 million Americans who care deeply about ecology and saving the planet; about relationships, peace and social justice; and about authenticity, self-actualization, spirituality and self-expression. In short, they are the most loyal and demanding naturals consumers."

Truth 10: Natural must mean effective. The Natural Marketing Institute (NMI) has reported that 28% of the general population desires natural personal care products fortified with functional ingredients. Merely calling something natural isn't enough. There must be results. Seeing is believing.

Truth 11: The rise of the do-it-yourself (DIY) culture is good news for the naturals segment. Young women are knitting again. They're making their own cosmetics. They can go online and design a personalized fragrance. The prevalence of this culture reflects consumers' desire to connect with the things they use and to take charge of their lives.

This trend has reached every kind of woman, from homemakers to punk rockers. Whether they're seeking independence or comfort, DIY consumers want to know where things come from and how they affect them. If you are what you buy, it goes double for what you make.

Truth 12: The media can be a tastemaker. Some time ago, the Chicago-based Smell and Taste Institute released study results that revealed that the scent of grapefruit can lead men to perceive women as being an average of five years younger. Never mind the particulars or the reproducibility of the results. The public now believes that grapefruit scent makes women look younger. I haven't seen any studies, but I imagine there's been a run on all things grapefruit-scented.

For better or worse, CNN, *Time* magazine, WebMD and other media representatives are the primary sources for medical, scientific and consumer information. Once a study makes headlines, it quickly becomes part of the public consciousness. This can work for and against the personal care and spa industries. You should constantly ask yourself: "Is the media working with me or against me, and how can I harness that power?" If you don't educate your consumer, someone else will.

Truth 13: Tell consumers a story. The Keebler Elves in their hollow tree, Cap'n Crunch defending the *SS Guppy* from Crunch Berry pirates, Juan Valdez questing for the perfect coffee bean—everyone loves a product with a back story. Spa and personal care offerings are no different. Are *you* selling a story? Do you know the whole story? Where do the naturals in your products come from? Isn't *Tahitian* vanilla more compelling than simply vanilla? What place does this material play in the local indigenous culture? Who produces the naturals? How are they cultivated? A story, among other things, is crucial to creating an emotional connection between consumers and your offerings, while ensuring the kind of transparency naturals buyers crave.

Recapping the Truths

So, what do the 13 truths tell us? In order to reach today's sophisticated naturals consumer, you must address the whole person—spiritually and emotionally—while delivering functionality.

In doing so, you must reach all consumers—from shortsighted teens to fussier cultural creatives. Give them guilt-free indulgence and a sense of self-determination. Educate them directly and through the media. Tell them a story about the origins of your products or services. This is the path to success in naturals.

Published March 2006 *Cosmetics & Toiletries* magazine

References

1. Helen Feygin, Creating Effective Natural Fragrances, *Perfumer & Flavorist*, May 2007
2. Organic foods not living up to firms' expectations, *Globe Newspaper Company*, March 11, 2007
3. Keep on booming: a generation turns 50 and heads to drug stores, *Drug Store News*, 42, May 2, 2005
4. Morality Drives Tom's Business, *Seacoast Online*, Feb 22, 2007

CHAPTER 12

The Blossoming of Naturals II: The Impact of Wellness/Naturals Globally

Karen A. Newman
GCI Magazine, Carol Stream, IL, USA

KEY WORDS: *statistics, cosmeceuticals, antiaging, international*

ABSTRACT: *Discussion of product categories such as skin care, sun care, fragrance and spa retail and sales of these categories around the world*

How many of you use natural skin care, hair care or other beauty products? How many of you regularly exercise—yoga included? How many of you consider yourself a *tree hugger*? Well, you don't have to be a tree hugger to embrace the naturals and wellness trend.

Statistics

The naturals and wellness trend has gone mainstream. It includes beauty, health and fitness and is expected to grow into a US$1 trillion business by 2010. The natural ingredients segment, targeting women 35–55 years and baby boomers, is growing with the rise of the wellness trend. Even 20-year-olds who want to postpone the aging process are discovering wellness.

Within the wellness trend, naturals have become a key element in marketing cosmetics and personal care products. Consumers are looking for safe products and naturals are associated with comfort and quality of life.

Few have embraced the wellness trends with such business savvy as Nicholas Perricone, M.D. Perricone recently opened his New York City wellness center where antioxidant teas, the Perricone antiaging diet, and his line of cosmeceutical skin care products are offered.

Looking at the numbers, in 2004 a total of 2,900 new cosmetics and personal care products containing natural or organic ingredients were launched worldwide.

Sales of natural and organic cosmetic items are expected to reach $5.8 billion by 2008, which means 9% annual growth. We are seeing naturally oriented launches across all categories: lip plumpers by Jasön, natural nail care by Laboratoires Sanoflore, and even baby care such as Little Me Baby Organics by Floraroma.

Brazil's number one cosmetic company, Natura, is a great example of a cosmetic manufacturer embracing the naturals trend. The company harvests most of its ingredients from the Amazon rain forest under strict guidelines for sustainable growth. The natural beauty care company is growing rapidly and will be present in all of Latin America by next year. In addition, the company recently opened a flagship store in the heart of Paris and soon will be landing on US shores.

Product Categories

Now, let's break it down into product categories. An important area for natural ingredients is in the global body care market. Some of the largest manufacturers have launched body soap blends of natural and synthetic ingredients. Among the recent launches are:

- Colgate-Palmolive's Softsoap Naturals
- Unilever's Suave Naturals
- Avon's Avon Naturals

The idea is that if the product at least sounds natural, it will appeal to consumers.

Skin care: The skin care category is huge and growing. It is expected to account for 60% of the cosmetic market by 2007. Products in this category include antiaging, acne, sun care and cosmeceuticals.

Cosmeceuticals: A total of 59% of all cosmeceuticals are in the skin care category. Cosmeceuticals are expected to continuing growing at 11% annually by 2008.

Antiaging: Natural antiaging products are on the rise with natural antiaging brands such as Reborn, targeting men and women of all ages.

Anti-cellulite: The fastest growth market is anticellulite products, which grew at a robust 14.2% in 2004. Seventy percent of women are said to suffer from cellulite and most products that show any promise in helping the appearance of cellulite contain caffeine. All topical anticellulite products offer only temporary improvement in appearance.

Sun care: A rise in awareness of the sun's damage is part of the wellness trend and boosted sun care sales to $4.8 billion in 2004.

Nutraceuticals: Wellness also is driving nutraceutical sales. In response to consumers looking to enhance their beauty from the inside out, major manufacturers such as P&G and L'Oréal have launched nutraceutical lines. Also, we are in the middle of a functional beverage boom. This segment grew by 18% in 2004 and currently is posting $1.8 billion in sales both in natural and conventional sales channels. Despite the high growth numbers, 50% of consumers feel manufacturers' claims about nutraceuticals are untrustworthy.

Fragrance: Perfumers constantly are experimenting with capturing and blending exotic fragrances. Natural ingredients are excavated worldwide for perfumes such as Prada's *Intense* Deluxe Natural Spray and Yves Rocher's *Neonatura Cocoon* Perfume.

Men's grooming: It might take time, but even men catch on, and they are catching on to wellness and skin care to a tune of $18 billion annually. Skin care for men is expected to grow 67% to become a $19.5 billion market. The spa industry is accommodating men, its fastest-growing segment, with his-and-her packages, shorter sessions for time-conscious males and retail products designed specifically for men. Natural male grooming products include Jane Iredale's His Excellency and Aubrey Organics' Men's Stock.

Spa retail: Spa retail is becoming an increasingly important distribution channel for beauty products and is expected to reach $700 million in sales by the end of 2005. Natural and wellness products are obvious winners in this sector.

Global Markets

Where in the world has the wellness trend caught on? The answer may surprise you.

Europe: Western Europe is the current leader based on product sales. Body care is its largest market at $3.3 billion. Anticellulite is its fastest growth market, expanding 112% between 1997 and 2004.

United States: In the United States, the demand for natural products in cosmetics and personal care is projected to increase 7.5% annually to $1 billion in 2008. The United States experienced the largest number of natural or organic launches in 2004 at 1,022.

Japan: Japan has the second largest skin care market in the world. Nutraceutical beauty beverages also are very popular in the East. One popular nutraceutical drink, Kaigen Fushin-san no Biyo Sogo, has a tagline that reads "drink to make a beautiful face."

China: China's $6.3 billion cosmetic market has averaged 20%–25% annual growth over the last five years and is expected to reach $36.2 billion, in sales by 2010.

India: Herbal is big in India's personal care market. Basic products such as toothpaste and creams often contain natural ingredients.

Conclusion

Opportunities abound for cosmetics and personal care products containing natural ingredients. Skin care, fragrance and men's grooming are among the categories showing promise for future growth.

Published June 2006 *Cosmetics & Toiletries* magazine

CHAPTER 13

The Blossoming of Naturals III: Raw Materials

Rachel L. Grabenhofer
Cosmetics & Toiletries magazine, Carol Stream, IL, USA

KEY WORDS: *definitions, nature-identical, botanicals, regulations*

ABSTRACT: *Discussion of concept of natural and a description of several ingredients with feel-good benefits*

Within the personal care industry, the term *natural* is controversial in that products touted as such tend to fall on a scale of how natural they are. For example, if an ingredient is taken from its original source but altered even physically, such as by crushing it into a fine powder, some individuals argue that the ingredient no longer is in its natural state and thus should not be considered natural. At another level, extracts derived from natural sources that contain synthetic solvents or carriers may no longer be considered natural. At the opposite extreme, some consider synthetic equivalents to naturally unchanged materials as natural.

A recent report about research conducted at the New Zealand-based life sciences company HortResearch put an even different twist on natural products by introducing the concept of combining biofermentation techniques with genetic engineering to match the flavor and fragrance genes of natural ingredients. Biofermentation techniques—essentially the same processes that help bread rise or turn grape juice to wine—could make it possible for the natural tastes and aromas of fruit and flowers to be re-created on a more massive scale and with less environmental impact, said the company. And because biofermentation uses the actual genes of the plants found in nature, the resulting flavor or fragrance compound claims to have the same molecular makeup. It is, as the report claims, *nature-identical*. Would this be considered *natural?*

In this discussion all levels of natural products will be considered—and a recent flux of newer launches have flooded the market—from flower, fruit and vegetable extracts to herb and stone extracts, among others.

Delivering Nature

To meet the demand of a growing green consciousness, raw material suppliers of natural ingredients have been faced with the challenge of designing products that are natural, yet equivalent in performance to the strongest synthetic actives. One raw material supplier has gone so far as to mimic the natural chemicals in snake venom for use in antiaging applications to induce paralyzing effects on expression wrinkles.

Another way to accomplish efficacy of naturals is through specialized delivery. For example, in the prestige market, Lancôme introduced a $Hydroxy_{(a)}$-Calcium complex with a delivery system including cyclodextrins containing a *bioassimilable* form of calcium, ginseng and yeast extract to reach targeted areas in the skin. Another form of delivery involves inducing micro-channels in the skin for enhanced delivery of naturals.

Emotional Investment

Somewhere in the middle, natural ingredients are beginning to prove more effective, which only leaves the consumer wanting more. So what is the next level of efficacy for ingredients? The answer moves from the physical to the emotional.

One concept being explored is the mind/spirit connection to beauty. Several recently launched ingredients claim to possess *feel-good* elements and have interesting properties. Many companies are selling *happy* toiletries derived from happy molecules. For example, one supplier developed a product based on a peptide found in the body that promotes the natural release of messengers to trigger happiness and feelings of well-being.

The whole "inside out" trend in beauty also relates to overall feelings of well-being. Terms such as *holistic*, *chi* (the balance of energy), increased skin *energy* and euphoria-like feelings are common buzzwords in products and raw materials.

So along with the physical benefits of a product, the consumer can expect psychological benefits. One tag line on a popular brand claims that massage plus technology equals plentiful skin energy (see **Neuronal Metabolism**). The research presented is based on the skin's energy conversion of glucose. The products also contain 75% more of what is known as the *energy* vitamin B3, according to the manufacturer.

Environmentally Sound

The wellness concept is not limited to the physical or the mental—it also can pertain to the soul and the wallet. Consumers feel good about buying products from sustainable resources; they feel they are giving back to the planet because the crops that are harvested are replenished and often assist local economies of impoverished countries by providing harvesting work. For example, Brazil-based Beraca Ingredients has developed a rain forest line of ingredients that contains a series of fruits, nuts, butters and vegetable oils with applications in dandruff, anti-acne and hair care products. But along with touting the benefits and properties of these ingredients, the company also prides itself in that it has been certified by both the Forest Stewardship Council (FSC) and for Good Manufacturing Practices—environmental seals of approval. Several other companies have jumped on board with harvesting sustainable resources that also enrich the indigenous cultures affected in those regions.

Neuronal Metabolism

Research into neuronal metabolism in the epidermis was presented at the Society of Cosmetic Chemists' Annual Scientific Seminar held in Boston in May 2006. James V. Gruber, Ph.D., and Robert Holtz described how two natural ingredients, *Rhodiola rosea* (0.01%) and a 1% aqueous extract of lyseed (*Saccharomyces cerevisiae*) (0.25%), were shown to increase nerve cell oxygen consumption.

Interesting Stories

Some ingredients are not only natural and have feel-good benefits, but also have an interesting story to tell. The following are only a few:

Marula oil: Also known as *the wonder oil,* marula oil is extracted from the seed kernels from the golden fruit of the marula tree and is a rich source of oleic acid, which is useful in preserving the health of the skin and minimizing moisture loss. This oil may be used in aromatherapy products in addition to massage lotions and oils, and is excellent in applications geared for dry skin. It is a perfect example of an ingredient that can make consumers feel as good about their purchase as it makes their skin feel. The harvesting and extraction process of this botanical provides both social and economical benefits to impoverished rural women in the Western Cape of Africa.

Rooibos extract: A quote about rooibos extract from one industry source offers an impressive claim: "New spa treatments for antiaging use rooibos extract from the South African red bush that has powerful antioxidant ingredients—50 times more effective than green tea."[1]

The rooibos shrub is a hot new ingredient in skin care. It first was used centuries ago by the indigenous Khoisan tribe as an herbal remedy and healing tea. Traditionally this tea was enjoyed by native South Africans for generations. The extract from this shrub is said to be brimming with flavonoids and is, as mentioned previously, more potent than green tea.

Rooibos grows in the arid conditions of the Cedarburg Mountains in the Western Cape of Africa. Its production boosts the economy of that region, which suffers from an 82% unemployment rate. As international demand for rooibos increases, nonprofit organizations have assisted farmers to implement methods of cultivation to compete in the world market. Most products containing rooibos originate outside of the United States in places such as Japan, South Korea and South Africa. Some examples of finished products include the Ginger with a Twist line, from Origins Japan; Natuer BE:, from Enprani in South Korea; and Repêchage Deep Relief Tea Gel, from Repêchage in the United States.

Monk's pepper: Berries from the Monk's pepper shrub, also known as the *chaste tree* from the Mediterranean region, are claimed to contain an endorphin-based ingredient that returns to the happy toiletry concept. In natural medicine practice, this berry has been used for centuries to regulate women's menstrual cycles and to relieve PMS, which supports the endorphinlike claims. It also is suggested that this berry stimulates cell growth. In fact, Mibelle AG Biochemistry of Switzerland has formulated a compound including Monk's pepper and has termed it Happybelle.

Seabuckthorn oil: Seabuckthorn oil appears to be an ideal ingredient for skin care. It is derived from a wild bush that grows in poor, arid soils like the Gobi Desert. Tibetan and Mongolian legend has it that Genghis Khan considered the oil and berries the key in making his army stronger than his enemies.

Seabuckthorn oil traditionally has been used in wound healing and is said to counter the effects of sun damage. The oil is processed from the seeds and berries and is the best source known for a bevy of vitamins, including vitamins E, C and beta-carotene. It also contains essential fatty acids, amino acids and flavonoids, and omega-3, -6 and -9, and is said to contain more potassium than sodium. The high content of its fatty acids is important to the claim that it can restore skin tissue. This ingredient is useful in antiaging and in sun care products.

Tomato extract: New active ingredients are being derived from colorless carotenoids in tomatoes (the precursors phytoene and phytofluene) by extracting them before the tomatoes can convert them into red pigment. These colorless carotenoids claim to have antioxidant, UV-protective, anti-inflammatory and anti-mutagenic properties.

Burt's Bees, for example, offers a Garden Tomato Complexion Soap that claims to naturally cleanse and balance oily facial skin, as well as balance the skin's pH with alpha hydroxy acids and lycopene. The soap also is said to refine enlarged pores and provide a soothing effect.

Algae extract: Algae extracts are potent cosmetic active ingredients that make it possible to create biologically active polysaccharides demonstrating effectiveness in the protection of microcapillary integrity. These extracts mainly target the cytokine VEGF and also modulate PGE2 activity—biochemical mediators that are unregulated in the skin during aging, exposure to UV and environmental insults. They also are associated with the phenomenon of microcapillary dilation and hyperpermeability.

Emu oil: Emu oil has been reported as useful in transdermal delivery applications. Data suggests that the delivery of nutrients by emu oil might be greater than other delivery systems, and cosmetic companies are using it in cosmetic bases as a natural ingredient for moisturizers, lotions and lip balms to penetrate the skin deeper and faster.

Hematite extract: Stone extract derived from hematite reportedly is rich in iron. Tests conducted on human fibroblasts indicate that the ingredient has a dose-dependent action that is 4–16 times more powerful than TGF ß, a benchmark growth factor that stimulates pro-collagen synthesis. This active increases the maturation of the pro-collagen by stimulating the activity of prolylhydroxylase. Its stimulating action on collagen synthesis is useful in filling in wrinkles for a plumping effect on the skin.

Circling Back

Europe's Registration, Evaluation and Authorization of Chemicals (REACH) program could force the personal care industry back to the basics of all things being truly natural. According to one industry expert, suppliers of raw materials are unsure about how REACH could affect the industry. The law requires companies that manufacture or import more than 1 ton of a certain chemical substance per year to register it in a centralized database. The intent of this program was to protect the environment and European citizens, as well as to boost competitiveness and innovation in the European chemical industry.

For the personal care industry, this puts more responsibility on suppliers regarding chemical risks and they will have to provide information about the safety of all chemical substances. For now, this legislation is rolling out only in Europe, but it has the potential to shift the industry away from synthetics and back to nature.

Published September 2006 *Cosmetics & Toiletries* magazine

References

1. Advances in Anti-aging Spa Treatments, Spa 20/20

CHAPTER 14

Navigating the Challenges of Formulating with Naturals

Lakshmi Prakash, PhD, and Muhammed Majeed, PhD

Sabinsa Corp., Piscataway, NJ, USA

KEY WORDS: *botanicals, Boswellia serrata, tetrahydrocurcuminoids, dispersibility, stability, skin permeation*

ABSTRACT: *Formulating with natural botanical extracts poses unique challenges to formulators such as color issues, ingredient instability, poor absorption of actives, dispersibility problems and quality, safety and efficacy concerns, all of which are discussed.*

A judicious blend of art and science is critical to creating natural cosmeceuticals for use in personal care products. The major challenge is finding ingredients that are compatible with existing formulations. Aesthetics is a particularly important concern. For example, while there is much interest in using natural botanical extracts in cosmetic preparations, a too-dark color, a gritty texture, ingredient instability, poor absorption of actives, or dispersibility problems could render the "healthy and natural" ingredient unattractive. Additionally, the safety and efficacy of natural ingredients need to be established in order to enable their use in finished personal care products.

Challenges in Innovating

Color issues: Natural ingredients for antiaging skin care are prepared from botanicals with a long history of traditional cosmeceutical use, such as skin lightening, skin smoothing and antimicrobial applications, although the term itself is of recent origin. Botanicals are rich in phenolic and other pigments including carotenoids, flavonoids and related compounds, and often some of the healthful properties of these natural materials reside in the pigments themselves. An example is turmeric, a culinary spice with a tradition of topical use in South Asia. The active compounds in this case are the yellow curcuminoids that also are used as a natural colorant. This brilliant yellow color, however, does not blend well with currently manufactured personal care products. The end user is concerned about the unappealing yellow color staining the skin.

Scientific developments such as extraction processes and derivatization techniques have enabled a method to extract the mixture of biologically active curcuminoids from turmeric roots and convert them into colorless biologically active tetrahydrocurcuminoids. Such a composition finds versatile applications in personal care products, particularly in the antiaging category.

Tetrahydrocurcuminoids have been found to efficiently inhibit protein cross-linking and provide skin-lightening action as well as provide antioxidant and bioprotectant properties. This discovery is the subject of a recently granted U.S. patent.[1]

Tetrahydrocurcuminoids offer additional functional antioxidant benefits in protecting fat-based compositions from oxidation. In laboratory studies,[2] tetrahydrocurcuminoids were found to quench free radicals more efficiently than the commonly used synthetic antioxidant, butylated hydroxytoluene (BHT).

From a safety point of view, the bioprotectant role of tetrahydrocurcuminoids is further enhanced by its low toxicity, (oral LD50 is 5000 mg/kg) with a 0.00 irritation score in a skin patch test.[3] Turmeric root, the source of tetrahydrocurcuminoids, is listed by the U.S. Food and Drug Administration (FDA) as an herb generally recognized as safe (GRAS) for its intended use as a spice, seasoning and flavoring agent.[4]

Dispersibility: Botanicals often are difficult to use in formulations because of their poor solubility or dispersibility in acceptable solvents. In such cases, the formulator faces a challenging task that sometimes requires modifications to the formulation process itself. The order of addition of ingredients, the type of solvents used, temperature and pH conditions, the nature of the mixing process and several other factors influence dispersibility.

Boswellia serrata, for example, has been used in the ayurvedic system of medicine to manage inflammatory conditions (see **Boswellia serrata in Antiaging**).

Boswellia serrata In Antiaging

Olibanum, the resin from the *Boswellia* species, has been used as incense for centuries. Its major use today is as a fixative in perfumes, soaps, creams, lotions and detergents. In India, the gum resin exudates of *Boswellia serrata* have been used in the ayurvedic system of medicine in the management of several inflammatory conditions.

Inflammation is considered to be the prime cause in aging; an inflamed site forms a micro-scar that over time develops into a wrinkle or blemish. Inflammatory mediators such as leukotrienes and prostaglandins, cytokines and growth factors target skin texture, integrity and tone. Containing inflammation at its roots is therefore an effective antiaging strategy.

The active boswellic acids reside in the gum resin from the tree, which is a difficult material to formulate, and the gum constituents may irritate the skin. Natural extract manufacturers have developed efficient extraction processes that produce a composition rich in boswellic acids in a powder form. Such an ingredient can be conveniently used in formulations for soaps, lotions and cosmetic creams as an anti-inflammatory ingredient (see **Formula 1**)—however, the powder must be dispersed well during the formulation process. Optimal proprietary methods for formulation have been developed after extensive experimentation.

Products tested containing 5% of a standardized extract from the gum resin[a] did not produce any irritation or sensitization in standard patch tests.[5]

Stability issues: Retaining the biological activity of natural ingredients through raw material preparation, processing, extraction, packaging and storage presents a myriad of challenges.

Nutrients in natural materials such as vitamins, growth factors, amino acids, flavonoids, pigments and essential oils are susceptible to degradation on contact with oxygen or exposure to suboptimal temperature and pH conditions.

[a] Boswellin (INCI: *Boswellia serrata* extract) is a registered trademark of Sabinsa Corp.

Formula 1. Cream formulation with Boswellia serrata extract

A. Water (*aqua*)	59%–60%
Carbomer	0.25%–0.27%
B. Glycerin	4.0
Methylparaben	0.2
Edetate sodium	0.01
C. Cetyl alcohol	3.5
D. Stearyl alcohol	3.5
Stearic acid	6.5
Glyceryl stearate	2.5
PEG-100 stearate	2.5
Isopropyl palmitate	6.0
Vitamin E acetate	1.0
Dimethicone	0.1
Propylparaben	0.1
Vitamin A palmitate	0.1
Ascorbyl palmitate	0.2
E. *Boswellia serrata* extract	5.0
F. Water (*aqua*)	2.0
Triethanolamine	0.4
G. Imidazolidinyl urea	0.3
Water (*aqua*)	1.0

Procedure: Mix A under propeller agitation until dissolved. Add B to A and blend. Begin heating to 72°C–77°C and continue mixing until completely dissolved. In a separate container, charge C and add D to C in order. Heat CD to 72°C–77°C until dissolved. Mix CD with AB, maintaining 72°C–77°C. Add E to batch under propeller agitation. In a separate container, combine F until dissolved and mix with batch. Keep mixing until completely dissolved while maintaining 72°C–77°C. In a separate container, combine G until dissolved and add to the main batch. Mix and cool to 35°C–40°C and package.

An example is young or "green" coconut water—a reservoir of nutrients and growth factors. Green coconut water is the liquid endosperm of coconut (*Cocos nucifera L*), which is a refreshing natural drink in the tropics and traditionally used as a health and beauty aid. Natural coconut water is rich in proteins, amino acids, sugars, vitamins, minerals and growth hormones that are essential to promote tissue growth. Laboratory researchers use the material as a supplement in media for the growth of plant tissue cultures.

Coconut water is useful in hair care formulations and in topical preparations to rejuvenate, nourish, condition, soothe and moisturize the tissues. However, its short shelf life and sensitive nature of the inherent actives make it difficult to use the material in cosmetic formulations. A freeze-drying process has been developed to retain the activity of coconut water components. The process produced a light tan-colored powder consisting of coconut water solids that readily blends into cosmetic preparations. In *in vitro* irritation studies, a product formulated with the ingredient[b] was found to be non-irritating.

Skin permeation: The efficacy of actives depends upon their skin permeation capabilities. Selective nutrient absorption by the skin is an important physical property of the skin. This selective process begins with the stratum corneum (SC). The function of this barrier is related to the unique composition of the lipid moiety in the epidermis. The intercellular lipids mediate transdermal delivery of both lipophilic and hydrophilic molecules. Research shows that regulating the composition of intracellular lipids in the skin can increase or decrease the bioavailability of nutrients.[6]

Besides the modification of skin lipid composition, there are several strategies to improve topical nutrient bioavailability. Improvement can be accomplished by supersaturation of the delivered ingredient. The delivery formulation also may contain ingredients that decrease the diffusional (electrostatic) resistance of the lipid bilayer to the passing molecule. Topical liposome preparations are effective penetration enhancers for the delivery of biological compounds, probably due to their role in increasing cell membrane fluidity. In addition, an increase in blood supply to the skin can enhance absorption of delivered nutrients.

Historically, a number of chemical-penetration enhancers have been used to enhance the uptake of actives. These include: solvents such as dimethyl sulfoxide (DMSO), ethanol and other alcohols; glycols such as propylene glycol; fatty acids such as oleic acid; and detergents such as sodium lauryl sulfate, polyoxyethylene lauryl ethers, and chaotropic agents such as thioglycolate, urea, and mercaptoethanol.

---

[b] Cococin (INCI: *Cocos nucifera* (coconut) fruit juice) is a registered trademark of Sabinsa Corp.

As such, they also have the potential to cause damage to the SC and to increase the probability of irritation. Most of these agents work by perturbation of the intercellular lipid bilayers present in the SC.

Therefore, there is a need for compounds of natural origin with low irritancy and minimal side effects that can be efficiently combined with nutrients to enhance the uptake and utilization of such active molecules.

An innovation in enhancing topical delivery of natural actives is available in the form of a proprietary extract obtained from black pepper fruits[c], a common culinary spice.

When added in small amounts (0.01%–0.1%) to cosmetic formulations, tetrahydropiperine, the active principle, enhances the uptake and delivery of other actives in the formulation. Poorly absorbed botanicals, therefore, can be made more "bioavailable" with this ingredient.[7]

Quality, safety and efficacy: Herbal raw materials available commercially as powders and extracts often do not meet global standards of quality, efficacy and safety. To preserve the authenticity and credibility of such products, it is important that the ingredients therein contain adequate amounts of biologically active principles that manifest the desired biological functions.

Plant materials pose several challenges in standardization. Natural products are complex matrices with a number of active principles varying widely in content and type, based on geographical origin, cultivation and collection practices, and processing and storage conditions. This often leads to variations in potency, label ambiguity and related problems in finished cosmetics.

Compositional consistency of botanical extracts in terms of active principles is the key factor in ensuring potency and sustaining consumer confidence. Marker compounds are chemicals proven to be characteristic of botanicals and endowed with validated health benefits. Chemical fingerprints using chromatography and spectrophotometric methods, in combination with bioassays, are the accepted methods to ensure the presence of marker compounds in botanical materials.

A botanical's active principle may concentrate in a specific location in the plant and manufacturers often use combinations of plant materials in preparing finished extracts. Contaminant levels, including heavy metals, pesticide residues, extraneous matter and genetic modification

[c] Cosmoperine (INCI: Tetrahydropiperine) is a registered trademark of Sabinsa Corp.

Organic vs. Natural

According to the U.S. Department of Agriculture's (USDA) National Organic Program (NOP), the term *organic* may be used on product labels when certain conditions are met.[1]

100% organic:
- This designation may be used for agricultural products that are composed of a single ingredient such as raw, organically produced fruits and vegetables and products composed of two or more organically produced ingredients, provided that the individual ingredients are, themselves, wholly organic and produced without any nonorganic ingredients or additives. (Only processing aids that are, themselves, organically produced, may be used in the production of these products.)

Organic:
- Products labeled or represented as *organic* must contain, by weight (excluding water and salt), at least 95% organically produced raw or processed agricultural product.
- Up to 5% of the ingredients may be nonagricultural substances and, if not commercially available in organic form, nonorganic agricultural products and ingredients in minor amounts (i.e., spices, flavors, colorings, oils, vitamins, minerals, accessory nutrients, incidental food additives).

Made with organic ingredients:
- Multi-ingredient products containing by weight or fluid volume (excluding water and salt) between 70%-95% organic agricultural ingredients may be designated as "made with organic [specified ingredients or food group(s)]." Up to three organically produced ingredients or food groups may be named in the phrase.

The term *natural*, according to the National Consumer's League (NCL), is not regulated by the FDA as far as the use of the word on personal care or cosmetic products.[2] The FDA's Office of Cosmetics and Colors has, however, produced consumer information regarding the *natural* claim for personal care products. Products claiming to be *all natural* or *plant-derived* may include more than just natural ingredients or plant products.

1. *Source: National Organic Program (NOP) Web site. Available at: www.ams.usda.gov/nop/NOP/standards/LabelPre.html. (Accessed Jan. 23, 2006)*

2 *Source: Naturally misleading: Consumers' understanding of "natural" and "plant-derived" labeling claims, National Consumers League (NCL) Web site. Available at: www.nclnet.org/naturalsreport.htm#_ednref5. (Accessed Jan. 23, 2006)*

aspects also need to be considered. The complexity of these challenges is exacerbated by mislabeling in the commercial marketplace.

Authentication of plant materials used to manufacture cosmetic ingredients is critical. Selecting appropriate extraction and purification processes is important as this reflects heavily on the quality of finished extracts. To avoid skin irritation and sensitization, solvent residues and other contaminant levels in finished extracts should be minimized.

Meeting These Challenges

In the rapidly growing market for natural antiaging cosmetics, application-oriented product development goes a long way in facilitating the introduction of traditionally used botanicals into conventional formulations. The initial challenge is to innovatively transform plant materials into safe and efficacious ingredients for functional cosmetics. Once this is achieved, the next step is to comprehensively address global regulatory issues and nurture consumer confidence through consistent quality management. Furthermore, in vitro testing methods for safety and efficacy need to be optimized to facilitate cruelty-free product development.

Nature provides a plethora of options to support healthy aging. Blending traditional knowledge with modern science results in innovative approaches to the effective use of plant-based materials in contemporary personal care formulations.

Published May 2008 *Cosmetics and Toiletries* magazine

References

1. US Patent 6,653,327, Cross-regulin composition of tumeric-derived tetrahydrocurcuminoids for skin lightening and protection against UVB rays
2. Research Reports 8–13, Sabinsa Corp. (1999)
3. Research Report, Sabinsa (1999)
4. Code of Federal Regulations Title 21, 100.0, 182.10, 182.20
5. Research Report, Sabinsa Corp. (Feb. 2000)
6. E Proksch, WM Holleran, GK Menon, PM Elias and KR Feingold, Barrier function regulates epidermal liquid and DNA synthesis, Br J Dermatol 128 (5) 473–482 (May 1993)
7. M Muhammad and L Prakash, THP: An all natural delivery system adjuvant, in Delivery System Handbook for Personal Care and Cosmetic Products: Technology, Applications and Formulations, MR Rosen, ed., William and Andrew Publishing (2005)

CHAPTER 15

Mildness Meets Greenness

Annette Mehling, Guadalupe Pellón and Hermann Hensen

Cognis GmbH, Düsseldorf, Germany

KEY WORDS: *alkyl polyglucosides, mildness, test methods, green concepts*

ABSTRACT: *Alkyl polyglucoside surfactants are obtained from renewable, plant-derived raw materials. Compatibility test results and exemplary formulations presented here show that alkyl polyglucosides enable cosmetic chemists to formulate mild body cleansing formulations that fulfill the new "green" formulation trend and enable the formulation of alkyl sulfate-free and ethoxylate-free cleansing concepts.*

Natural-sourced, plant-based renewable raw materials are the key drivers influencing the modern day chemicals-based market. They offer innovative possibilities to connect with consumers and their expectations for sustainable and "green" chemicals in the personal care segment. This chapter demonstrates that alkyl polyglucosides are green; i.e., natural-sourced, plant-based and renewable, in addition to being mild, as demonstrated here in screening tests and formulations.

Alkyl Polyglucosides

Alkyl polyglucosides (APGs)[a] are sugar-based nonionic surfactants. They can be differentiated by their alkyl chain length (**Figure 1**) and they generallyvary in distribution and content, with chain lengths of C8 to C16 being the predominant lengths found in consumer products.

The surfactant properties of APGs are based on the amphiphilic character of the molecule. The hydrophobic (or lipophilic) hydrocarbon chain is formed by a fatty alcohol obtained from palm kernel oil or coconut oil. The hydrophilic part of the molecule is based on glucose obtained from starch.

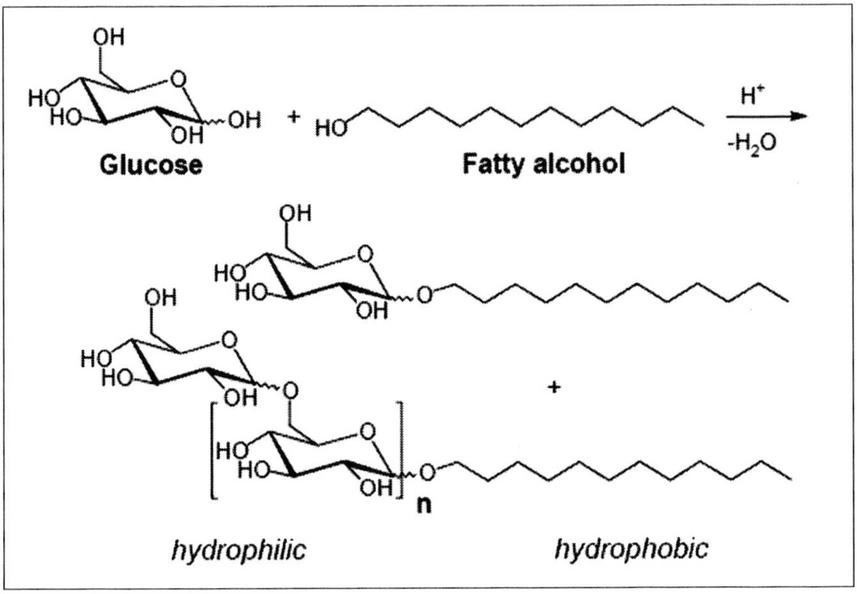

Figure 1. A schematic of the synthesis of alkyl polyglucosides by acid-catalyzed acetalization of glucose in molar excess of fatty alcohol and removal of water

The irritation potential of surfactants is in part attributed to their ability to interact with the proteins of the skin, which in turn leads to corneocyte swelling and irritation. Due to the large hydrophilic head groups, interaction between the APGs and the amino acid side chains is impeded and corneocyte swelling reduced. In addition, in combination with other surfactants, such as fatty alcohol ether sulfates (SLES), the nonionic APGs reduce the electrostatic repulsion of the anionic head groups of the SLES. This results in the formation of larger micelles with a rod-like structure. These micelles penetrate less easily into the skin, further decreasing interactions with the skin proteins and subsequent development of irritation.

Most consumers associate greenness with safeness for their health and the environment. APG surfactants are obtained from natural, renewable, plant-derived raw materials, such as coconut oil and starch. They have been extensively tested in various eco-toxicological and toxicological studies. Linear APGs are completely and rapidly biodegradable regardless of whether they are tested in seawater or freshwater as well as being biodegradable under both aerobic and anaerobic conditions. Compared to other surfactants, APGs can be more easily removed from the wastewater in sewage treatment plants and they are well-tolerated by aquatic organisms.[1] In a nutshell: They are natural-based surfactants from renewable sources and have a good environmental compatibility profile.

Screening for Mildness

Shampoos and body washes inevitably come into contact with the skin, eyes and mucous membranes. It is therefore essential that the surfactants chosen have a minimal irritation potential. Assessment of ocular/mucous membrane and dermal irritation plays a role in both occupational hazard assessment and classification as well as in consumer product development. In the former, the product is typically tested undiluted and the pH is not adjusted. This reflects the situation of some types of industrial uses, such as transport or storage of the raw materials. In contrast to consumer products, many of these bulk materials will be adjusted so their pH is very high or low to prevent microbial contamination in the absence of preservatives. For a bulk raw material, a high concentration of the surfactant is used to facilitate transport and to further impede growth of microorganisms.

APGs are examples of a raw material that needs pH adjustment and diluting. Typically, the pH of the raw material is adjusted to approximately 12 and the material will have an active substance (AS) content of approximately 50%. Because the irritation potential of a surfactant or a formulation is markedly dependent on its pH and the concentration at which the surfactant is used, higher concentrations or an extreme pH make irritation more probable. In personal care formulations, however, mildness is essential. In consumer products, the pH is usually within a range of the physiological pH of the skin and is adjusted to pH 5–8. Therefore, when performing comparative testing of the compatibility of products or substances, in order to assess the mildness under use conditions, it is essential that within any one test the surfactants be tested at the same pH and the same AS content. Surfactant concentrations and pH levels are also essential when assessing compatibility during product development.

Various methods are commonly used to differentiate between surfactants with respect to their potential irritancy.

Ocular/mucous membrane and dermal irritation: The Draize eye irritation test has been the gold standard for testing eye irritation for many years. Concerns for animal welfare have led to the development of alternative methods such as the red blood cell (RBC) test[2,3] and the hen's egg test—chorioallantoic membrane (HET-CAM) test,[4,5] to assess the mucous membrane/ocular irritation potential of surfactants and other substances.

Primary skin irritation is assessed in humans using epicutaneous patch testing (ECT), in which substances are occlusively applied to the backs of volunteers for 24 hr and reactions monitored for 3 days following removal of the patch.

To evaluate the relative irritation potential of one of the APGs, the authors used HET-CAM, RBC and ECT to compare decyl glucoside with other surfactants typically used in cosmetics (**Table 1**). Within each method, all the surfactants were used at the same AS and pH, as shown in **Table 2**.[6]

Comparative testing of the exemplary APG, decyl glucoside, with other surfactants typically used in cosmetics using the above-mentioned methods and the same AS and pH within each method has been reported previously[6] and is summarized here in **Table 3**.

Table 1. Surfactants tested

INCI	Surfactant type	Chemical description
Decyl glucoside	nonionic	alkyl-polyglucoside
Disodium laureth sulfosuccinate	anionic	alkyl-ether-sulfosuccinate
Disodium cocoamodiacetate	amphoteric	alkyl-amphoacetate
Cocamidopropyl betaine	amphoteric	alkyl-amidobetaine
Sodium lauryl sulfate	anionic	alkyl-sulfate
Sodium laureth sulfate	anionic	alkyl-ethersulfate
Ammonium lauryl sulfate	anionic	alkyl-sulfate
Disodium cocoyl glutamate	anionic	acyl-glutamate

With the exception of the disodium laureth sulfosuccinate with respect to skin irritation (ECT), the results of all other tests indicate that the APGs have a lower irritation potential than the other surfactants, thus underlining the mildness of APGs.

Table 2. pH and concentration (active substance or AS) of the surfactants used in the four tests in this study

Test	Surfactant pH	Surfactant AS
RBC	7.4	1.0%[a]
HET-CAM	6.5	3.0[b]
ECT	6.5	2.0[c]
SCT	6.5	1.0[d]

[a] Starting concentration
[b] The positive control, Texapon ASV 50 (INCI: Sodium laureth sulfate (and) sodium laureth 8-sulfate (and) magnesium laureth sulfate (and) magnesium laureth 8-sulfate (and) sodium oleth sulfate (and) magnesium oleth sulfate), is a product of Cognis GmbH and was tested at 5% AS.
[c] The positive control SLS was tested at 0.5% active substance content.
[d] The positive control SLS was tested at 0.2% active substance content.

Cumulative irritation potential: The skin plays a principal role in protecting the body against water and heat loss as well as in forming a defensive barrier against harmful agents and unwanted influences from the environment. The barrier function of the skin is mainly attributed to its outermost layer, the stratum corneum. It is often described using the "bricks and mortar" model in which the bricks are the corneocytes and the mortar is made up of the intercellular lipids. If the barrier function is compromised, water loss through the epidermis increases.

The ability of surfactants to emulsify and to reduce the surface tension of water means they can remove lipids from the skin during the washing process. This can result in dryness and roughness of the skin. In addition, due to the damage to the lipid barrier, an increase in transepidermal water loss (TEWL) is usually observed.[7,8]

The soap chamber test (SCT) according to Frosch and Kligman[9] is the method of choice for testing the cumulative irritation potential of surfactants and includes assessments of both dryness and skin

Table 3. Irritant potential of the tested surfactants in three ocular/mucous membrane and dermal irritation tests (HET, RBC, ECT) and two cumulative irritation tests (dryness, TEWL). For each test, higher numbers indicate higher irritancy potential, except for RBC where the reverse is true.

HET = Hen's egg chorioallantoic membrane test

ECT = 24-hr occlusive epicutaneous patch test (n = 21)

TEWL = Soap chamber test: TEWL on Day 8

RBC = Red blood cell test

Dryness = Soap chamber test: Dryness on Day 8

	Ocular/Mucous Membrane and Dermal Irritation Tests			Soap Chamber Tests[a] for Cumulative Irritation	
	HET (Q)[b]	RBC (H_{50}/DI)	ECT (%)[c]	Dryness (d8) (mean values)	TEWL[d] (d8) ($g/m^2/hr$)
Decyl glucoside	0.59	342.76	6.1	0.05	9.32
Disodium laureth sulfosuccinate	0.72	2.66	5.1	0.09	11.92
Disodium cocoamodiacetate	0.63	7.77	14.1	0.00	10.49
Cocamidopropyl betaine	2.05	7.87	13.5	0.32	11.82
Sodium lauryl sulfate	2.59	0.22	104.3	3.86	27.44
Sodium laureth sulfate	1.56	0.17	58.0	1.35	16.04
Ammonium lauryl sulfate	3.02	0.14	82.0	3.68	19.16
Disodium cocoyl glutamate	1.16	23.68	9.4	0.12	11.31
Sodium lauryl sulfate, 0.2%	-	-	-	2.55	24.50
Water (aqua)	-	-	-	0.07	9.00

a For soap chamber tests the positive control SLS was tested at 0.2% AS content. All other test materials were tested at 1% AS content.

b Irritation Index relative to 5% AS Texapon ASV 50 (INCI: Sodium laureth sulfate (and) sodium laureth 8-sulfate (and) magnesium laureth sulfate (and) magnesium laureth 8-sulfate (and) sodium oleth sulfate (and) magnesium oleth sulfate), a product of Cognis GmbH

c Total irritation score relative to 0.5% sodium lauryl sulfate (analysis grade)

d TEWL adjusted to baseline

barrier function. The substances are occlusively applied to the ventral forearm of human volunteers for 24 hr on the first day and for 6 hr each day for the next 4 days. Irritation is evaluated via visual assessment of the parameters erythema, dryness and fissure. Changes in skin barrier function are assessed by TEWL.

The authors performed an SCT with various surfactants.[6] Skin dryness was assessed on day 8. The TEWL values obtained on day 8, following a three-day regeneration phase, were used to assess skin barrier function. The TEWL results for day 5, the last day of treatment, have been reported previously.[6] The results for both dryness and TEWL on day 8 are summarized in **Table 3**, which shows that the potential of APGs to irritate the skin or to compromise the skin barrier is clearly lower than that of SLS or SLES. This has also been shown to be the case in a study conducted by Löffler et al.,[10] who reported that the kinetics of the skin barrier regeneration after 24 hr of occlusive patch testing (ECT) depend on the concentration of the surfactant (SLS, SLES, APG) used. Furthermore, the results of the SCT by the current authors indicate that the reported lipid solubilization may not accurately represent the actual effects on human skin induced by these surfactants because skin dryness can be induced by the solubilization of the intercellular lipids.

Formulating for Mildness

In addition responding to the green market drivers, formulators in the personal care market are sometimes challenged with eliminating alkyl-sulfates or ethoxylates from formulations. On the basis of the skin compatibility of alkyl polyglucosides, mild body wash preparations can be formulated. These formulations will fit well into the green and alkyl sulfate-free formulation concept.

Formula 1 describes a body wash gel formulation based on the alkyl-sulfate-free surfactants lauryl glucoside, sodium lauryl glucose carboxylate, cocamidopropyl betaine and disodium cocoyl glutamate. The dermatological and ocular compatibility of this formulation was assessed by performing an ECT and an RBC test, respectively. Body wash formulations found in the market were used as benchmarks. A 1% AS aqueous solution of SLS also was tested as the positive control. In both ECT and RBC tests, the green formulation proved to have a lower irritation potential than the benchmarks (**Tables 4** and **5**), indicating a mildness exceeding that of these market body wash products for babies.

Formula 2 is a moisturizing shower gel formulation with a surfactant matrix based on cocamidopropyl betaine and lauryl glucoside, along with a lipid layer enhancer composed of glyceryl oleate and coco glucoside. The formulation of this gel is in line

---

Formula 1. Body wash gel

Lauryl glucoside (Plantacare 1200 UP, Cognis)	11.7% w/w
Cocamidopropyl betaine (Dehyton PK 45, Cognis)	11.7
Sodium lauryl glucose (and) carboxylate (and) lauryl glucoside (Plantapon LGC Sorb, Cognis)	9.7
Disodium cocoyl glutamate (Plantapon ACG 35, Cognis)	3.2
Coco glucoside (and) glyceryl oleate (Lamesoft PO 65, Cognis)	3.0
Fragrance (*parfum*)	qs
Preservative	qs
Citric acid	qs
Water (*aqua*)	qs to 100.0

Properties: Viscosity 4000 mPas; pH 5.2

Table 4. ECT assessment of skin compatibility of body wash formulations. The total irritation scores of the 24-hr occlusive epicutaneous patch test are shown. Higher irritation scores indicate higher irritation potential. (n=22; 20% product dilution)

Product	ECT Irritation Score
Test body wash gel (**Formula 1**)	0.9
Benchmark A (marketed body wash for babies)[a]	2.5
1% AS Sodium laureth sulfate	6.6

[a] *Benchmark A surfactant system is polysorbate 80, sodium laureth sulfate, cocoamidopropyl betaine, PEG-150 distearate and sodium lauroamphoacetate.*

with the formulation guidelines issued by Ecocert, the France-based certification and control organization. Ecocert works to promote organic products in more than 80 countries by providing much respected and internationally recognized certification standards for organic and natural personal care products.

Table 5. RBC assessment of ocular compatibility of body wash and shampoo formulations. Higher H_{50}/DI readings indicate lower irritation potential.

Product	RBC (H_{50}/DI)
Test body wash gel (**Formula 1**)	431
Benchmark B (marketed baby shampoo)[b]	22
Benchmark A (marketed body wash for babies)[a]	10

[a] *Benchmark A surfactant system is polysorbate 80, sodium laureth sulfate, cocoamidopropyl betaine, PEG-150 distearate and sodium lauroamphoacetate.*
[b] *Benchmark B surfactant system is polysorbate 20, sodium laureth sulfate, sodium lauroamphoacetate, PEG-150 distearate and cocoamidopropyl betaine.*

Formula 2. Moisturizing shower gel

Cocamidopropyl betaine (Dehyton PK 45, Cognis)	12.60% w/w
Lauryl glucoside (Plantacare 1200, Cognis)	18.50
Coco glucoside (and) glyceryl oleate (Lamesoft PO 65, Cognis)	2.50
Fragrance (*parfum*)	0.20
Water (*aqua*)	55.05
Rosa damascena distillate (Eau de Rose HYRO23, Fytosan)	10.00
Citric acid, 50%	0.60
Sodium benzoate	0.55
	100.00

Properties: Viscosity 2500 mPas (Brookfield, RVT, spindle 4, speed 20, 25°C) pH 5.2

Formula 2, diluted to 16%, was tested with seniors in a 24-hr occlusive ECT to evaluate its irritation potential. A green concept benchmark found in the market was tested at the same dilution in order to compare its irritation potential with that of **Formula 2**.

According to the INCI declaration, the benchmark contained a surfactant system based on coco glucoside, caprylyl/capryl glucoside and sodium lauryl sulfoacetate. With respect to skin compatibility, the APG-based green body wash formulation (**Formula 2**) with an irritation score of 0.82 exhibited superior mildness compared with the benchmark formulation with an irritation score of 2.73.

Conclusions

APG surfactants are obtained from renewable, plant-derived raw materials, such as coconut oil and starch. Their environmental and skin compatibility profiles fit in well with consumer demands for green products, mildness to human skin and safety for human health. Compatibility test results and exemplary formulations presented here show that the surfactant group of alkyl polyglucosides enables cosmetic chemists to formulate modern, mild, body-cleansing formulations that fulfill the new green formulation trend and enable the formulation of alkyl sulfate-free and ethoxylate-free cleansing concepts.

Published June 2008 *Cosmetics and Toiletries* magazine

References

1. A Willing, H Messinger and W Aulmann, Ecology and toxicology of alkyl polyglucoside, in *Handbook of Detergents*, U Zoller, ed, New York: Marcel Dekker (2004) pp 487–521
2. WJ Pape et al, COLIPA validation project on in vitro eye irritation tests for cosmetic ingredients and finished products (phase I): The red blood cell test for the estimation of acute eye irritation potentials. Present status, *Toxicol in Vitro* 13 343–354 (1999)
3. Red Blood Cell Test System, Protocol No 37, InVittox Web site, available at: *www.invittox. com* (Accessed May 5, 2008)
4. W Steiling, M Bracher, P Courtelemont and O de Silva, The HET-CAM, a useful in vitro assay for assessing the eye irritation properties of cosmetic formulations and ingredients, *Toxicol in Vitro* 13 375–384 (1999)
5. HET-CAM Test, Protocol No. 96, InVittox Web site, available at: *www.invittox.com* (Accessed May 5, 2008)
6. A Mehling, M Kleber and H Hensen, Comparative studies on the ocular and dermal irritation potential of surfactants, *Food Chem Toxicol* 45 747–758 (2007)
7. F Bartnik and K Künstler, Biological effects, toxicology and human safety, Chapter 9 in *Surfactants in Consumer Products*, J Falbe, ed, Berlin: Springer Verlag (1987) pp 475–503
8. H Löffler, I Effendy and R Happle, Die irritative Kontaktdermitits, *Hautarzt* 51 203–215 (2000)
9. PJ Frosch and AM Kligman, The soap chamber test. A new method to assess the irritancy of soaps, *J Am Acad Dermat* 1 35–41 (1979)
10. H Löffler and R Happle, Profile of irritant patch testing with detergents: sodium lauryl sulphate, sodium laureth sulphate and alkyl polyglucoside, *Contact Derm* 48 26–32 (2003)

CHAPTER 16

Vernix Caseosa: The Ultimate Natural Cosmetic?

Johann W. Wiechers, PhD
JW Solutions

Bernard Gabard, PhD
Iderma

KEY WORDS: Vernix Caseosa, *natural, barrier formation, wound healing*

ABSTRACT: *Summarizes the current knowledge of* vernix caseosa *and discusses the underlying principles by which* vernix caseosa *operates; this can be applied in moisturizing and barrier-enhancing products.*

Many research articles have been published since the turn of this century investigating the origin, composition, function and potential benefits of *vernix caseosa.* Not only does this research provide an understanding of the formation of perfect young skin, some of it can be translated into benefits for the cosmetic industry. The present review summarizes the current knowledge of *vernix caseosa* and discusses the underlying principles by which *vernix caseosa* operates; this can be applied in moisturizing and barrier-enhancing products, although the proteolipid biofilm itself cannot be used directly on the human body. The most important characteristic of *vernix caseosa* is its controlled degree of occlusivity—neither too much nor too little.

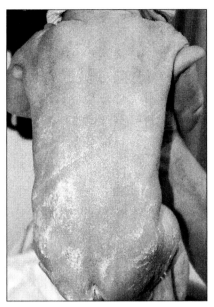

Figure 1. A newborn is often covered in a creamy white, cheesy biofilm called *vernix caseosa*. During the last trimester of gestation, this biofilm covers the skin of the fetus and after delivery, it dries. The boy pictured is Tristan Le Dévédec, son of Robert Rissmann, PhD, on whose thesis this review article is partly based. Reproduced with the kind permission of the father.

Vernix caseosa

Vernix caseosa is the creamy white, viscous biofilm that surrounds a newborn's body during birth (see **Figure 1**). The Latin words *vernix caseosa* mean *varnish* and *cheese-like*, respectively, and indeed, sometimes the whole body is covered in this whitish cream during delivery. The *vernix caseosa* is produced during the last trimester of gestation as a remnant of the original periderm. It provides a temporary skin barrier that is suitable for the aqueous environment in utero, with active transport mechanisms between the amniotic fluid and embryo by virtue of its microvilli situated at the top of its surface.

Periderm cells are replaced continuously until 21 weeks of gestation when they are completely shed and replaced by the stratum corneum (SC). The shed periderm cells are mixed with secretions from the sebaceous glands within the epithelial walls to form *vernix caseosa*.[1] At the same time, the fetal lungs mature, which requires amniotic surfactant levels to increase. This in turn causes the *vernix caseosa* to detach from the fetal skin surface, contributing to the turbidity of the amniotic fluid at the end of pregnancy.[2]

While the exact function of *vernix caseosa* is still under debate, a multitude of different functions have been suggested, and in some cases identified. These can be divided into prenatal, during birth and postnatal functions. Prenatal functions include: waterproofing, since due to the low surface energy, *vernix caseosa* is highly unwettable;[3] the facilitation of the skin formation in utero;[1] and protection of the fetus from acute or sub-acute chorioamnionitis (an inflammation of the outer (chorion) and inner (amnion) fetal membranes due to a bacterial infection).[4,5] During delivery, *vernix caseosa* acts as a lubricant while postnatally, it exhibits antioxidant, skin cleansing,[6] temperature-regulating[7] and antibacterial properties.[8]

Other possible prenatal roles have been suggested, such as facilitating the colonization of skin with microorganisms after birth,[3,9] but for the cosmetic formulator, the most interesting properties of *vernix caseosa* are its skin moisturizing and skin barrier-enhancing properties. While a previous column linked the presence of orthorhombic skin lipid packing with good skin hydration,[10] this column steps further back to examine how young, healthy skin is created.

Vernix caseosa Composition: The 'Inside' Story

The typical composition of *vernix caseosa* is 10% lipid, 10% protein and 80% water. The water is mainly present within the keratinocytes as identified with cryo-scanning electron microscopy coupled with X-ray beam analysis.[11] Although the protein content is not as well-characterized as its lipid constituents, a plethora of antimicrobial peptides have been recently identified.[2,5,8,9] Much more is known about the lipid composition of *vernix caseosa*. Recent analyses of the lipid constituents have been published[12-15] and these results are compared in **Table 1** with the typical composition of SC lipids and skin surface lipids, also previously published.[12,14,15]

Table 1 groups together typical skin barrier lipids (ceramides, cholesterol and free fatty acids) as well as those originating from the sebaceous glands. Comparing these groups, one can clearly see that the SC and sebaceous glands produce completely different lipids. However, the lipids found in *vernix caseosa* are a mixture of skin barrier and sebaceous lipids (also see **Table 1**). Scientists have used this profile as a way to establish the origin of *vernix caseosa*. Its high content of squalene and wax esters originally suggested that the lipids in *vernix caseosa* were derived mainly from fetal sebaceous glands. Stewart et al., for instance, demonstrated in the early 1980s that the lipids in *vernix caseosa* were most likely derived from the sebaceous gland via the fatty acid composition of wax esters in this biofilm.[16] Later studies, however, demonstrated the presence of all major SC lipids in *vernix caseosa*.[12]

Table 1. A comparison of the lipid components of *vernix caseosa*, stratum corneum and skin surface (sebaceous) lipids, expressed as percentage of total weight of lipids.

Lipid Class		Vernix caseosa				Stratum corneum			Skin surface
		Sumida[12]	Hoeger[13]	Tansiri-kongkol[14]	Rissmann[15]	Sumida[12]	Tansiri-kongkol[14]	Rissmann[15]	Sumida[12]
Skin barrier lipids	Ceramides	17.9	7.7	18	4.9	40	40	36	
	Cholesterol	7.5	12.1	8	4	25	25	18.9	
	Free fatty acids	6.5	6.6	7	2	25	25	23.6	18.4
	Cholesterol sulfate	0.3	nr*	0.3	nr*	10	10		
Sebaceous lipids	Cholesterol esters	30.6	nr*	42	42				3
	Wax esters	6							20.3
	Triglycerides	15.1	nr*	15	35.9				41.8
	Squalene	4	nr*	4	5				12.2
	Diols	nr*			6				
	Alkane	-			-				2.8
	Phospholipids	6.1	4.4	6	nr*				1.5

*nr = Not reported

Hoeger et al.[13] refined this picture and demonstrated that the composition pattern of the ceramides found in *vernix caseosa* mirrored that of mid-gestational fetal epidermis, therefore representing what they called a *homologous* substitute for the immature epidermal barrier in fetal skin. Combine this with the fact that the periderm, mentioned above, is shed as the fetal sebaceous unit is developing, and this composition is explained.

If all the usual SC lipids including ceramides, cholesterol and free fatty acids are present in *vernix caseosa*, does this mean that *vernix caseosa* also fulfills a barrier function for the unborn child? In order to address this question, two other issues must first be addressed. Apart from having ceramides, cholesterol and free fatty acids present, the ceramide profile (i.e., *which* ceramides are present) and the packing state of the lipids (i.e., *how* they are grouped) need to meet certain requirements.

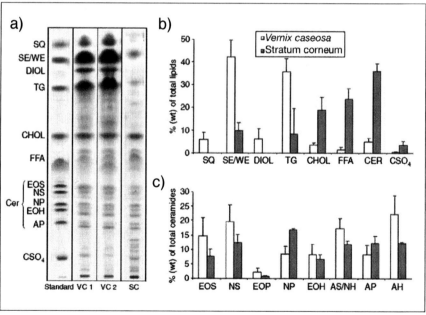

Figure 2. a) Lipid analyses of a standard solution (STD), two **vernix caseosa** (VC) samples and one stratum corneum (SC) sample by HPTLC; b) quantitative analysis of the free lipid extracts for all **vernix caseosa** compounds; c) quantitative analysis of ceramides only. Results are shown as weight percentage ± standard deviation.
SQ = squalane; SE = sterol esters; WE = wax esters; DIOL = dihydroxy WE;
TG = triglycerides; CHOL = cholesterol; FFA = free fatty acid; Cer = ceramides (EOS-1, NS-2, NP-3, EOH-4, AS-5, AP-6, AH-7, NH-8, EOP-9); CSO4 = CHOL sulfate;
reproduced with permission from Reference 15.

Hoeger et al.[13] and Rissmann et al.[15] both describe the complete ceramide profile of *vernix caseosa*. Whereas the former states that the ceramide profile is identical to mid-gestational and immature SC of a developing fetus, the latter states that although the levels of ceramides present in mature SC and the *vernix caseosa* are very different, their profiles are very similar (see **Figure 2**). Most abundant is CER(AH) at 22.0 ± 6.6% (formerly known as Ceramide 7); followed by slightly lower levels of CER(NS) (Cer 2, 19.5 ± 5.9%); CER(AS/NH) (Cer 5/8, 17.3 ± 3.3%); and CER(EOS) (Cer 1, 14.8 ± 6.0%).

When it comes to studying the structural packing of the *vernix caseosa* lipids, the available literature is scarce. In 2000, Pickens et al. had already described the *vernix caseosa* as a mobile or fluid phase SC, suggesting hardly any barrier function at all.[11] This was confirmed by the work of Rissmann et al.,[15] who concluded—based on small angle X-ray diffraction work—that there was no well-defined, long-range ordering, such as the occurrence of lamellae stacks, visible in the *vernix caseosa* samples they studied. However, a small population of lipids formed a long-range ordering at room temperature that, in a later article from the same group, was shown to disappear at elevated temperatures; these changes were found to be reversible.[17]

Finally, Rissmann et al. describe, in a third article, that *vernix caseosa* lipids are able to form the long periodicity phase with similar spacing to the human SC.[18] This phase has been shown by Bouwstra et al. to be essential for the barrier function of the SC.[19] But the temperature required for the formation of the long periodicity phase is different for *vernix caseosa* than SC barrier lipids, which can be most likely attributed to the different fatty acid chain composition (especially the presence of branched fatty acid chains) and the resulting difference in physicochemical properties.[18] From this, one can conclude that the barrier function of *vernix caseosa* in the womb is definitely different from and less pronounced than the SC, and possibly only functions via the waterproofing mechanism described by Youssef et al.[4] However, once the baby is delivered, the barrier function of the *vernix caseosa* changes again, as will be discussed next.

Vernix caseosa Water-holding Capacity: The 'Outside' Story

Once a baby is delivered, *vernix caseosa* has two important external functions. First, it must regulate the newborn's transepidermal water loss (TEWL) and second, it must maintain its body temperature. Most babies, however, are immediately cleaned after delivery—and rumor has it that midwives apply some of the *vernix caseosa* they remove to their own hands, rendering them soft and well-hydrated. This suggests good hydrating properties of *vernix caseosa.* As was demonstrated in a previous column, however, good skin hydration is not just a matter of sufficient water in the skin; hydration also relates to optimized barrier function.[10]

The SC of a newborn baby is still in the process of adapting to extra-uterine life[20] and has therefore not yet matured. At certain body sites, this may manifest itself in excessive water loss, leading not only to a reduced enzymatic activity in the skin, but also a reduced body temperature. It must be mentioned here, however, that other investigators state that term newborns have a functionally superb epidermal barrier.[21]

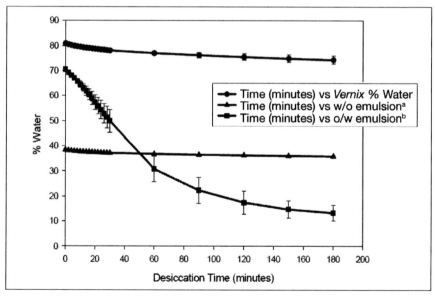

Figure 3. Water loss profiles of **vernix caseosa**, w/o emulsion[a] and o/w emulsion[b] films (applied at a rate of 3 mg/cm[2]) for 3 hr; note that the three films have different initial water contents (82.1%, 37.4% and 70.0%, respectively); reproduced with permission from Reference 25; later re-published in Reference 26.

Over the last decade, many investigators have studied the water-holding capacity of *vernix caseosa*.[22-28] This bio-film indeed has a unique water-holding capability. Despite its high water content (about 80%), water is released slowly from *vernix caseosa*, which is comparable to the release of water from a water-in-oil emulsion, as shown in **Figure 3**. Here, the loss of water is measured as a function of time from *vernix caseosa*, a water-in-oil emulsion[a] and an oil-in-water emulsion[b].

Vernix caseosa released water at roughly the same rate as the w/o emulsion. At the end of 3 hr, *vernix caseosa* and the water-in-oil emulsion lost 8.1% and 6.6% of their original water content, respectively.[26] In contrast, the o/w emulsion released as much as 30% of its total water content within the first 30 min of the experiment and 81% by the end of the experiment.[25]

The water release rate depends on the thickness of the layer of *vernix caseosa* applied. Gunt showed that the percentage of water lost from *vernix caseosa* films decreases with an increase in film thickness.[25] In addition, the water loss profile depends on the relative humidity of the external environment—at a higher relative humidity, more water is retained within *vernix caseosa*, yet the difference in water loss in the range of 82% to 98% relative humidity is dramatic, relative to the losses measured in the range of 35% to 82% relative humidity (see **Figure 4**).

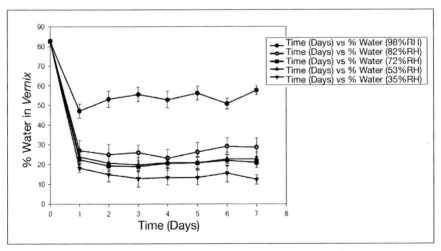

Figure 4. Water loss profiles of **vernix caseosa** films applied at a rate of 2.5mg/cm² as a function of relative humidity; reproduced with permission from Reference 25.

Tansirikongkol et al. took this experiment one step further and measured sorption-desorption curves at different relative humidities. They assessed the equilibrium water content in native *vernix caseosa* and *vernix* corneocytes and compared this to the SC.[27] The equilibrium water content for native *vernix* and *vernix* corneocytes decreased with decreasing water activity (desorption study) and increased with increasing water activity (sorption study). Native *vernix caseosa* released and absorbed water at a very low level at low relative humidities. Once the humidity reached approximately 90%, the sorption and desorption curves rose dramatically (see **Figure 5a**).

Similarly, the sorption and desorption of water in *vernix caseosa* corneocytes occurred in low levels at low humidities. However, compared to native *vernix*, isolated *vernix* corneocytes exhibited unusually high water sorption at the 75% relative humidity condition, resulting in a 5- to 7-fold increase over the water content at 64% relative humidity (see **Figure 5b**).[27]

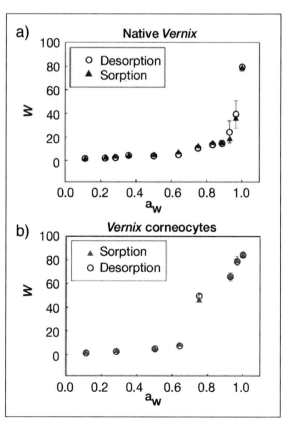

Figure 5. Equilibrium water sorption-desorption curves of a) native **vernix caseosa** (n = 4) and b) vernix corneocytes (n = 6), expressed as % w/w water in the tissue (mean ± SD) versus water activity; reproduced with permission from Reference 27.

When this data is compared with similar curves established for SC by Kasting and Barai,[29] it can be seen that native *vernix caseosa* showed the most similar water sorption profile to the profile of human SC. This combination of graphs suggests that when the relative humidity is lowered, as happens during delivery, water is released from the *vernix* corneocytes into the *vernix* and therefore to the SC. In doing so, it ensures that the imperfect SC of the newborn baby will have sufficient water for all its enzymes to function properly, so that a proper barrier can be formed.

Barrier Formation and Wound Healing

Summarizing the discussion thus far, immediately after birth, *vernix caseosa* is involved in maintaining the water balance in the skin of a newborn and in that way, helps to maintain skin temperature as well as the right water activity in the skin for optimal skin barrier formation. This suggests that *vernix caseosa* could also have a skin repairing effect when applied to damaged skin (i.e., wounds, scars) as well as dry skin.

Wound treatment and management is an important aspect of curing hospital patients that either are admitted with existing wounds or who obtain new wounds from surgical procedures. The healing of open cutaneous wounds has been divided into three overlapping phases: inflammation, re-epithelization and wound contraction. A moist environment was found to be optimal for wound healing, particularly during the inflammatory and proliferative phases, whereas enhanced cell migration, which is part of the re-epithelization process, has also been facilitated by moist conditions.[30] Occlusive dressings have therefore become increasingly popular since they enhance wound healing primarily by preventing wound desiccation and by creating this moist environment.

However, when comparing fully occlusive foils to semi-occlusive foils, Schunck et al.[30] found that wounds treated with semi-occlusive foils reduced wound contraction but enhanced cell migration and re-epithelization without irritation. This finding matches the observations of Visscher et al., who found that wounds treated with semi-permeable membranes undergo a more rapid barrier recovery than either non-occluded wounds or wounds under complete occlusion. Coverings that produce intermediate levels of skin hydration during recovery produced the highest barrier repair rates.[31]

These results suggest that barrier repair is augmented because semi-permeable membranes provide an optimal water vapor gradient during the wound healing process. Unfortunately, the optimal water gradient for wound care was not investigated but studies in the SC have shown that there is a critical range of water activities of 80% to 95% relative humidity, which permits filaggrin proteolysis to take place.[32]

The ideal water vapor transport rate through *vernix caseosa* and its implications for barrier repair were presented by Gunt et al. in 2002.[33] The flux of water was measured as a function of time through an artificial membrane[c] that was chosen because it had a water vapor transport profile in the same range as that of preterm infant or wounded skin.

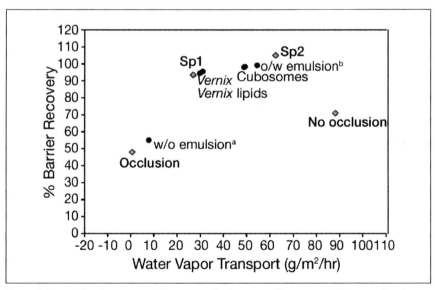

Figure 6. Percent barrier recovery after tape stripping versus film permeability; reproduced with permission from Reference 33; later re-published in Reference 25.

This data was combined with the SC barrier recovery following tape stripping assessed previously,[31] and the resulting graph is shown in **Figure 6**. This shows that optimal barrier recovery is obtained when the water vapor transport rate is in the range of 25–65 g.m^{-2}.h^{-1}. In this experiment *vernix caseosa* has a water vapor transport rate of 25 g.m^{-2}.h^{-1} and 70 g.m^{-2}.h^{-1}, depending on the thickness of the layer of *vernix caseosa* applied, avoiding both total occlusion of the skin surface and total free transport of water, where the barrier recovery rate is significantly lower.[33]

These findings make *vernix caseosa* a perfect candidate as a therapeutic to be applied topically to impaired and/or damaged human skin, but because it is a biological material of human origin, and because of its less favorable cosmetic properties—e.g., cheesy appearance, odor, consistency, potential presence of blood and skin cells—its use is not widespread. The scientific literature references a limited number of research papers where *vernix caseosa* has been tested on human skin. In one Russian study, for example, *vernix caseosa* exhibited wound healing properties in adults treated for trophic ulcers of the lower extremities.[34] In another, Moraille et al.[6] investigated the skin cleansing properties of *vernix caseosa* on the volar forearm of human subjects. A study by Bautista et al. measured baseline surface hydration, moisture accumulation and TEWL, concluding that *vernix caseosa* treated skin had a significantly higher water-holding capacity, which was provisionally attributed to the absorption of water by the fetal corneocytes;[23] similar work was conducted by Gunt.[25]

A fifth study by Barai using *vernix caseosa* on human skin in vivo measured the speed of barrier repair of tape stripped volar forearm skin that showed an intermediate water vapor permeability, resulting in a rapid increase in barrier recovery between days 3 and 5, following tape stripping.[35] Interestingly, the *vernix caseosa* samples were sterilized by gamma radiation after collection[6, 23, 35] and before application to the skin of the newborn's mother.[35]

The biological origin of *vernix caseosa* has led to two types of current research. First, it is being used in cultured skin substitutes that serve as wound healing models to study fundamental skin biology.[36] In addition, synthetic analogues of *vernix caseosa* are being developed in an attempt to obtain its beneficial properties from a non-biological origin; after all, this is where great potential is, as Haubrich states: "Application of the fetal/neonatal skin science findings (of *vernix caseosa*) to the adult burn population offers the potential for a clinically relevant homologous substitute for impaired integrity."[37] Therefore, the last section of this review will evaluate current attempts to mimic *vernix caseosa* and identify the criteria for success, to give cosmetic formulators some guidance as to how to make a perfect skin repair cream.

How to Mimic *Vernix caseosa*

Understanding the physical chemistry and biology of *vernix caseosa* poses a significant challenge to the cosmetic scientist. Hoath et al.[38] list the functions and characteristics that should be fulfilled by a synthetic analogue of *vernix caseosa*. These include considerations such as being: "structurally similar to the stratum corneum, which it intimately covers; *vernix caseosa* lacks lipid lamellae [although Rissmann et al. recently did find some[18]] and desmosomal contact. Uniquely human, *vernix caseosa* is multifunctional: a skin cleanser, moisturizer, anti-infective and antioxidant, which works in both aqueous and non-aqueous environments.

"In utero, its rheological properties are modified by extracutaneous secretions such as pulmonary surfactant. Detached *vernix* is swallowed by the fetus. *Vernix* contributes to the electrical isolation of the fetus and has osmoregulatory capability. At the time of birth, its water content precisely matches the cube of the golden section ratio. Following tactile spreading, polygonal *vernix* corneocytes orient parallel to the skin surface. The hydrophilic (intracorneocyte) and hydrophobic (external lipid) domains of *vernix* contain a plethora of biologically active, small molecules in a complex, structured array.

"Cleansing studies[6] support ready entry of applied *vernix* into surface pores such as hair follicles. *Vernix* has a nongreasy feel and its physical properties hypothetically contribute to the panoply of sensory cues, which attract caregivers to the skin of the newborn. The possibility that vernix contains pheromones, like mother's milk, is open to investigation. *Vernix* facilitates acid mantle formation and presumably contributes to optimal bacterial colonization of newborn skin after birth."

Imagine getting such a product brief from marketing!

From all of the above, it is clear that a synthetic analogue of *vernix caseosa* cannot simply mimic all its biological and physical characteristics. Formulators have therefore focused on a few main points, including the water-holding capacity and the water vapor transport rate; more recently, the skin barrier effect has become another focus. Papers describing synthetic analogues of *vernix caseosa* include the following, discussed in chronological order of publication:

Sumida 1998: Sumida et al.[12] were (one of) the first to describe a pseudo *vernix caseosa* formulation and found that the skin's hygroscopicity and water-holding ability markedly improved after application of a test cream, even after washing with water. The authors suggested that the liquid crystalline structure of both the *vernix caseosa* and pseudo *vernix caseosa* formulation contributed water-absorption ability to these lipid mixtures.

The next six publications describing synthetic analogues for *vernix caseosa* all come from the University of Cincinnati School of Pharmacy, or the Skin Science Institute at the Cincinnati Children's Hospital Research Foundation, which clearly made this into a research theme for almost a decade. It started with a poster of Bautista et al.[22] in which *vernix caseosa* was compared with a petrolatum and mineral oil-based ointment[d] and petrolatum. Initially, the comparisons were only conducted with oil-based formulations but over the course of approximately seven years, more complex formulations were studied.

Bautista 1999: In the first poster from Bautista et al.,[22] three test creams were applied to the volar skin surface of adult volunteers following cleansing; these contained *vernix caseosa*, a petrolatum- and mineral oil-based ointment[d] and petrolatum. Results indicated an increase in skin surface hydration on the sites where barrier creams had been applied—but not on the *vernix caseosa*-treated control sites. The researchers concluded that there are major differences between *vernix caseosa* and the o/o ointments.

Youssef, Bautista 2000: Youssef et al.[24] compared the in vitro tritiated water flux through layers of varying thickness of *vernix caseosa*, a petrolatum- and mineral oil-based ointment[d] and petrolatum, and found that the permeability coefficient of water through a film of *vernix caseosa* with a thickness of 20 μm was significantly higher than that through both the petrolatum and mineral oil ointment (2-fold) and petrolatum alone (25-fold). This supported the hypothesis that *vernix caseosa* does not act as a totally occlusive biofilm *in utero* but rather forms a semi-occlusive barrier overlaying the developing SC.

Also in 2000, Bautista et al.[23] published the first full paper on the comparison between *vernix caseosa* and standard oil-based ointments, of which the conclusions were, as might be expected, similar to the 1999 poster. In this paper, a petrolatum-, mineral oil- and lanolin alcohol-based w/o emulsion[e] also was included. Given the lipid constituents of *vernix caseosa*, the researchers anticipated that it would function as a hydrophobic barrier to prevent water loss and thereby act in a similar manner to hydrophobic ointments.

Surface electrical capacitance and TEWL experiments were conducted as indices of surface hydration. Sorption-desorption profiles were taken to determine skin surface hydrophobicity and immediately after the application of *vernix caseosa*, an increase in the rate of water loss from the skin surface was noted. Relative to control skin and the skin treated with the ointments and w/o emulsions, the application of *vernix caseosa* to freshly bathed human skin resulted in a unique profile of temporal change in baseline surface hydration, moisture accumulation and water-holding capacity (see **Figure 7**). These results, however, indicated major differences between human *vernix caseosa*, standard ointments and w/o emulsions, especially in their time profiles.[23]

Gunt 2002: The next publication was a thesis from Gunt.[25] Apart from studying fundamentals such as the influence of film thickness and relative humidity (see **Figure 4**), Gunt was the first to measure the water loss profiles of: *vernix caseosa*; the w/o emulsion[a]; o/w emulsion[b] (see **Figure 3**); and cubosomes. Cubosomes, or cubic liquid crystalline nanoparticles, have a bicontinuous liquid phase structure wherein both the water and lipid domains are continuous.

The lipid bilayer forms the building block of the bicontinuous cubic phase and is arranged in periodic three-dimensional structures.[39] Glycerol mono-olein-water, for instance, exhibits a bicontinuous cubic phase. These systems are highly viscous, clear, and have a high surface area.

Gunt's in vivo findings suggested that cubosome formulations did not impede water loss and the rate of moisture accumulation for cubosome formulas was higher than that of petrolatum or petrolatum-, mineral oil- and lanolin alcohol-based w/o emulsions[d], suggesting that more moisture was built up with cubosome formulas than occlusive petrolatum and petrolatum-based products.

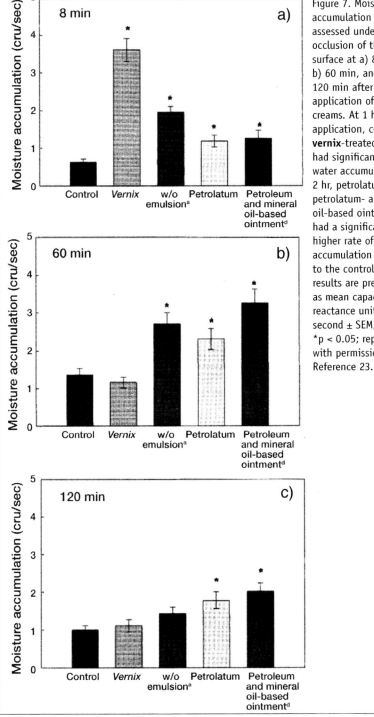

Figure 7. Moisture accumulation was assessed under probe occlusion of the skin surface at a) 8 min, b) 60 min, and c) 120 min after topical application of barrier creams. At 1 hr after application, control and **vernix**-treated sites had significantly lower water accumulation; at 2 hr, petrolatum and petrolatum- and mineral oil-based ointment had a significantly higher rate of moisture accumulation relative to the control site. All results are presented as mean capacitance reactance units per second ± SEM, *p < 0.05; reproduced with permission from Reference 23.

Both the *vernix caseosa* and cubosome formulations, which showed increased hydration at raised ambient humidity in vitro, also showed a higher water-holding capacity in vivo. From the water vapor transport data, Gunt concluded that the lipid fraction of *vernix caseosa* is primarily responsible for providing a controlled water vapor transport, whereas the role of cellular components of *vernix caseosa* is still unclear.

Since the increase in hydration at raised humidity is due to the entire *vernix caseosa* composition, however, one cannot exclude *vernix caseosa* cells from the material. These studies supported the view that topical application of *vernix caseosa* may provide the optimum water gradient required for restoration and development of the stratum corneum barrier by allowing the generation of NMF; the cubosomes were able to provide this both in vitro and in vivo.

Barai 2006: While the work of Gunt in 2002 identified that cubosomes were the best synthetic analogues of *vernix caseosa* so far, Barai assessed the effects of *vernix caseosa* and synthetic analogues on barrier repair in 2006.[35] These results, described above, identified that the semi-permeability or semi-occlusivity of *vernix caseosa* was an essential requirement for its biological benefits, since the effect of the petrolatum- and mineral oil-based ointment[d] and other barrier creams were too occlusive.

Tansirikongkol 2006-07: The last work on *vernix caseosa* synthetic analogues from the University of Cincinnati was conducted by Tansirikongkol[14, 26] and focused on high internal phase emulsions— i.e., w/o emulsions with an internal aqueous phase, as high as 78% (see **Figure 8**). This work aimed to simulate the water/lipid ratio and water-handling properties of native *vernix caseosa* by combining the slow water release profile of w/o emulsions with the high water content of o/w-emulsions. Initially the oil phase contained conventional, non-*vernix caseosa*-like lipids but later, more *vernix caseosa*-like lipids were used.

Preparations with *vernix caseosa*-like lipids demonstrated water release profiles closer to that of native *vernix caseosa* than those with conventional lipids. The remainder of Tansirikongkol's work focused more on the protective function of *vernix caseosa* against the enzymes present in the amniotic fluid, such as the chymotryptic enzyme, and excrements[21] than on the development of synthetic analogues of *vernix caseosa.*

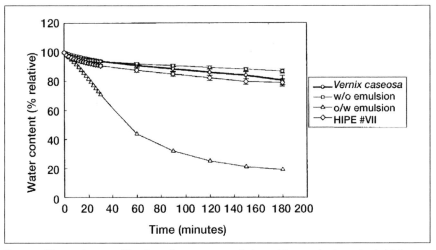

Figure 8. Water release profile of **vernix caseosa**, typical emulsions and selected w/o high internal phase emulsion (HIPE) based on 100% initial water content; reproduced with permission from Reference 26.

Erdal and Araman, Bouwstra, Hennink 2007: The children's hospital and university in Cincinnati were not the only groups working on *vernix caseosa* imitations. Erdal and Araman from Istanbul University, for instance, suggested to be working on the same but results were not provided.[40] As indicated above, Gunt had already identified that the total composition was important, not just the *vernix caseosa* lipids.[25] However, it was when Bouwstra, PhD, of the University of Leiden, Netherlands, and Hennink, PhD, of the University of Utrecht, Netherlands, began to collaborate that a fundamentally different approach to *vernix caseosa* imitation emerged based on creating "cell-like" structures containing water in a lipid base formation rather than an o/w or w/o emulsion.

While Rissmann, PhD, worked with Bouwstra and Ponec, PhD, to characterize the lipids in *vernix caseosa* to study their packing and structure, Oudshoorn, PhD, worked with Hennink, on mimicking the *vernix caseosa* corneocytes. All literature cited until now has stated that water is present in the *vernix caseosa* corneocytes, and that *vernix caseosa* is different in that it can take up water at high relative humidities, but apart from the cubosomes, no formulation was capable of mimicking this.

Methacrylated hyperbranched polyglycerol microparticles with uniform sizes and shapes were prepared using photolithography, resulting in a size range of 30 μm to 1,400 μm.[41] For the synthetic variant of *vernix caseosa* corneocytes, hexagons with a diameter of 30 μm were prepared, similar to the size of human corneocytes, which were loaded with FITC-dextran and coated with lipids (see **Figure 9**). Next, a lipid mixture mimicking the intercellular lipid composition and organization of *vernix caseosa* was prepared—similar to that reported in **Table 1** for *vernix caseosa*, from Rissmann et al.[15]—and mixed in different ratios with the microparticles. Subsequently, the water-handling properties were measured gravimetrically and compared to native *vernix caseosa* in a dehydration study over P_2O_5. The result of this experiment is shown in **Figure 10**.[28]

Vernix caseosa is characterized by an initial rapid water loss prior to a sustained, steady dehydration at room temperature. Of all the synthetic analogues developed, the one labeled B2c (see **Figure 10**) was closest to native *vernix caseosa*; this sample included coated particles and had an initial water content of 80%; the particle/lipid ratio was 2:1. With these modifications, the researchers were able to extend the water release from 24 hr to 140 hr.[28] This of course raised the question of whether or not the synthetic *vernix caseosa* also had a superb barrier repair mechanism, which was the subject of later papers.

First, a tape-stripping model on mouse skin was developed in which skin was stripped to a specific level (79 ± 6 g/m²/hr), where a crust was formed and almost complete recovery (~90%) was obtained within only 8 days. The topical application of *vernix caseosa* considerably increased initial and long-term recovery, promoted a rapid formation of the SC, and prevented epidermal thickening.[42]

Second, this model was treated with the same synthetic biofilms as well as oil-based ointments and the skin barrier recovery was compared to native *vernix caseosa*. Application of all tested formulations improved the skin barrier recovery and reduced crust formation and hyperproliferation but remarkably, the best-performing biofilm was the one containing *uncoated* particles with 50% (w/w) initial water content and a particle/lipid ratio of 2:1. The fact that the water profile experiments depicted in **Figure 10** were the most similar to *vernix caseosa*, in which the initial water content was 80%,

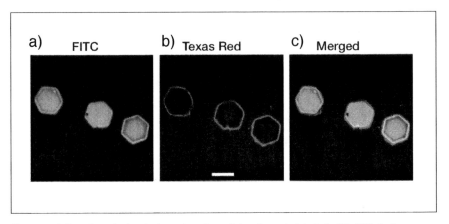

Figure 9. a) Hyperbranched polyglycerol methacrylate microgels labeled with FITC-dextran and b) the coating lipids, labeled with Texas Red, surrounding the microgels as visualized by confocal laser scanning microscopy. Confocal laser scanning microscopy was performed with 488 nm and 543 nm excitation wavelengths for a) and b), respectively. Scale bar represents 25 μm; reproduced with permission from Reference 28.

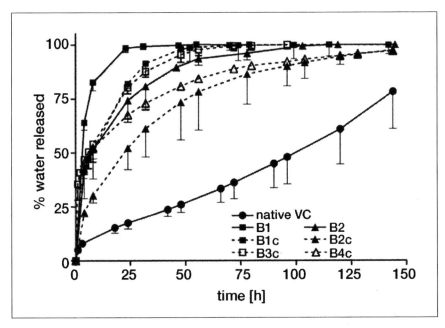

Figure 10. Water release profiles of native VC (●) and various biofilms obtained by monitoring the weight loss of the specimen in a desiccator over P_2O_5 at room temperature. Various parameters were changed in the formulations: the initial water content of the particles was either 50% (■,□) or 80% (▲,△). The particles were coated with lipids (dashed lines) or were kept uncoated (solid lines) prior to embedding in the synthetic biofilm lipid matrix. The particle/lipid ratio was either 2:1 (■,▲) or 5:1 (□,△). Data is presented as mean (w/w) − S.D. (n = 3); reproduced with permission from Reference 28.

indicated that the amount of lipids might play an important role in the skin barrier recovery.

This raised the question of how important water-handling properties, as well as the presence of corneocytes, are for barrier recovery. Synthetic lipid mixtures with and without barrier lipids were therefore included in the study. The skin barrier repair results for a water and particle-free formulation with barrier lipids were very similar to those observed for native *vernix caseosa.* This demonstrated that the lipids, including barrier lipids, play a more prominent role in barrier recovery than the water content and presence of corneocytes. The latter, however, may be beneficial for increasing skin hydration and act as a drug delivery reservoir.[43]

Vernix caseosa: The Ultimate Natural Cosmetic?

Scientific research of the last decade has provided sufficient evidence for the beneficial properties of *vernix caseosa* as a barrier cream that not only corrects moisturization levels within the skin, but also improves skin barrier recovery by creating and maintaining a water activity level that allows all enzymes to function properly. However, its availability is insufficient to address the needs of the world of products that can restore skin barrier function and moisturization. Synthetic analogues have therefore been created and tested, and such *vernix caseosa* substitutes must meet only one criterion to be successful.

While the necessity of water in such a formulation is still debated (for instance, see Reference 43), the semi-permeable nature of the product is absolutely essential, since both fully occlusive and non-occlusive products function far less well; and indeed there are already a few cosmetic ingredients[44] as well as formulated products on the market that meet this requirement.

Published September 2009 *Cosmetics and Toiletries* magazine

References

1. G Singh, and A G, Unraveling the mystery of *vernix caseosa, Ind J Dermatol* 53 54–60 (2008)
2. HT Akinbi, V Narendran, A Kun Pass, P Markart and SB Hoath, Host defense proteins in *vernix caseosa* and amniotic fluid, *Am J Obstet Gynaecol* 191 2090–2096 (2004)
3. MO Visscher et al, *Vernix caseosa* in neonatal adaptation, *J Perinatol* 25 440–446 (2005)

4. W Youssef, RR Wickett and SB Hoath, Surface free energy characterization of *vernix caseosa*. Potential role in waterproofing the newborn infant, *Skin Res Technol* 7 10–17 (2001)

5. G Bergsson et al, Antimicrobial components of *vernix caseosa*, *Pediat Res* 56 469, Poster 30, presented at the European Society for Pediatric Research, Stockholm, Sweden (Sep 19-22, 2004)

6. R Moraille, WL Pickens, MO Visscher and SB Hoath, A novel role for *vernix caseosa* as a skin cleanser, *Biol Neonate* 87 8–14 (2005)

7. C Saunders, The *vernix caseosa* and subnormal temperature in premature infants, *Br J Obstet Gynaecol* 55 442–444 (1955)

8. M Tollin et al, *Vernix caseosa* as a multi-component defense system based on polypeptides, lipids and their interactions, *Cell Mol Life Sci* 62 2390–2399 (2005)

9. H Yoshio, H Lagercrantz, GH Gudmundsson and B Agerberth, First line of defense in early human life, *Sem Perinatol* 28 304–311 (2004)

10. JW Wiechers, Orthorhombic phase stabilization for internal occlusion: A new mechanism for skin moisturization, *Cosmet & Toilet* 124 (6) 45–50 (2009)

11. WL Pickens, RR Warner, YL Boissy, RE Boissy and SB Hoath, Characterization of *vernix caseosa*: Water content, morphology, and elemental analysis, *J Invest Dermatol* 115 875–881 (2000)

12. Y Sumida, M Yakumaru, Y Tokitsu, Y Iwamoto, T Ikemoto and K Mimura, Studies on the function of *vernix caseosa*—The secrecy of baby's skin, *Proceedings of the 20th IFSCC Congress*, P201, Cannes, France (Sep 14-18, 1998)

13. PH Hoeger, V Schreiner, IA Klaassen, CC Enzmann, K Friedrichs and O Bleck, Epidermal barrier lipids in human *vernix caseosa*: Corresponding ceramide pattern in vernix and fetal skin, *Br J Dermatol* 146 194–201 (2002)

14. A Tansirikongkol, Development of a synthetic *vernix* equivalent and its water-handling and barrier protective properties in comparison with *vernix caseosa*, doctoral thesis, University of Cincinnati, College of Pharmacy, Division of Pharmaceutical Sciences, Cincinnati, OH, USA (2006)

15. R Rissmann, HWW Groenink, AM Weerheim, SB Hoath, M Ponec and JA Bouwstra, New insights into ultrastructure, lipid composition and organization of *vernix caseosa*, *J Invest Dermatol* 126 1823–1833 (2006)

16. ME Stewart, MA Quinn and DT Downing, Variability in the fatty acid composition of wax esters from *vernix caseosa* and its possible relation to sebaceous gland activity, *J Invest Dermatol* 78291–295 (1982)

17. R Rissmann et al, Temperature-induced changes in structural and physicochemical properties of *vernix caseosa*, *J Invest Dermatol* 128 292–299 (2008)

18. R Rissmann, G Gooris, M Ponec and JA Bouwstra, Long periodicity phase in extracted lipids of *vernix caseosa* obtained with equilibration at physiological temperatures, *Chemi and Phys of Lipids* 158 32–38 (2009)

19. JA Bouwstra, GS Gooris, FE Dubbelaar, AM Weerheim, AP IJzerman and M Ponec, Role of ceramide 1 in the molecular organization of the stratum corneum lipids, *J Lipid Res* 39 186–196 (1998)

20. G Yosipovitch, A Maayan-Metzger, P Merlob and L Sirota, Skin barrier properties in different body areas in neonates, *Pediatrics* 106 105–108 (2006)

21. A Tansirikongkol, RR Wickett, MO Visscher, and SB Hoath, Effect of *vernix caseosa* on the penetration of chymotryptic enzyme: Potential role in epidermal barrier development, *Pediatr Res* 62 49–53 (2007)

22. MI Bautista, WL Pickens, MO Visscher and SB Hoath, Characterization of *vernix caseosa* as a natural biofilm: Hydration effects and comparison to Aquaphor, *Pediat Res* 45 4; part 2; 185A, abstract 1081; poster 26 (1999)

23. MI Bautista, RR Wickett, MO Visscher, WL Pickens and SB Hoath, Characterization of *vernix caseosa* as a natural biofilm: Comparison to standard oil-based ointments, *Pediat Dermatol* 17 253–260 (2000)

24. W Youssef, SB Hoath and RR Wickett, In vitro water transport through *vernix caseosa* compared to Aquaphor and petrolatum, *AAPS Journal*, 2000 (S1) (2000) 2206, available at *www.aapsj.org/abstracts/AM_2000/2206.htm* (accessed May 11, 2009)

25. HB Gunt, Water-handling properties of *vernix caseosa*, *M.Sc. Thesis*, University of Cincinnati, OH, USA (2002)

26. A Tansirikongkol, MO Visscher and RR Wickett, Water-handling properties of *vernix caseosa* and a synthetic analogue, *J Cosmet Sci* 58 651–662 (2007)

27. A Tansirikongkol, SB Hoath, WL Pickens, MO Visscher and RR Wickett, Equilibrium water content in native *vernix* and its cellular component, *J Pharm Sci* 97 985–994 (2008)

28. R Rissmann, MHM Oudshoorn, R Zwier, M Ponec, JA Bouwstra and WE Hennink, Mimicking *vernix caseosa*—Preparation and characterization of synthetic biofilms, *Int J Pharm* 372 59–65 (2009)

29. G Kasting and N Barai, Equilibrium water sorption in human stratum corneum, *J Pharm Sci* 92 1624–1631 (2003)

30. M Schunck, C Neumann and E Proksch, Artificial barrier repair in wounds by semi-occlusive foils reduced wound contraction and enhanced cell migration and reepithelization in mouse skin, *J Invest Dermatol* 125 1063–1071 (2005)

31. MO Visscher, SB Hoath, E Conroy and RR Wickett, Effect of semipermeable membranes on skin barrier repair following tape stripping, *Arch Dermatol Res* 293 491–499 (2001)

32. IR Scott and CR Harding, Filaggrin breakdown to water-binding compounds during development of the rat stratum corneum is controlled by the water activity of the environment, *Dev Biol* 115 84–92 (1986)

33. HB Gunt, RR Wickett and MO Visscher, Water vapor transport through *vernix caseosa*—Implications in barrier repair, Poster 4 at the Annual Scientific Seminar of the Society of Cosmetic Chemists, San Antonio, TX, USA (May 9-10, 2002)

34. BN Zhukov, EI Neverova, KE Nikitin, VE Kostiaev and PN Myshentsev, A comparative evaluation of the use of *vernix caseosa* and solcoseryl in treating patients with trophic ulcers in the lower extremities, *Vestn Khir Im I I Grek* 148 339–341 (1992) (article in Russian without English abstract)

35. ND Barai, Effect of *vernix caseosa* on barrier repair in tape-stripped forearm skin, *in: Effect of* vernix caseosa *on epidermal barrier maturation and repair: Implications in wound healing*, Dissertation, University of Cincinnati, College of Pharmacy, Division of Pharmaceutical Sciences, Cincinnati, OH, USA, ch 5, pp 81–101 (2006)

36. ND Barai, Effect of *vernix* on barrier maturation in cultured skin substitutes, *in: Effect of* vernix caseosa *on epidermal barrier maturation and repair: Implications in wound healing*, *Dissertation*, University of Cincinnati, College of Pharmacy, Division of Pharmaceutical Sciences, Cincinnati, OH, USA, ch 4, pp 53–80 (2006.)

37. KA Haubrich, Role of *vernix caseosa* in the neonate. Potential application in the adult population, *AACN Clinical Issues* 14 457–464 (2003)

38. SB Hoath, WL Pickens and MO Visscher, The biology of *vernix caseosa*, *Intl J Cosmet Sci* 28 319–333 (2006)

39. PT Spicer, K Hayden, ML Lynch, A Ofori-Boateng and JL Burns, Novel process for producing cubic liquid crystalline nanoparticles (Cubosomes) *Langmuir* 17 5748–5756 (2001)

40. MS Erdal and A Araman, *Vernix caseosa*'nin ínsan derisi ile etkilesiminin biyofiziksel yöntemler arastirilmasi—Investigation of the interaction of *vernix caseosa* with human skin using biophysical methods, *Turkiye Klinikleri J Dermatol* 17 171–179 (2007)

41. MHM Oudshoorn, R Penterman, R Rissmann, JA Bouwstra, DJ Broer and WE Hennink, Preparation and characterization of structured hydrogel microparticles based on crosslinked hyperbranched polyglycerol, *Langmuir*, 23 11819–11825 (2007)

42. MHM Oudshoorn, R Rissmann, D van der Coelen, WE Hennink, M Ponec and JA Bouwstra, Development of a murine model to evaluate the effect of *vernix caseosa* on skin barrier recovery, *Exp Dermatol* 18 178–184 (2009)

43. R Rissmann, MHM Oudshoorn, D van der Coelen, WE Hennink, M Ponec and JA Bouwstra, Effect of synthetic *vernix* biofilms on barrier recovery of damaged mouse skin, *Exp Dermatol* in press (2009); also available at *https://openaccess.leidenuniv.nl/bitstream/1887/13664/12/chapter+9.pdf* (Accessed Aug 6, 2009)

44. WO/2007/039149, Method and composition comprising squalane and/or squalane for treating burn, Unichema Chemie BV, FJ Groenhof and JW Wiechers (Apr 12, 2007)

CHAPTER 17

A 'Green' Microemulsion for Improved Conditioning Performance of Shampoos

Matthias Hloucha, Hans-Martin Haake and Guadalupe Pellón

Cognis GmbH, Düsseldorf, Germany

KEY WORDS: *shampoo, hair care, performance, microemulsion, renewable, ethoxylate- and sulfate-free*

ABSTRACT: *In the present chapter, a renewable ingredient microemulsion is formulated that is free from ethoxylates and sulfate groups. Used as an additive, the material boosts the conditioning performance of shampoos and improves wet-combing performance by affecting phase separation. In addition, base formulas for standard and "green" shampoos are discussed.*

Consumers are more and more interested in living a "green" lifestyle and have come to understand the impact of the products they use on society, the environment and on themselves. Despite this eco-friendly consciousness, however, consumers are generally unwilling to sacrifice product performance; thus, they seek eco-conscious products that provide the same or better performance levels.

Naturally sourced ingredients offer formulators innovative possibilities to develop products that fulfill these consumer expectations by combining performance benefits with environmental compatibility. Modern consumers expect more than one function from a cosmetic product. For example, shampoo should have an appealing appearance—i.e., it should be clear or pearlescent—with good cleansing and hair conditioning properties as well as fast foam generation.

A pearlescent appearance can be achieved by adding well-known pearlescent agents such as glycol distearate; cleansing and foam performance are dominated by the surfactant system, which is usually a synergistic combination of two or more surfactants such as fatty alcohol ether sulfate, cocamidopropyl betaine (CAPB) and alkyl polyglucoside (APG)[a].

The most difficult task is to develop a product with the described properties and good hair conditioning performance at the same time. To achieve this, conditioning cationic polymers are used in combination with silicone oils that form a substantive hair gel or coacervate phase during the application.[1] While this is a smart technology, it is limited by patents for silicones in cosmetic compositions. Moreover, it is not compatible with the eco-friendly trend.

The present paper describes current research to evaluate whether a nature-based composition can be used to improve hair combability after the hair is washed to increase its compatibility with natural raw materials. This study investigates the conditioning performance of a silicone-free shampoo when a microemulsion[b] is added to it. The microemulsion is characterized and its effect on the phase behavior of a shampoo is described, followed by hair conditioning performance data.

Microemulsion Characteristics

Emulsions are dispersions of two immiscible liquids such as oil and water. Usually, they are thermodynamically unstable, which means that Ostwald ripening, coalescence and phase separation occur. Thus, these so-called *macroemulsions* need kinetic stabilization by surfactants, cosurfactants and rheological modifiers.

Microemulsions, on the other hand, are defined as being thermodynamically stable, which can otherwise be achieved only in optimized surfactant, cosurfactant and oil combinations where the interfacial tension is extremely low.[2] The result is usually a clear product with a nanosized emulsion structure.

---

[a] APG is a registered trademark of Cognis GmbH. It is also a commonly used abbreviation for alkyl polyglucoside in the personal care industry and beyond, and it is in that common use sense that it appears in this article.

---

[b] Plantasil Micro (INCI: Dicaprylyl Ether (and) Decyl Glucoside (and) Glyceryl Oleate) is a product of Cognis GmbH, Monheim, Germany.

Many different microemulsion systems have been described so far.[2] The focus of the present work was to develop a microemulsion based on renewable and nature-based ingredients that is free of ethoxylate and sulfate groups. The starting point was a previously published phase diagram for emulsion compositions that consisted of sodium laureth sulfate (SLES), APG, glycerol monooleate (GMO), dicaprylyl ether and octyl dodecanol.[3] In general, a phase diagram represents the appearance of an emulsion based on the interaction between its components. In multicomponent systems, it is necessary to fix some concentrations in order to get a graphical picture; here, the water content is set to 60% (see **Figure 1**).

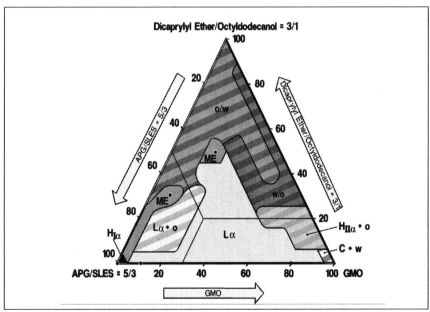

Figure 1. Phase diagram for a fixed water content of 60%; reproduced with permission from Reference 3

Liquid crystalline phases and macro-emulsion regions occur in this phase diagram. In addition, two regions where microemulsions are formed can be seen. In the lower left corner of **Formula 1**, where there is maximum surfactant content, the oil is solubilized. It is interesting how the other region is shifted toward the center of the phase diagram, which means that a higher amount of oil is incorporated into the microemulsion.

Formula 1. Shampoo with microemulsion

Sodium laureth sulfate (Texapon N70, Cognis GmbH)	12.9% w/w
Cocamidopropyl betaine (Dehyton PK 45, Cognis GmbH)	7.5
Dicaprylyl ether (and) coco glucoside (and) glyceryl oleate	
(Plantasil Micro, Cognis GmbH)	0–6.0 (varied)
Polyquaternium-10 (Dekaquat 400, Jan Dekker)	0.2
PEG/PPG-120/10 trimethylpropane trioleate (and) laureth-2	
(Arlypon TT, Cognis GmbH)	1.44
Sodium chloride	1.0
Fragrance (*parfum*)	qs
Preservative	qs
Citric acid	qs
Water (*aqua*)	qs to 100.00

Viscosity: 4000 mPas; PH: 5.0

To achieve a microemulsion with a high oil content, the addition of the synergistic cosurfactant, glycerol monooleate, is necessary. However, the development of a "green" shampoo formula with a natural-based microemulsion requires a different surfactant than SLES because its raw material base is partly originated from petrochemical products.

This surfactant exchange has an influence on the hydrophilic-lipophilic balance of the whole system. Therefore, the system must be counterbalanced by making the oil phase less polar. This can be achieved by taking out the octyl dodecanol. The result of this approach is a clear, eco-friendly microemulsion that is based only on APG, GMO and dicaprylyl ether (see **Figure 2**).

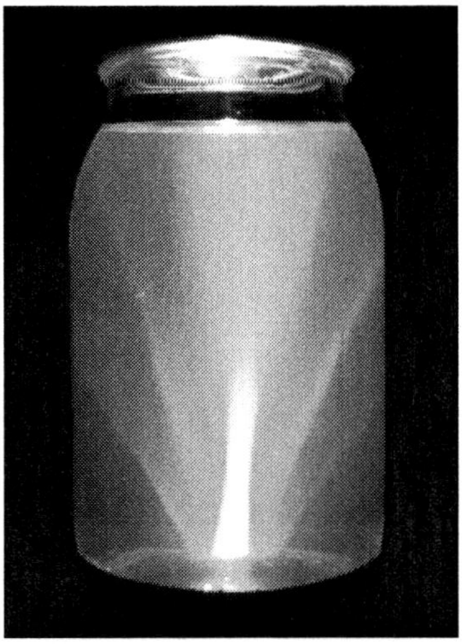

Figure 2. Clear, eco-friendly microemulsion based only on APG, GMO and dicaprylyl ether

If a bright, LED light beam is passed through the sample, a blue light scattering effect can be seen (the Tyndall effect). This is due to the nanosized structure of the microemulsion, which has an average particle size of less than 100 nm.

The raw material bases for these substances are vegetable oil and starch. The active matter of this microemulsion is approximately 44–48%; the pH is set to 3.8–4.5, which fits well with modern shampoo formulations. This microemulsion also is compatible with standard surfactant systems for shampoos, such as SLES and CAPB. For example, it can be added in any ratio to a 12% SLES/CAPB (3:1) solution. The addition is possible in a cold process and gentle stirring is enough to produce a clear final product.

Chemistry of Shampoos Containing Microemulsion

Shampoos with conditioning properties typically contain anionic surfactants in combination with cationic polymers, such as poly-quaternium-10 (PQ-10), a polymeric quaternary ammonium salt of hydroxyethylcellulose reacted with a trimethyl ammonium substituted epoxide. These shampoos exhibit a phase transition during application by the consumer. On dilution during washing, the one-phase micellar solution of the shampoo crosses a phase boundary to a two-phase region where a second gel phase is formed.[4] A microscopy image of this phase is shown in **Figure 3**.

The formation of gel-like particles can be seen in the range of 10–50 µm. The refractive index of the two phases is similar; therefore, the interface between the gel particles and the continuum phase is diffuse. The formation of such a gel phase, also called *coacervate* or *precipitate*, can be monitored by the measurement of the transmittance of the shampoo on dilution. The method[c] for turbidity titration is calibrated by water, where the transmittance is arbitrarily set to 100%; if no light passes through a sample, the transmittance is 0%.

Thus, the decrease of the transmittance on dilution is a measure for the formation of a turbid phase. The following discussion examines how the phase separation of shampoos during their application is influenced by the addition of the microemulsion.

---

[c] The experimental setup used, T50, is from Mettler Toledo in Germany.

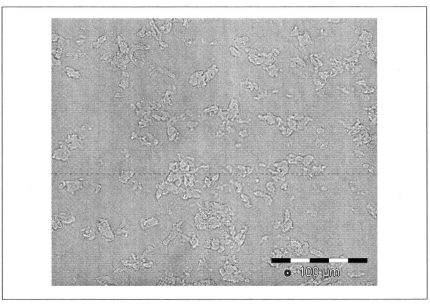

Figure 3. On dilution during washing, the one-phase micellar solution of the shampoo crosses a phase boundary to a two-phase region where a second gel phase is formed.

Materials and Methods

The shampoo base tested is shown in **Formula 1**. SLES and CAPB were used as the surfactant base, and salt and a polymer were used for thickening purposes. The cationic polymer PQ-10 is a standard polymer used in shampoos. Different levels (1–6%) of the described microemulsion were added to this shampoo; for comparision a shampoo without microemulsion was also tested. To investigate the phase behavior of these formulas, the following procedure was used: to 30 mL of the shampoo, initially 15 mL of deionized water was added, at which point all shampoos stayed clear. Then, titration with water as described in the experimental setup above was initiated. Results from these shampoos are shown in **Figure 4**.

The horizontal axis of this graph shows the amount of added water; the vertical axis shows the transmittance of the sample. For all tested shampoos, the same general pattern can be seen. With the addition of up to 25 mL of water, the shampoo remains clear; after further addition of water, a sharp decrease in the transmittance can be seen, which indicates the formation of a gel phase. For all shampoos, the minimal transmittance was reached at the addition of approximately 60–65 mL of water. This equals a dilution of the shampoo by a factor of 3.0–3.2.

After further addition of water, the transmittance increases again, showing that the turbid shampoo is now being diluted without the generation of more gel phase. The main differences between the curves are seen at the point of minimum transmittance (60–65 mL). The addition of the microemulsion led to a decrease of the minimum transmittance, meaning a larger amount of the gel phase was formed. As more microemulsion was added, this effect became more pronounced. In summary, the phase separation of a shampoo during application was enhanced by the addition of the microemulsion.

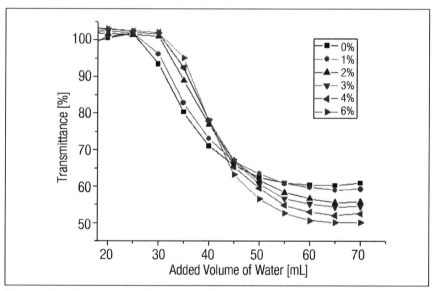

Figure 4. Transmittance versus dilution curves for shampoos with different levels of added green microemulsion

Conditioning of Shampoos with Microemulsion

Next, the wet-combing performance of standard shampoos with the microemulsion was investigated (see **Formula 1**). The wet-combing performance was determined using an automated system, as shown in **Figure 5**. Ten dark brown European hair strands per shampoo formulation were bleached with hydrogen peroxide and baseline combing forces were recorded. From the force versus path curves of the comb through the hair, the combing work was calculated by integration. The combing forces and work of treated hair strands were determined after a twofold application of 0.25 g shampoo per 1 g hair with standardized rinsing in between and after the second application. For each strand, the residual combing work was calculated according to:

Residual combing work = $\dfrac{\text{Combing work after treatment}}{\text{Combing work before treatment}}$

Table 1 shows the results for the residual combing work of standard shampoos with different levels of the microemulsion.

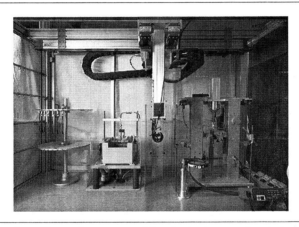

Figure 5. The wet-combing performance was determined using an automated system.

Table 1. Residual Wet-combing Work for Standard Shampoos with Added Microemulsion

Microemulsion [%]	Residual wet-combing work [%]
0.0	77 (6)*
1.0	68 (7)
2.0	58 (2)
3.0	54 (4)
4.0	47 (4)
6.0	42 (3)

*Numbers in parenthesis indicate statistical error.

The addition of the microemulsion significantly lowered the wet-combing work. The statistical significance of this effect was checked by a *t*-test ($p < 0.05$). In **Figure 6**, the residual wet-combing work is plotted as a function of the minimum transmittance of the investigated shampoos. A direct correlation between the physical chemistry and the wet-combing performance of the shampoos can be seen. The stronger the phase separation during application, the better the conditioning performance of the shampoo.

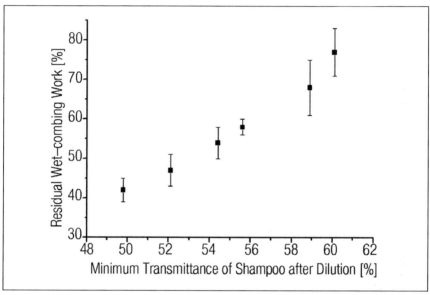

Figure 6. Residual wet-combing work plotted as a function of the minimum transmittance of the investigated shampoos

Improving Eco-friendly Conditioning

One well-known challenge to formulators is achieving performance with eco-friendly or natural based formulations. In general, such formulations show poor conditioning performance when compared with standard shampoos. However, adding this eco-friendly microemulsion to a selected "green" benchmark formulation can significantly improve its wet-combing results (see **Table 2**).

To test the effects of the microemulsion on an eco-friendly formula's stability, a different shampoo base was developed (see **Formula 2**). The stability was evaluated by a three-month storage test at 5°C, room temperature and 40°C. During this period the samples were visually checked for phase separations. In contrast to the first formula, this formula incorporates surfactants and a cationic polymer that are free of ethoxylated groups. The stability results of shampoos with increasing amounts of the microemulsion are shown in **Table 3**.

Table 2. Residual Wet-combing Work for 'Green' Benchmark Shampoo with Microemulsion

Formulation	Residual wet-combing work [%]
Benchmark shampoo	89 (11)*
Benchmark shampoo with 3.6% microemulsion	70 (13)
Benchmark shampoo with 17.9% microemulsion	61 (4)

*Numbers in parenthesis indicate statistical error.

Formula 2. Eco-friendly shampoo with microemulsion

Decyl glucoside (Plantacare 2000UP, Cognis GmbH)	15.4% w/w
Sodium coco-sulfate (Sulfopon 1216G, Cognis GmbH)	5.2
Cocamidopropyl betaine (Dehyton PK 45, Cognis GmbH)	5.2
Dicaprylyl ether (and) coco glucoside (and) glyceryl oleate (Plantasil Micro, Cognis GmbH)	0–18.0 (varied)
Hydroxypropyl guar hydroxypropyltrimonium chloride (Jaguar C162, Rhodia)	0.2
Xanthan gum (Keltrol CG-SFT, CP Kelco)	1.0
Fragrance (*parfum*)	qs
Preservative	qs
Citric acid	qs
Water (*aqua*)	qs to 100.00
Viscosity: 3600 mPas; PH: 5.0	

Naturally based shampoos with cationic polymers and xanthan thickeners often are unstable. This was also the case for **Formula 2** without the microemulsion and therefore, measurement of the combability work was not meaningful. However, the addition of the microemulsion did have a positive impact on the stability of the benchmark "green" shampoo described above, which made it possible to record performance measurements. Compared with the described "green" benchmark shampoo, **Formula 2** including the microemulsion achieved better conditioning performance. Also, the addition of large amounts of the microemulsion led to a significant reduction in the residual wet-combing work. Although, in comparison with the standard shampoo (**Formula 1**), higher amounts of the microemulsion were necessary since the overall performance of the eco-friendly shampoo is lower.

Table 3. Residual Wet-combing Work for Formula 2 with Microemulsion

Microemulsion [%]	Residual wet-combing work [%]
0.0	Formulation not stable; measurement insignificant
7.0	58 (9)*
11.0	57 (6)
14.0	53 (6)
18.0	50 (8)

*Numbers in parenthesis indicate statistical error.

Conclusion

Addition of the described eco-friendly microemulsion to a shampoo base was shown to improve its performance and conditioning properties. However, although it is also possible to formulate eco-friendly shampoo variants with improved performance, the authors note that performance levels did not reach those of an SLES/CAPB/PQ-10 shampoo. Thus it is suggested that in the end, the decision is up to consumers regarding how "green" they want to be and how much performance they expect from a product. For manufacturers interested in developing products with good performance that are highly nature-based, the addition of the described microemulsion offers a viable option.

Published May 2009 *Cosmetics and Toiletries* magazine

References

1. RY Lochhead and LR Huisinga, A brief review of polymer/surfactant interactions, *Cosmet Toil* 119 37–45 (2004)

2. C Stubenrauch (ed.), *Microemulsions: Background, new concepts, applications, perspectives*, Oxford, UK: Blackwell (2009)

3. T Förster, B Guckenbiehl, A Ansmann and H Hensen, Neuartige Körperpflegemittel auf Basis von Mikroemulsionen und Alkylpolyglucosiden, *SÖFW* 122 746-753 (1996)

4. TV Drovetskaya, RL Kreeger, JL Amos, CB Davis and S Zhou, Effects of low-level hydrophobic substitution on conditioning properties of cationic cellulosic polymers in shampoo systems, *Int J Cosm Sci* 55 195–205 (2004)

CHAPTER 18

Antiaging Benefits of French Rose Petal Extract

Sonia Dawson, Cara Eaton, Laurie B. Joseph, PhD
Croda Inc., Edison, NJ, USA

Christine Bertram
Crodarom S.A.S, Chanac, France

KEY WORDS: *premature skin aging, UVA/UVB cell damage, DNA protection, free-radical scavengers, glutathione production,* Rosa gallica, *French Rose, environmental stress*

ABSTRACT: *Botanicals are re-emerging as key ingredients in the defense against premature skin aging. French rose petal extract, when used in a cosmetic formulation, can help decrease the damage of ultraviolet light and other environmental stresses that can cause premature aging of the skin.*

Environmental stress leads to cellular oxidation and signs of aging. Certain botanicals, such as French rose petal extract, can protect skin cells from oxidative damage. This extract and its benefits are described in this chapter.

Oxidative Stress

Overexposure to sunlight has been linked to cutaneous aging through the production of reactive oxygen species (ROS) that can activate matrix metalloproteinases, enzymes involved in the breakdown of the dermal proteins, such as collagen and elastin.[1] The degradation of these proteins is a primary contributor to wrinkle formation and loss of skin elasticity.

The skin has a complex defense mechanism to guard against UV-induced oxidative stress, but excessive amounts of ROS can overwhelm the body's natural defenses and lead to premature skin aging, evidenced by wrinkle formation and age spots. Further damage results in immunosuppression, and ultimately, skin cancer.[2-4]

Several studies have confirmed that sun exposure is responsible for the development of at least two-thirds of all skin cancers. The American Academy of Dermatology (AAD) estimated that 80% of a person's lifetime sun damage occurs before the age of 18, a significant portion of which occurs during peak sun hours in the summer. This combination of intense, intermittent sun exposure and sunburn has been shown to increase a child's risk for developing melanoma.[5-8]

The result is an increasing awareness of the need for sun protection, as evidenced by the promotion of the use of sun protection products year-round with an emphasis on protection for infants and children. Sun protection products also have evolved to do more than form a barrier against UV radiation, but also to assist in handling and eliminating any damaging byproducts formed by UV radiation's interaction with the skin. Some interesting results are shown with products that contain new actives drawn from nature (see **Formula 1**).

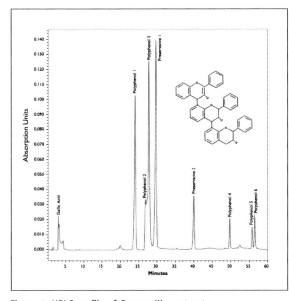

A French Rose Petal Extract

Rosa gallica, commonly known as French rose, has been used in traditional healing to alleviate a multitude of maladies, including skin disorders. Based on this history, it was chosen for this study. The effect of French rose petal extract was evaluated

Figure 1. HPLC profile of *Rosa gallica* extract

on the generation of intracellular oxidants, in particular to determine if its water-soluble tannins and proanthocyanidins enhance the response of keratinocytes to oxidative stress (see **Figure 1**). The data presented in this chapter will show that *Rosa gallica* extract[a] (RGE) increases the natural cellular response to oxidation while also inhibiting free radical production and protecting DNA from UVA and UVB damage.

Formula 1. SPF 15 day cream

A. Water (*aqua*)	53.35% w/w
Xanthan gum	0.2
Disodium EDTA	0.1
Glycerin	2.0
B. Cetearyl alcohol	1.5
PPG-3 Benzyl ether myristate	3.0
Di-PPG-3 Myristyl ether adipate	5.0
Cetearyl ethylhexanoate	3.0
PPG-2 Myristyl ether propionate	3.0
Cetearyl alcohol (and) dicetyl phosphate	
(and) ceteth-10 phosphate	6.0
Steareth-2	0.5
Steareth-10	1.0
Ethyl hexyl cinnamate	7.5
Avobenzone	2.0
Oxybenzone	3.0
Sucrose polysoyate	2.0
C10-30 Cholesterol/lanosterol esters	1.0
Microcrystalline wax	0.75
C. Sodium hydroxide, 10%	qs to pH 6± 0.5
D. Water (*aqua*) (and) butylene glycol (and) *Rosa gallica*	5.0
Methylisothiazolinone	0.1

Procedure: Combine A and heat to 75–80°C. In a separate vessel, combine B and heat to 75–80°C. Add B to A while mixing. Add C to batch. Allow emulsion to cool while mixing. When emulsion temperature reaches 40°C, add D in order. Mix until cool. pH: 6.5; Viscosity: 90,000 cps (TE@10 rpm, 1 min)

Cellular Detoxification

Cellular detoxification is the process by which the body removes cellular and DNA damaging materials that are responsible for adverse effects on skin. In response to sunburn, the skin produces ROS that can modify cellular function.

Catalase and glutathione: The natural antioxidants catalase and glutathione exist within cells. They assist in limiting ROS levels since an overabundance will negatively impact the integrity of the cells. Catalase inhibits the production of ROS following UV exposure, while glutathione's primary function is to remove free radicals from the cell.

Glutathione (GSH), often called the master antioxidant, is a tripeptide consisting of cysteine, glycine and glutamic acid, which acts as a donor of sulfhydryl (-SH) groups essential for cellular detoxification. Cellular GSH levels increase in the presence of oxidizers, such as hydrogen peroxide and UV radiation, and then become covalently bound to cysteine residues in proteins through a process referred to as glutathionylation.[9,15]

Cellular detoxification by GSH involves two phases: Phase I involves the activation of toxic substances, and in Phase II, the activated substances are bound to glutathione and excreted through urine and perspiration.[11–14]

GSH plays a crucial role in guarding against cellular damage, particularly oxidation of lipids, proteins and nucleic acids.[11,12] Unfortunately, as the body ages, GSH production decreases resulting in an impaired ability of the body to protect itself from ROS.[10]

Effect of RGE: The effect of RGE on the natural cellular detoxification mechanism was examined using PAM 212 murine (mouse) keratinocytes[b], shown in **Figure 2**.

The cells were labelled with ^{35}S-cysteine and then incubated with 0.03% decaffeinated green tea (approximately 700 ppm polyphenols neat), 0.03% RGE (approximately 300 ppm polyphenols neat), or the matched butylene glycol control for 30 minutes (min). Green tea was included as a reference of high antioxidant activity. These samples then were incubated for 10 min with and without hydrogen peroxide (H_2O_2).[16]

---

[b] PAM 212 Murine Keratinocytes were provided by Dr. Stuart Yuspa, National Cancer Institute, National Institutes for Health, Bethesda, MD, USA.

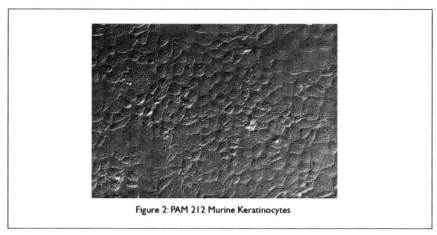

Figure 2: PAM 212 Murine Keratinocytes

Figure 2. PAM 212 murine keratinocytes

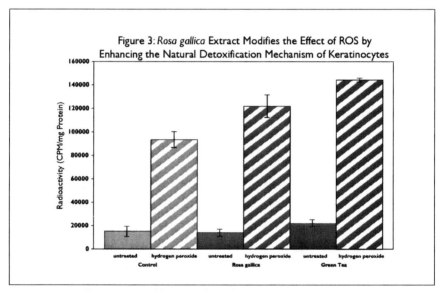

Figure 3. *Rosa gallica* extract modifies the effect of ROS by enhancing the natural detoxification mechanism of keratinocytes.

Under nonstimulated conditions (without H_2O_2), no difference was observed between the control, RGE, or green tea, in the amount of glutathione bound to damaged proteins, as shown in **Figure 3**. Upon addition of H_2O_2, there was an increase in the glutathionylation of proteins for all three samples.

From this data, RGE is shown to have activity similar to green tea (30% increase in GSH-protein expression in RGE-treated cells vs. 40% GSH-protein expression in green tea-treated cells). Interestingly, RGE has 90% of the activity of green tea with less than half the polyphenol content.

Inhibition of Cellular Oxidant Production

Catalase inhibits the production of ROS following UVB exposure,[17] thereby preventing oxidative damage to skin cells. UVB is absorbed by catalase and converted to reactive chemical intermediates that are detoxified by cellular antioxidant enzymes such as GSH.[18] Since overexposure to UV radiation is so common, further inhibition of oxidant production is greatly desirable. In order to determine if RGE retarded ROS formation, keratinocytes were incubated with, or without, 1% RGE and exposed to 10 mJ/cm² UVB and treated with 2′,7′-dichlorofluorescein diacetate, a hydroperoxide-sensitive dye. The treated cells then were analyzed on a Coulter Epics II Profile flow cytometer for fluorescent shift, monitored at 525 nm.

The fluorescent intensity is directly proportional to the production of H_2O_2. The more cells were oxidized, or damaged, the more fluorescence was observed and depicted on the x-axis, as seen in **Figure 4**. UVB exposure shifted the fluorescent profile of the PAM cells by 100 fold (blue line vs. yellow line). Addition of the RGE to the keratinocytes (red line), before UVB exposure, showed a return in the fluorescent profile back toward the untreated control (blue line), demonstrating that RGE decreased UVB-induced oxidant damage in keratinocytes. This indicates RGE can enhance cellular defense against UVB damage.

Inhibition of Hydroxyl Damage

Peroxides such as UV contribute to cellular damage via the formation of ROS, and therefore, preventive measures need to be taken to guard against oxidant production.

To determine the effect of RGE against peroxide-induced hydroxyl damage, terephthalate, iron chloride ($FeCl_3$), ethylenediaminetetraacetic acid (EDTA) and H_2O_2 were incubated with RGE in increasing concentrations (0–1.0%). Methanol was added to each sample, and all were analyzed for 2-OH-terephthalate production, an indicator of hydroxyl damage. Terephthalate, when hydroxylated on the second position, becomes fluorescent when excited at 315 nm. Fluorescence of 2-OH-terephthalate was measured by HPLC.

As seen in **Figure 5,** increasing amounts of RGE significantly reduced the production of 2-OH-terephthalate, signifying its ability to inhibit damage caused by peroxides.

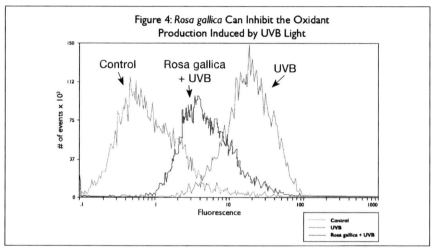

Figure 4. *Rosa gallica* can inhibit the oxidant production induced by UVB light.

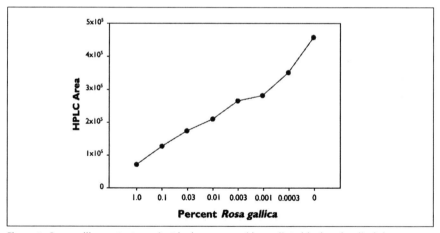

Figure 5. *Rosa gallica* protects against hydrogen peroxide-mediated hydroxyl radical damage.

A similar experiment was conducted in which terephthalate, $FeCl_3$ and EDTA were incubated with increasing concentrations of RGE (0–1.0%) and irradiated with 50 mJ/cm^2 UVB (see **Figure 6**). Methanol was added and the samples were analyzed by HPLC for 2-OH-teraphthalate production. RGE decreased UVB mediated hydroxyl damage, in a dose-dependent manner.

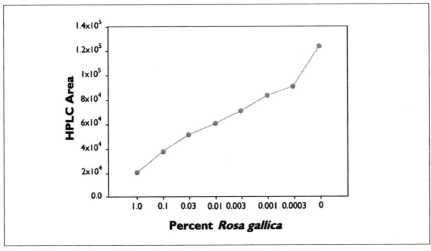

Figure 6. *Rosa gallica* protects against UVB-mediated hydroxyl radical damage.

Protection of Plasmid DNA from UV Damage

No induced DNA strand breaks: UV radiation (UVA/UVB) has been shown to induce a wide range of DNA damage, such as protein-DNA cross-links and single strand breaks6 that have been linked to skin cancer.7 To determine RGE's ability to protect DNA from UVA damage, supercoiled plasmid DNA (PzeoSV) was incubated with RGE (0.001–10 micrometers μm, or 4,5´,8-trimethylpsoralen (TMP, 0.001–1.0 μm), with and without UVA (1.4 J/cm2). Psoralens, such as TMP, are phenolic structures that are used in combination with UVA to treat eczema and psoriasis. DNA damage is a direct result of psoralen activation by UVA, evidenced by strand breaks. The activated TMP was used as the positive control in this experiment.

As seen in **Figure 7**, RGE was compared to TMP to determine the effect of the phenolic compounds on DNA.

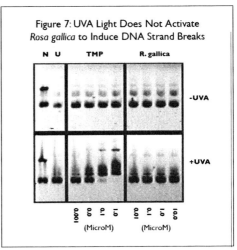

Figure 7. UVA light does not activate Rosa gallica to induce DNA strand breaks.

Examples of nicked (N) DNA and untreated (U) DNA were included as references. UVA plus RGE did not increase the number of DNA strand breaks, whereas UVA plus TMP caused numerous strand breaks, thereby demonstrating that RGE did not cause DNA damage.

Plasmid DNA protected: Supercoiled plasmid DNA (pcdna3.1v5hisA), treated with $FeCl_3$ and EDTA, was incubated with RGE (0.001–1.0%) in the absence or presence of UVB (50 mJ/cm^2). This assay is used to determine the presence of damaged and undamaged DNA upon exposure to UVB.

As shown in **Figure 8**, the top band is an indicator of the presence of undamaged DNA while the bottom band denotes the nicked (damaged) DNA. Exposure to UVB alone resulted in complete degradation of the DNA. In the samples treated with RGE, the amount of undamaged DNA increased with increasing concentrations, showing RGE protected DNA from UVB damage in a dose-dependent manner.

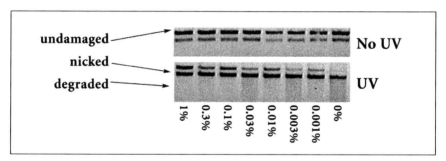

Figure 8. Rosa gallica protects plasmid DNA against UVB damage in the presence of iron/EDTA.

Conclusion

The mystery of botanicals now is being unlocked and is turning folklore into innovation. Botanicals, such as RGE, are leading the way for a new age of protection against cellular oxidation. *Rosa gallica* extract protects skin cells from oxidative damage that increases premature aging.

Overproduction of ROS from UVA exposure has been associated with the breakdown of the dermal matrix that leads to wrinkle formation, while UVB has been demonstrated to induce skin cancer. With a more rapidly depleting ozone layer, the need for sun protection is greater than ever. Sunscreens provide an effective barrier to block harmful UV rays (UVA/UVB), but this barrier only *physically* hinders the UV damage. A second line of defense is imperative into inhibit the negative effects of UV radiation.

The presented data suggests that the use of RGE in skin care formulations can prevent damage due to environmental stresses that can lead to premature aging of the skin.

Published May 2008 *Cosmetics and Toiletries* magazine

Acknowledgments

The authors wish to thank Jeffrey Laskin, PhD; Diane Heck, PhD; Josh Gray, PhD; Adrienne Black of Rutgers University Department of Pharmacology and Toxicology; and Nigel Langley, PhD of Croda Inc. The authors also wish to thank Crodarom SAS for the development of the Rosa gallica extract and Technical Services at Croda Inc. for preparation of the sunscreen formulation.

References

1. Jones, MD, PhD, Reactive oxygen species and rosacea, *Cutis* 74 (2004)
2. DP Steenvoorden, GM van Henegouwen, The use of endogenous antioxidants to improve photoprotection, *J Photochem Photobiol B* 41(1–2) 1–10 (1997)
3. SR Pinell, Cutaneous photodamage, oxidative stress, and topical antioxidant protection, *J Am Acad Dermatol* 48 1–19 (2003)
4. SK Katiyar, F Afaq, A Perez and H Mukhtar, Green tea polyphenol (-)-epigallocatechin-3-gallate treatment of human skin inhibits ultraviolet radiation-induced oxidative stress, *Carcinogenesis* 22(2) 287–294 (2001)
5. LJ Shapiro and Associates, Children at risk: Protecting our children from skin cancer, Telephone survey, American Academy of Dermatology (2000)
6. BK Armstrong, A Kricker, DR English, Sun exposure and skin cancer, *Australas J Dermatol* 38 Suppl 1: S1–6 (Jun 1997)
7. KH Kraemer, MM Lee, AD Andrews, WC Lambert, The role of sunlight and DNA repair in melanoma and nonmelanoma skin cancer: the xeroderma pigmentosum paradigm, *Arch Dermatol* 130 (8) 1018–1021 (Aug 1994)
8. BK Armstrong, A Kricker, The pidemiology of UV induced skin cancer, *Journal of Photochemistry and Photobiology* 63 1: 8–18 (11) (Oct 2001)
9. JO Moskaug, H Carlsen, MCW Myhrstad and R Blomhoff, Polyphenols and Glutathione Synthesis Regulation, *Am J Clin Nutr* 81 277S–83S (2005)
10. KJA Davies and F Ursini, eds, *The Oxygen Paradox*, Padova, Italy CLEUP University Press (1995) pp 413–424
11. P Perera, IB Weinstein, Molecular Epidemiology: Recent Advances and Future Directions, *Carcinogenesis* 21(3) 517–524 (2000)
12. L Van Iersel, H Verhhagen et al, The role of biotransformation in dietary (anti) carcinogenesis, *Mutation Research* 443(1–2) 259–270 (1999)
13. C Willet, Diet, nutrition and avoidable cancer, *Environmental Health Perspectives* 103(8) 165–170 (1995)
14. Lutz, Carcinogens in the diet vs. overnutrition: Individual dietary habits, malnutrition and genetic susceptibility modify carcinogenic potency and cancer risk, *Mutation Research* 443 251–58 (1999)

15. Ogawa, M Matsumoto, H Ito, K Henmi, The physiological role of glutathionylation of plastidic fructose-1,6-bisphosphate aldolase in *Arabidopsis thaliana, Proceedings of American Society of Plant Biologists: Minisymposium 28—Photosynthesis II*, July 2005
16. DE Heck, DL Laskin, CR Gardner and JD Laskin, *J Biol Chem* 267(30) 21277–21280 (1992)
17. Heck, AM Vetrano, TM Mariano, and JD Laskin, *J Biol Chem* 278(25) 22432–22436 (2003)
18. Monks, MW Anders, W Dekant, JL Stevens, SS Lau and PJ van Bladeren, *Toxicol Appl Pharmacol* 106(1) 1–19 (1990)

CHAPTER 19

Developing a Long-Lasting Tyrosinase Inhibitor from *Morus alba* L.

Michelle Kim, Xiaofeng Meng, PhD, and Abraham Kim
Time and Cross Inc., North Brunswick, NJ, USA

Mingfu Wang, PhD
Hong Kong University, Hong Kong, Japan

James E. Simon, PhD
Rutgers State University, New Brunswick, NJ, USA

KEY WORDS: *skin whitening, tyrosinase, melanin, Morus alba, mulberroside A*

ABSTRACT: *By using solvent fractionation and column chromatography, a purified extract of Morus alba L. can be obtained that demonstrates the ability to perform as a melanogenesis inhibitor, and therefore, a potential new whitening agent.*

There are various causes for the darkening of skin color, UV rays considered the primary source. When skin is exposed to UV rays, melanin is synthesized in melanocytes and released to darken the skin. Melanin pigmentation in human skin is a major defense mechanism against UV light from the sun, but abnormal pigmentation such as freckles or chloasma can be a serious aesthetic problem. Tyrosinase and other proteins, such as tyrosinase-related protein 1 (Tyrp-1) and tyrosinase-related protein 2 (Tyrp-2, Dopachrome tautomerase), are responsible for the biosynthesis of melanin.

Among these enzymes, tyrosinase plays the most important role in melanin synthesis.[1]

Tyrosinase is a copper-containing enzyme and is expressed exclusively in melanocytes, the melanin-producing cells in the epidermis. Tyrosinase itself can produce melanin pigments in the absence of other melanogenic enzymes. In fact, fibroblast cells transfected with tyrosinase cDNA produce melanin in their lysosome-like structures. It is not fully understood how the expression of tyrosinase is regulated. Studies are being conducted to discover melanogenic inhibitory compounds to prevent or to cure these hyperpigmentary disorders with tyrosinase as the major target.

In the process of melanogenesis in melanocytes, tyrosinase reacts on tyrosine in the cell to yield dopaquinone and it goes through sequential oxidation to form dopachrome and then 5,6-dihydroxyindole (DHI) [the 5,6-dihydroxyindol-2-carboxylic acid (DHICA)], the monomers of melanin, which are polymerized with each other to provide a co-polymeric black pigment—melanin.

Most whitening agents have an inhibitory effect on tyrosinase (see **Tyrosinase-Inhibiting Agents**).

Tyrosinase-Inhibiting Agents

Kojic acid: Strong inhibitory activity is shown on tyrosinase, but stability problems occur.

Arbutin: Shown to inhibit melanin synthesis by inhibition of tyrosinase activity but it has very weak antioxidant activity.

Hydroquinone: Exhibits high efficacy but its skin-bleaching mechanism may cause serious skin irritation; its use in cosmetic products is prohibited in many countries including Japan and the European Union.

Vitamin C: Effectiveness as whitening agents is questionable due to the low stability of the molecule and a low whitening effect.

Licorice extract: Strongly inhibits tyrosinase activity of melanocytes with no cytotoxicity but has stability issues; exhibits difficulty in delivering the extract to the skin.

Morus alba L extract: Provides long-lasting skin lightening effect and removes dark spots from the skin; can be formulated into creams and lotions at low percentages of 1%-5%.

Currently, research to develop an agent with tyrosinase-inhibiting activity is intensive. Representatives of tyrosinase-inhibiting agents include: kojic acid, arbutin, hydroquinone, vitamin C and licorice extract. Among these, kojic acid forms a chelate with a copper ion at the active site of tyrosinase to inhibit the enzyme activity. Although strong inhibitory activity is shown on tyrosinase, stability problems occur during the process of blending it into cosmetic formulations.

Hydroquinone is undesirable for use in cosmetic materials because it strongly irritates the skin and the use of hydroquinone in cosmetic products now is prohibited in several countries including the European Union, some African countries, and countries in Asia including Japan and Korea. As for vitamin C and its derivatives, their effectiveness as whitening agents is questionable due to the low stability of the molecule and a low-whitening effect.

Materials extracted from various plants have attracted interest. In the present study, extracts of *Ramulus mori*, young twigs of *Morus alba* L, showed inhibition activity in tyrosinase and melanin synthesis in B-16 melanoma cells, and oxyresveratrol was identified as one of the active ingredients.[2] In the present study, in addition to oxyresveratrol, mulberroside A[a] was isolated from the extract of *Morus alba* and has shown potential as a skin-whitening agent based on in vitro studies.

Identification of Mulberroside A

Dried *Morus alba* plant was purchased and extracted with 70% ethanol to obtain *Morus alba* extract. Mulberroside A-enriched fraction was prepared from *Morus alba* extract by polyamide-6 column chromatography or solvent partition, while oxyresveratrol was prepared mainly with solvent partition. In brief, *Morus alba* extract (20 g) was dissolved into 200 ml methanol/water (40:60, v/v) and directly loaded to a 30 g of polyamide-6 column. The column first was eluted by 600 ml of methanol/water (40:60, v/v) to obtain yellow-red mulberroside A–enriched liquid fraction. The liquid fraction then was evaporated to dryness under reduced pressure to produce mulberroside A-enriched

[a] WITESKIN Mulberroside A (INCI: Morus alba bark extract) is a product of Time and Cross Inc.

powder. For the preparation of oxyresveratrol, 10 g of *Morus alba* extract was suspended in 200 g of water and partitioned with chloroform (200 ml) three times. The water layer was then extracted by 200 ml of ethyl acetate three times. The ethyl acetate solution was evaporated to dryness under reduced pressure to obtain oxyresveratrol-enriched powder. The final water solution was evaporated to dryness to produce mulberroside A-enriched powder. The mulberroside A-enriched powder typically contained 2%–50% of mulberroside A.

Further isolation and purification of mulberroside A and oxyresveratrol were carried out using thin layer chromatography (TLC), silica gel column chromatography and Sephadex LH-20 gel filtration chromatography. For example, 20 g of mulberroside A-enriched powder was loaded directly onto a silica gel column filled with 300 g of silica gel and eluted by chloroform-methanol-water(2.5:1:0.1) to produce five subfractions. The fifth subfraction was repurifed by Sephadex LH-20 column to obtain 700 mg of pure mulberroside A. The structures of these two compounds were confirmed by MS and NMR spectra (**Figure 1**).

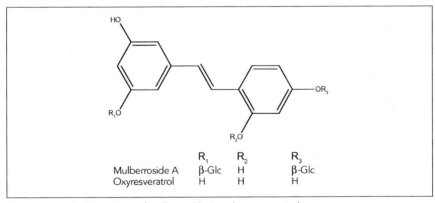

	R_1	R_2	R_3
Mulberroside A	β-Glc	H	β-Glc
Oxyresveratrol	H	H	H

Figure 1. Chemical structures of mulberroside A and oxyresveratrol

Biological Activities of Mulberroside A and Oxyresveratrol

Inhibitory effects on mushroom tyrosinase: Purified tyrosinase from mushroom[b] was used in for this test.

L-Tyrosine, the substrate of tyrosinase, was dissolved in sodium phosphate buffer (50 mM, pH 6.8) to a concentration of 0.1 mg/ml.

[b]Mushroom tyrosinase (Cat# T7755) was obtained from Sigma-Aldrich Co.

Each compound was dissolved in dimethyl sulfoxide (DMSO) at a concentration of 1 mg/ml. The test mixture was incubated at 37°C for 15 min, which consisted of 100 µl of L-tyrosine solution, 100 µl of sodium phosphate buffer (50mM, pH 6.8) with or without test compounds, and 10 µl of tyrosinase (200 U/ml). The amount of dopachrome generated after the reaction was measured by a spectrophotometer with wavelength setting of 490 nm. The mushroom tryosinase-inhibiting activities of the test samples were plotted as a function of concentration.

As shown in **Figure 2**, *Morus alba* extract showed similar inhibitory activity as kojic acid against mushroom tyrosinase. The inhibitory activities of mulberroside A and oxyresveratrol are presented in **Figure 3** with kojic acid and arbutin as positive controls.

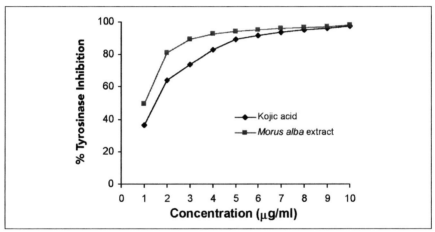

Figure 2. Inhibitory effects on mushroom tyrosinase

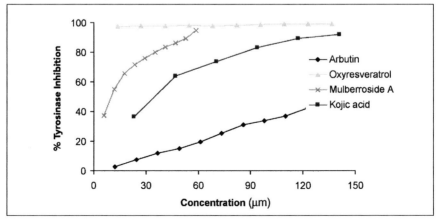

Figure 3. Inhibitory effect of **Morus alba** extract and kojic acid on mushroom tyrosinase

Oxyresveratrol and mulberroside A demonstrated much stronger inhibitory activities than kojic acid and arbutin. *Morus alba* extract, oxyresveratrol, mulberroside A, kojic acid and arbutin each showed dose-dependent inhibitory effects on mushroom tyrosinase activity. The concentrations of each sample that inhibited 50% of the enzyme activity (IC_{50}) are summarized in **Table 1**.

Table 1. Inhibitory effects on mushroom, murine and human tyrosinases

Compounds	Mushroom Tyrosinase IC_{50} (μM)	Murine Tyrosinase IC_{50} (μM)	Human Tyrosinase IC_{50} (μM)
Arbutin	144.6	>500	>500
Kojic acid	34.7	402	421
Morus alba extract	1.3 μg/ml	39.5 μg/ml	47.2 μg/ml
Oxyresveratrol	2.4	42.5	57.4
Mulberroside A	9.5	61.5	76.8

The IC_{50} values for oxyresveratrol, mulberroside A, *Morus alba* extract, arbutin and kojic acid were determined to be: 2.4 μM, 9.54 μM, 1.3 μg/ml, 144.6 μM and 34.7 μM, respectively.

Inhibitory effects on murine tyrosinase: Murine tyrosinase was prepared from melanoma B-16. Murine melanoma B-16 cells were grown in DMEM (13.4 mg/ml of Dulbecco's modified Eagle's medium, 24 mM NaHCO3, 10 mM n-(2-Hydroxyethyl) piperazine-n´-2-ethanesulfonic acid (HEPES), 143 units/ml of penicillin G potassium, 160 μg/ml of streptomycin sulfate, pH 7.1) containing 10% fetal bovine serum (FBS) with 5% CO_2 at 37°C. When the cells were confluent, melanoma cells were removed from culture dishes and washed once with phosphate buffer saline (PBS) buffer. The cell suspension was centrifuged at 250x g for 10 min at 4°C. The cell pellet was suspended in 0.5 ml of 50 mM sodium phosphate buffer (pH 6.8) containing 0.1 mM phenylmethylsulfonyl fluoride (PMSF) and 0.5% detergent[c].

---

[c] Triton X-100 (Cat# T9284-1L) was obtained from Sigma-Aldrich Co.

183

Developing a Long-Lasting Tyrosinase Inhibitor from *Morus alba* L.

The cell suspension was sonicated six times for 30 sec each with 1-min intervals and then incubated at 4°C for 1 h to solubilize the tyrosinase. After centrifugation at 50,000× g for 20 min at 4°C, supernatant was dialyzed against 50mM sodium phosphate buffer (pH 6.8) and then used as a source of murine tyrosinase.

Inhibitory activities on murine tyrosinase by test samples were measured following the same procedure described above and the results also are presented in Table 1. Similarly, *Morus alba* extract, oxyresveratrol and mulberroside A showed much stronger inhibitory activities against murine tyrosinase than kojic acid and arbutin. *Morus alba* extract, mulberroside A and oxyresveratrol showed IC_{50} value of 39.5 µg/ml, 61.5 µM, and 42.5 µM on the murine tyrosinase system, respectively.

Inhibitory effects on human tyrosinase: Human tyrosinase was prepared from HM3KO human melanoma cell line. HM3KO cell lines were cultured in modified Eagle's medium supplement with 10% fetal-calf serum. Cultured HM3KO cells were removed from culture dishes and washed once with PBS buffer. After centrifugation, the cell pellets were sonicated in 100 mM sodium phosphate buffer (pH6.8) containing 0.1 mM PMSF and 1% Triton X-100, and then incubated in ice for 1 h to solubilize the tyrosinase. After centrifugation, supernatant was dialyzed against 50 mM sodium phosphate buffer (pH 6.8) and then used as a source of human tyrosinase.

Inhibitory activities on human tyrosinase by test samples were measured similarly (see **Table 1**). *Morus alba* extract, mulberroside A and oxyresveratrol showed IC_{50} value of 47.2 µg/ml, 76.8 µM, and 57.4 µM on the the human tyrosinase system, respectively. Arbutin and kojic acid exhibited weak inhibitory activities.

Effect on melanin production and cell viability in cultured melanoma B-16: Commercially available B-16 melanoma (ATCC CRL6323) cell line mouse-derived was used as melanocytes. The melanoma mouse-derived cell line was grown in DMEM culture medium containing 4.5 g of glucose/l, 10% fetal bovine serum and 1% antibiotic agent and cultivated at 37°C under a condition of 5% CO_2. The cell suspension was inoculated into a 50 ml T-flask (3×10^5 cells/ml) and the cells were allowed to completely adhere to the plate for 24 h. Then, test samples diluted in DMEM medium as

concentration of 1, 5, 10, 50, and 100 µg/ml were added to the cultivated cells, and the mixture was cultivated at 5% CO_2 and 37°C for
3 days. After cultivation, culture medium thoroughly was removed
and the cells were isolated through trypsin treatment. The suspensions then were centrifuged for 5min to collect cells. The obtained
cells were treated with 5% trichloroacetic acid (TCA), stirred and
centrifuged. Then, precipitated melanin was washed with PBS, and
treated with 1 N NaOH to dissolve melanin therein. Absorbance at
475 nm was measured. Melanin concentration was determined from
a standard concentration curve of synthetic melanin.

The percentage of viable cells was determined by MTT assay.
After cultivation was completed, the cultivation solution was added
with MTT solution and incubated at 37°C for 4 h. After incubation,
culture medium thoroughly was removed, and the residue was
treated with DMSO and shaken for 20 min. The optical density at
580 nm was measured by a 96-well microplate reader. The results are
shown in the **Table 2**.

Treatment of *Morus alba* extract, oxyresveratrol and mulberroside
A resulted in a significant reduction in melanin production (76.9% of
Morus alba extract at 100 µg/ml, 80.5% of oxyresveratrol at 100 µg/ml
and 78.2% of mulberroside A at 100 µg/ml) in melanoma B-16 cells.
The cell viability results indicated that oxyresveratrol started to induce
cytotoxicity at the concentration of 10 µg/ml, while *Morus alba* extract
and mulberroside A did not show significant cytotoxicity even at
100 µg/ml.

***Effect on melanin production and cell viability in cultured
melan-a cell line:*** Melan-a cells were grown in 10 ml of RPMI 1640
medium supplemented with antibiotics, 10% FBS, and 20 nm tissue
plasminogen activator (TPA). The cells suspension was inoculated
into a 24-well plate (10^5 cells/ml) and the cells were allowed to completely adhere to the plate for 24 h. Then, test samples dissolved in
DMSO were added to the plate and incubated at 37°C for 72 h in
a CO_2 incubator. After cultivation, culture medium was thoroughly
removed and the cells were isolated through trypsin treatment. The
suspensions then were centrifuged for 5 min to collect cells. The
obtained cells were treated with 5% TCA, stirred and centrifuged.
Then, precipitated melanin was washed with PBS, and treated with
1 N NaOH to dissolve melanin therein. Absorbance at 475 nm was

185

Developing a Long-Lasting Tyrosinase Inhibitor from *Morus alba* L.

Table 2. Effects of *Morus alba* extract, oxyresveratrol and mulberroside A on cell viability and melanin production of murine melanoma B16 cells

Compounds	Concentration (µg/ml)	Melanin production (%)	Cell viability (%)
Arbutin	1	99.4±2.1	102.4±5.3
	5	100.8±4.5	100.1±7.8
	10	103.2±1.9	98.5±6.3
	50	98.9±8.2	96.6±8.0
	100	98.2±6.9	93.2±5.6
Kojic acid	1	102.4±4.7	95.2±8.3
	5	98.2±7.1	97.2±7.6
	10	96.5±3.7	96.2±5.0
	50	94.1±5.2	86.7±3.4
	100	91.6 ±7.1	81.7±8.5
Morus alba extract	1	97.2±5.3	105.6±1.3
	5	93.3±9.2	103.0±2.6
	10	90.4±6.3	98.7±6.9
	50	64.2±7.6	96.1±7.5
	100	23.1±7.2	94.5±8.1
Oxyresveratrol	1	94.3±7.7	99.5±5.4
	5	90.8±4.4	97.4±5.9
	10	87.5±6.9	95.3±7.6
	50	57.3±8.1	66.2±8.3
	100	19.5±8.2	23.1±4.8
Mulberroside A	1	98.3±1.0	103.2±1.5
	5	92.4±2.1	101.1±3.8
	10	91.2±7.3	98.7±8.4
	50	59.8±9.0	97.1±5.9
	100	21.8±5.4	94.0±6.4

measured. Melanin concentration was determined from a standard concentration curve of synthetic melanin.

After incubation, similar MTT assay procedures were applied and the results are shown in the **Table 3**.

Similar to melanoma B-16 cell system, treatment of *Morus alba* extract, oxyresveratrol and mulberroside A resulted in a significant reduction of melanin production (75.1% of *Morus alba* extract at 100 µg/ml, 79.4% of oxyresveratrol at 100 µg/ml and 76.3% of mulberroside A at 100 µg/ml in melan-a cell system). The cell viability results indicated that oxyresveratrol started to induce cytotoxicity at the concentration of 10 µg/ml. Kojic acid and arbutin did not show inhibitory effects of melanin production at any concentrations.

Lasting effect on tyrosinase inhibition: In order to examine whether test sample exhibits maintained inhibitory effect on tyrosinase activity, the reaction mixture containing test sample was kept at 37°C according to the method of tyrosinase inhibition. Each whitening agent was dissolved in DMSO at a concentration of 1 mg/ml. The L-tyrosine solution (100 µl) was introduced into a test tube and 100 µl of 50 mM sodium phosphate buffer (pH 6.8) with or without test samples were added thereto. Then, 10 µl of 200 U/ml tyrosinase were mixed and incubated at 37°C. The amount of dopachrome in the reaction mixture was determined. Absorbance was measured at a wavelength of 490 nm by using a spectrophotometer. The inhibitory effect on tyrosinase activity was measured over 24 h. The results are shown in the **Figure 4**.

Most of melanogenesis inhibitors lose the inhibitory activity on tyrosinase within 1–2 h of the reaction time. At the concentration of 2 µM, arbutin loses its inhibitory activity on tyrosinase in 1 h and kojic acid in 2 h. *Morus alba* extract, oxyresveratrol and mulberroside A exhibited the longest lasting inhibitory effect on tyrosinase. After 20 h of reaction, *Morus alba* extract, oxyresveratrol and mulberroside A still exhibited a significant inhibitory activity on tyrosinase. Among them, oxyresveratrol kept 90% inhibition on tyrosinase activity for the whole test period.

RT-PCR analysis of tyrosinase mRNA: mRNAs from cultured cells were isolated using a polytract system 1000 mRNA isolation kit[d].

---

[d] Promega polytract system 1000 mRNA isolation kit was obtained from Promega.

187

Developing a Long-Lasting Tyrosinase Inhibitor from *Morus alba* L.

Table 3. Effects of *Morus alba* extract, oxyresveratrol and mulberroside A on cell viability and melanin production of melan-a cell line

Compounds	Concentration (μg/ml)	Melanin production (%)	Cell viability (%)
Arbutin	1	104.2±3.2	104.2±7.2
	5	103.7±4.6	105.2±8.3
	10	102.0±5.7	100.7±5.0
	50	100.4±4.0	98.3±7.7
	100	99.5±7.2	93.8±5.6
Kojic acid	1	103.4±5.4	95.3±8.0
	5	100.5±8.2	96.8±4.7
	10	99.4±7.1	95.1±9.0
	50	95.1±6.7	84.2±8.2
	100	92.4±8.0	80.5±8.3
Morus alba extract	1	98.0±3.2	103.8±2.8
	5	94.2±5.3	102.1±6.1
	10	90.1±7.1	99.4±7.4
	50	68.3±8.9	96.9±8.2
	100	24.9±6.8	95.2±6.9
Oxyresveratrol	1	95.1±3.1	99.0±5.8
	5	90.2±6.4	96.9±7.9
	10	88.5±7.4	94.7±4.2
	50	60.3±9.1	68.5±5.5
	100	20.6±4.9	27.3±7.8
Mulberroside A	1	98.5±7.2	100.1±6.0
	5	93.6±4.8	99.2±7.6
	10	92.8±6.5	99.0±9.2
	50	61.2±8.0	97.3±8.4
	100	23.7±3.8	95.4±7.3

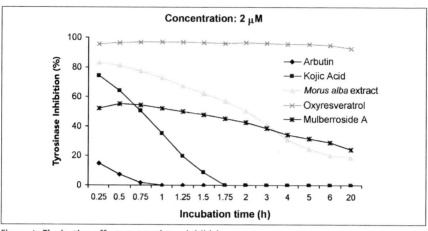

Figure 4. The lasting effect on tyrosinase inhibition

Finally 80 ~ 100 µg of mRNA was isolated from 10^8 cells. Primers used for reverse transcription polymerase chain reaction (RT-PCR) analysis of tyrosinase mRNA are as follows: 5´GACCTCAGTTC-CCCTTCAAA3´ (197 ~ 216 from ATG start codon), 3´ primer; 5´TCTCATCCCCAGTTAGTTCT3´ (669 ~ 688 from ATG start codon). These primers were synthesized. For cDNA synthesis, 20 ng of mRNA was reverse transcribed in 20 µl of a reaction mixture containing 2 µl of 10x reverse transcription buffer, 2 µl of 10mM $MnCl_2$, 0.2mM of each dNTPs, 50pmole of 3´ primer and 5 U of rTth DNA polymerase[e].

This enzyme reversely transcribes RNA in the presence of Mn^{2+}. Reverse transcription reaction mixture was incubated at 94°C for 1 min, at 55°C for 30 sec and at 72°C for 10 min. For PCR amplification of cDNA, 80 µL of PCR mixture containing 8 µl of 10x chelating buffer, 1mM $MgCl_2$ and 50 pmole of 5´ primer was added to RT reaction mixture. DNA amplification was performed by using a gene amp PCR system[f] 2400 thermal cycler. The PCR cycle conditions were melting for 30 sec at 94°C, annealing for 30 sec at 55°C, and extension for 1 min at 72°C. Reaction mixtures were cycled for 28 cycles. PCR products (492 bp) were analyzed by using 2% agarose gel electrophoresis. As internal control, mouse β-actin mRNA was also amplified by using mouse β-actin amplimer set[g].

[e] 5 U of rTth DNA polymerase was obtained from Perkin Elmer.
[f] The gene amp PCR system is manufactured by Perkin Elmer.
[g] The mouse β-actin amplimer set was obtained from Clontech, USA.

The results are shown in **Figure 5**.

In **Figure 5,** comparison of the bands of tyrosinase and β-actin mRNA on agarose gel shows that *Morus alba* and mulberroside A selectively inhibited the production of tyrosinase mRNA, while little effect was observed for the production of β-actin mRNA. The inhibitory effects of *Morus alba* and mulberroside A are shown in a dose-dependent manner and presented in **Figure 5a.**

To elucidate the mechanism by which *Morus alba* extract and mulberroside A exerts its effect, RT-PCR analysis was performed. *Morus alba* extract and mulberroside A decreased the amount of tyrosinase mRNA in a dose-dependent manner. *Morus alba* extract and mulberroside A had a melanogenesis inhibitory activity by downregulation of tyrosinase mRNA with inhibitory activity on tyrosinase.

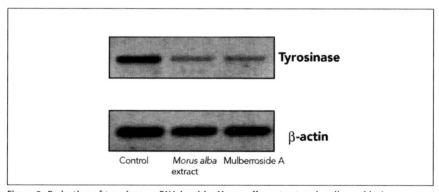

Figure 5. Reduction of tyrosinase mRNA level by **Morus alba** extract and mulberroside A

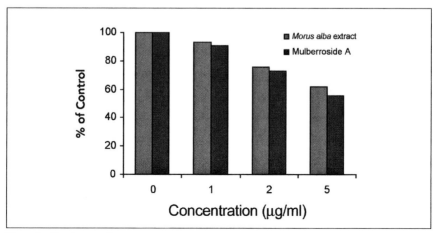

Figure 5a. Band comparison

Discussion

Compounds purified from different parts of *Morus alba*, such as oxyresveratrol and mulberroside F, have been reported to have inhibitory effect on melanin biosynthesis with tyrosinase as the main target.[2,3] Mulberroside A also was isolated from the root bark of the cultivated mulberry tree[4] and rhizomes of *Schoenocaulon officinale*,[5] but the report on its biological effect is scarce. During the screening for skin whitening agents, mulberroside A and oxyresveratrol were isolated from *Morus alba* and tested for their potential as skin-whitening agents.

Although oxyresveratrol has been demonstrated to have tyrosinase-inhibitory activity, this study presents the long-lasting effect of oxyresveratrol as a potential skin-whitening agent. This long-lasting efficacy is an attractive claim since it leads to less daily application and shorter time to reach the expected skin-lighting results.

In vitro enzymatic models and cell culture models suggest that mulberroside A acts as a potent melanogensis inhibitor. Although not as potent as oxyresveratrol, mulberroside A showed much lower cytotoxicity in cell culture models. Further studies of this compound as a new whitening agent and its application in cosmetics are warranted.

Published May 2008 *Cosmetics and Toiletries* magazine

Reference

1. S Ito, The IFPCS presidential lecture: A chemist's view of melanogenesis, *Pigment Cell Res* 16 3 230–6 (2003)
2. KT Lee et al, Inhibitory effects of *Ramulus mori* extracts on melanogenesis, *J Cosmet Sci* 54 2 133–42 (2003)
3. SH Lee et al, Mulberroside F isolated from the leaves of *Morus alba* inhibits melanin biosynthesis, *Biol Pharm Bull* 25 8 1045–8 (2002)
4. K Hirakura et al, Two phenolic glycosides from the root bark of the cultivated mulberry tree (Morus Lhou), *J Natural Products*, 49 2 218–224 (1986)
5. Kanchanapoom et al, Stilbene and 2-arylbenzofuran glucosides from the rhizomes of *Schoenocaulon officinale*, *Chem Pharm Bull* (Tokyo), 50 6 863–5 (2002)

CHAPTER 20

Grapefruit Extract Cream: Effects on Melanin and Skin

Naveed Akhtar, Gulfishan and Mahmood Ahmed
The Islaima University of Bahawalpur, Bahawalpur, Pakistan

Nazar M. Ranjha
BZ University, Multan, Pakistan

Ahmad Mahmood
University of the Punjab, Lahore, Pakistan

KEY WORDS: *grapefruit extract, stability, emulsion, melanin, erythema*

ABSTRACT: *The current work aimed to formulate a stable w/o emulsion containing grapefruit extract by entrapping the extract in the inner aqueous phase. The final formula was found to have skin-whitening, moisturizing, cleansing and antiwrinkle effects, among others.*

Emulsions are thermodynamically unstable systems defined as microscopic dispersions of liquid droplets contained within another liquid, with a diameter ranging from 0.5 μm to 100 μm.[1] Emulsions usually consist of mixtures of an aqueous phase with various oils or waxes. The liquid that is broken up into droplets is termed the *internal* or disperse phase, whereas liquid surrounding the droplets is known as the *external* or continuous phase. Both phases are stabilized by a third component, the surfactant.[2]

The two most familiar types of emulsions are readily distinguished as o/w and w/o.[3] The majority of skin care products and a significant percentage of toiletry products are emulsions.[4] The basic components of these formulations are emulsifiers, emollients and consistency enhancers.[5] Additional value can be given to these formulations by including active ingredients with specific cosmetic or dermatological effects.[4] Particularly advantageous cosmetic emulsion preparations are obtained when antioxidants are used as active ingredients.[6]

Based on a perceived safety benefit, the worldwide trend toward using natural additives has spurred interest in natural antioxidants found in plants.[7] Extract from grapefruit is rich in natural antioxidants[8] and provides some cosmetic benefits for the skin such as reduction in skin melanin, increase in skin moisture and antiwrinkle effects.[7] The best natural antioxidants present in grapefruit extract are ascorbic acid or vitamin C,[9] flavonoids,[10] beta carotene and lycopene.[11] Thus, the current work aimed to formulate a stable w/o emulsion containing grapefruit extract by entrapping the extract in the inner aqueous phase. Tests were performed on sample formulations to measure their effects on different physiological characteristics such as melanin, erythema, moisture, sebum, pH and TEWL.

Materials

Paraffin oil was used in the oily phase of a test formulation containing 1% grapefruit extract, as well as in the control (see **Formula 1**). Paraffin oil is a synthetic that is often preferred because of its benefits including being nontoxic and nonirritant to skin, as well as its ability to form an elegant white emulsion. It is a mixture of refined liquid saturated aliphatic (C_{14}–C_{18}) and cyclic hydrocarbons obtained from petroleum.[12]

In addition to the paraffin, cetyl PEG/PPG-10/1 dimethicone[a] was chosen as the lipophilic emulsifier to form a w/o emulsion in both the test formulation and the control.[13]

Beeswax was incorporated in both formulas to increase the consistency of the cream and to stabilize the w/o emulsion.[14]

Grapefruit extract is water-soluble and thus was used as an aqueous extract in the test formula. During this study, 30 different test formulations were prepared but in the present work, data is presented comparing only one test formulation with the control.

---

[a] Abil-EM 90 (INCI: Cetyl PEG/PPG-10/1 dimethicone) is a product of Evonik.

Formula 1. Control and test emulsions used in the described study

	Control formula	Test formula
Oil Phase		
Paraffin oil	20.00% w/w	20.00% w/w
Cetyl PEG/PPG-10/1 dimethicone		
(Abil-EM90, Evonik)	4.00	4.00
Beeswax	4.00	4.00
Aqueous phase		
Grapefruit extract	---	1.00 (concentrated)
Glycerin	1.00	1.00
Water (*aqua*)	qs to 100.00	qs to 100.00
Citric acid	qs to 100.00	qs to 100.00

Preparing the Emulsion

The w/o test emulsion was prepared by adding the aqueous phase incorporating the grapefruit extract to the oily phase with continuous agitation (see **Formula 1**).[15]

The oily and aqueous phases were separately heated to 75C ± 1C, and one to two drops of citric acid were added to the aqueous phase to adjust the pH before heating. After heating, the aqueous phase was added to the oily phase, drop by drop.

Stirring was continued at 2000 rpm by the mechanical mixer for about 10 min until the complete aqueous phase was added. Two to three drops of lemon oil were added during this stirring time to give the emulsion a fragrance.

After complete addition of the aqueous phase, the speed of the mixer was reduced to 1000 rpm for homogenization for a period of 5 min, then the speed was further reduced to 500 rpm for another 5 min for complete homogenization, until the emulsion cooled to room temperature. The control formula, without grapefruit extract, was prepared in the same manner.

Emulsion Analysis

The test and control emulsions were visually analyzed both orga-
noleptically to test color, thickness, look and feel, and physically to
measure creaming and phase separation.

Stability: In the cosmetics industry, product stability is one of the
most important quality criteria.[16] Final acceptance of an emulsion
by the consumer depends on its stability and appearance,[17] and one
readily apparent requirement in a well-formulated emulsion is that
the emulsion possesses adequate physical stability.[18]

In the present study, the base and test formulation each were
divided into four samples separately and these samples were kept at
different storage conditions—i.e., at 8°C in a refrigerator, at 25°C,
40°C, and at 40°C + 75% relative humidity (RH) in stability cham-
bers. These samples were observed with respect to change in color,
liquefaction and phase separation for a period of 28 days at definite
time intervals.

Color: The freshly prepared base and test formulation appeared
elegant white in color and no change in color was observed for
either the control or test formula, up to an observation period of
28 days. This showed both emulsions were stable at the different
storage conditions throughout the 28 days.

Liquefaction: The viscosity of an external oil phase is the key factor
contributing to the formation of stable emulsions.[19] According to
Stoke's law, increased viscosity of the external phase is associated
with an improved shelf-life of emulsions.[20] Cosmetic creams appear
as stable, concentrated emulsions[21] but as soon as an emulsion has
been prepared, time- and temperature-dependent processes occur to
affect its separation, leading to the decreased viscosity, which results in
increased liquefaction.[18]

No liquefaction was observed with the naked eye in the control
and test formulation samples stored at 8°C and 25°C during the
28 days but slight liquefaction occurred in the samples of the control
kept at 40°C and 40°C + 75% RH from the 21st day of observation.
No further increase in liquefaction was noted until the end of the
study. On the other hand, a slight liquefaction was observed in test
formulation samples stored at 40°C and 40°C + 75% RH at the 28th
day of the observation period.

Stoke's law states that the rate of creaming is inversely proportional to the viscosity. As creaming increased, the viscosities of the base and the formulation gradually decreased at rising temperatures, resulting in liquefaction.[20]

Phase separation: The instability of emulsions is explained by phase separation,[16]—i.e., any emulsion reverts back to the separate bulk phases. The separated phase can either cream or sediment.[18] Destabilization is compounded mostly by coalescence and gives a first indication through extension of droplets.[16] The two instability processes, coalescence and Ostwald ripening, result in droplet size growth with time.[2] According to Stoke's law, larger droplets cream much more rapidly than smaller particles.[20] The concentration of the disperse phase and the droplet size are key parameters in determining the type and time scale of the instability process.[2]

In the case of the control and test formulations, no phase separation was observed in any of the samples up to 28 days, indicating their stability.

Centrifugation: Centrifugation, if used judiciously, is an extremely useful tool for evaluating and predicting the shelf-lives of emulsions.[18] The cream volume or the separation of phases at a given time is taken as a measure of the physical stability of emulsion.[21] However, these are examples of situations that exist in any accelerated test—namely the tendency to "overkill" emulsions because the tests used introduce a new mechanism of instability by causing unreasonably high stress.[18]

In the described study, 5–10 g samples of the test and control formulas were rotated at 5000 rpm for 5 min. The test was performed for the formulations kept at the different storage conditions for up to 28 days at definite time intervals. No phase separation on centrifugation was noted in any of the samples thus indicating that both the test and control emulsions were stable for 28 days.

Electrical conductivity: Conductivity differences arise when an emulsion creams, the proportion of oil increases in the separated upper portion of the emulsion, and the proportion of water increases in the lower part of the emulsion. By measuring conductivity differences in the upper and lower parts as a function of storage time, instability can be determined.[21] Conductivity tests are also used to distinguish between emulsion types[22]—o/w emulsions will conduct because water is the continuous phase, and since oils are poor conductors, w/o emulsions conduct poorly.[23]

In the present study, a conductivity test was performed for all samples of the control and test formulation. No change in electrical conductivity was noted.

pH: pH is a significant parameter in so far as the effectiveness of the cream is concerned, and it can be used as an indicator of emulsion stability.[16] For the formation of stable emulsions, the pH value of the aqueous phase is a key factor.[19] The pH of skin ranges between 5 and 6; 5.5 is considered the average pH level. Therefore, formulations for application to skin should have pH close to this range.

In the present study, the pH of the freshly prepared control and test formulations was found to be 5.79 and 5.97, respectively (see **Table 1**).

The pH values decreased continuously from the first to the last day. On the 28th day, the pH levels of the control formulation samples were 4.45, 4.39, 4.35 and 4.27, respective to the different storage conditions. The pH of the control samples stored in different conditions showed slight variations with time, and slightly increased at the end of the study period. This could have been due to the production of metabolites; no such tendency is inherent in emulsions, but it can occur.

The pH values of the test formulation measured 6.09, 5.86, 5.35 and 5.85 on the 28th day, respective of their storage conditions—i.e., at 8°C in a refrigerator, at 25°C, 40°C, and at 40°C + 75% RH.

By using a two-way Analysis of Variance (ANOVA) technique at 5% level of significance, the change in pH of the samples of control formulation, at different levels of time and temperature, was found to be significant but there was an insignificant difference in changes of pH for samples of the test formulation.

A Least Significant Difference (LSD) test also was applied to determine the individual average effects of the pH levels of the control and test formulas at different temperatures with the passage of time. From this test it was concluded that at different storage conditions, a significant change occurred in the pH of the control formula but an insignificant change was observed in the test formulation samples.

Table 1. pH values of control (Ctrl) and test (Test) formulas stored at 8°C, 25°C, 40°C and 40°C + 75% RH

Time	8°C		25°C		40°C		40°C+ 75% RH	
	Ctrl	Test	Ctrl	Test	Ctrl	Test	Ctrl	Test
0 hr	5.97	5.79	5.97	5.79	5.97	5.79	5.97	5.79
12 hr	5.94	5.81	5.92	5.82	5.74	5.58	5.68	5.83
24 hr	5.76	5.95	5.64	5.81	5.58	5.96	5.53	5.98
36 hr	5.57	5.86	5.41	5.63	5.01	5.67	5.05	5.82
48 hr	4.96	5.84	4.87	5.49	4.74	5.04	4.61	5.06
72 hr	4.86	6.62	4.78	5.93	4.6	5.47	4.65	5.84
7 days	4.69	6.62	4.58	5.84	4.51	5.75	4.47	5.93
14 days	4.62	6.01	4.56	5.5	4.43	5.33	4.39	5.69
21 days	4.56	6.07	4.47	5.85	4.41	5.26	4.36	5.84
28 days	4.45	6.09	4.39	5.86	4.35	5.35	4.27	5.85

Dermatological Tests

Patch test: Before application of the control and test formulations to a total of nine male and female human volunteers aged 20–25, patch tests for melanin and erythema were performed and the values measured are shown in **Table 2.**

After performing the patch test for 24 hr, the test and control formulations were found to produce no skin irritation; thus both creams were deemed safe for in vivo evaluation. This lack of irritation could have been attributed to the presence of a good emollient in both formulas—i.e., glycerin[24]—or ascorbic acid, a natural antioxidant present in the formula from the grapefruit extract,[25,26] which has been shown to reduce skin erythema.[27,28]

Table 2. Percent change in melanin and erythema for control (Ctrl) and test (Test) formulas after a 24-hr patch test

Volunteer #	Melanin		Erythema	
	Ctrl	Test	Ctrl	Test
1	-22.35	-6.60	-4.64	0.54
2	-11.64	-10.32	13.76	-23.78
3	-11.38	-2.48	-3.78	-41.12
4	-0.94	-1.97	-11.62	-1.923
5	-1.69	-2.89	-1.89	-15.49
6	-2.48	-4.70	-6.76	3.51
7	-16.38	-12.83	-12.89	-2.33
8	3.83	-21.33	-3.62	-13.11
9	8.88	-6.76	-23.00	2.90
Mean ± SEM	-6.02 ± 3.36	-7.76 ± 2.09	-6.05 ± 3.31	-10.09 ± 4.98

Melanin

Melanocytes are present in the basal layer of the epidermis and they manufacture melanin, which is responsible for the color of skin. Melanin is formed through a series of oxidative reactions involving the amino acid tyrosine in the presence of the enzyme tyrosinase. Tyrosinase catalyzes three different reactions in the biosynthetic pathway of melanin in melanocytes.[29]

Antioxidants have important physiological effects on skin.[30] Their main role is to scavenge free radicals such as peroxides[27] that contribute to tyrosinase activation and melanin formation.[31] As previously mentioned, grapefruit extract is rich in natural antioxidants[32] that capture free radicals, resulting in the inhibition of melanogenesis.[30]

In the present study, the effect of the control and the test formulations on the production of skin melanin was examined. The amount of melanin was measured[b] for four weeks at different time intervals in each test subject after application of the control and test formulation.

It was found that the control formulation increased melanin content in the skin until the end of the 28-day test period, while the test formulation incorporating grapefruit extract decreased the melanin content throughout the study (see **Table 3**).

Table 3. Percent change in melanin content of the skin after application of the control (Ctrl) and test (Test) formulas

Volunteer #	First week		Second week		Third week		Fourth week	
	Ctrl	Test	Ctrl	Test	Ctrl	Test	Ctrl	Test
1	-5.11	-11.00	4.80	-12.62	17.42	-14.24	10.21	-20.71
2	5.34	-0.47	9.16	-3.50	13.99	-7.24	16.03	-9.35
3	-8.26	-0.32	-1.18	-8.06	5.31	-14.52	5.90	-19.03
4	0.96	-2.40	-2.30	-5.21	-1.54	-9.62	15.16	-10.62
5	-11.90	-1.04	-13.18	-5.19	-5.14	-7.27	15.11	-14.19
6	18.36	-2.03	12.46	-5.76	11.15	-13.90	5.57	-19.66
7	9.97	-12.67	13.90	-13.50	7.85	-10.47	16.62	-16.25
8	-6.80	-2.13	3.97	-3.66	-0.28	-7.93	-4.53	-9.15
9	-10.10	-11.01	1.63	-13.10	-0.98	-14.88	1.95	-27.98
Mean	-0.84	-4.79	3.25	-7.85	5.31	-11.12	9.11	-16.33
± SEM	± 3.42	± 1.72	± 2.79	± 1.38	± 2.61	± 1.09	± 2.47	± 2.08

An ANOVA test found the control and test formulations to produce statistically significant effects on skin melanin content in volunteers; a paired sample t-test showed a significant difference in the melanin effects of the control versus the test formulation from the second week, lasting to the fourth week of the study, confirming the two creams had different effects on melanin.

Researchers concluded that the decreased melanin content after application of the test formulation could have been attributed to the antioxidant activity of the grapefruit extract—particularly its potent antioxidant vitamin C that causes inhibition of melanogenesis.[9,30,31]

Erythema

Skin irritation is caused by the direct toxicity of chemicals on cells or blood vessels in the skin and is different from contact allergy, which is caused by an immune response.[28]

In the described in vivo study, irritation also was monitored weekly throughout the test period for both formulations. Erythema was measured[b] and found to be slightly increased after application of the control formula for the first week but almost no change was observed during the second week, and a pronounced decrease was observed at the third and fourth week.

In comparison, after application of the test formulation, erythema was slightly increased after the first week; however, decreased at the second and fourth week.

An ANOVA test confirmed statistically that the control and test formulation produced insignificant effects on skin erythema. A paired sample t-test showed a significant variation in irritation with respect to the control and test formulation at the first and second week (see **Table 4**).

It was thus concluded that both the test and control formulations decreased erythema at the end of the study period and the overall effect of the test formulation on erythema was insignificant; thus it could be used safely without irritating skin. In addition, the active ingredient in grapefruit extract is a good source of vitamin C,[33] which is used as an anti-inflammatory,[28] and topical vitamin C is claimed to inhibit UV-radiation-induced damage to porcine skin since it functions as a biological co-factor and an antioxidant.[29]

Moisture Content

Moisturizing treatments involve factors such as repairing the skin barrier; retaining/increasing water content; reducing TEWL; restoring the lipid barrier's ability to attract, hold and redistribute water; and maintaining skin integrity and appearance.[34]

Table 4. Percent change in skin erythema content, or potential of a substance to produce irritation, after application of control (Ctrl) and test (Test) formulas

Volunteer #	First week Ctrl	Test	Second week Ctrl	Test	Third week Ctrl	Test	Fourth week Ctrl	Test
1	-4.87	-1.17	1.87	-2.92	-4.87	-9.75	-17.42	2.14
2	-10.60	-3.75	-12.90	-5.93	-15.82	-3.16	-30.41	-2.77
3	-7.92	15.64	-1.58	8.06	1.23	43.60	-5.46	9.72
4	-3.36	-2.39	-4.53	-3.75	-7.21	-4.78	-0.34	-12.12
5	2.47	5.80	-16.92	-2.46	11.79	10.71	-14.83	1.79
6	5.30	-0.19	2.65	-0.78	0.00	-1.75	-7.94	-7.60
7	29.00	-0.97	25.34	-1.93	25.34	1.16	23.52	8.12
8	19.47	6.13	7.00	-10.94	10.72	0.66	6.56	-9.41
9	-4.70	3.71	0.00	10.35	-22.82	8.20	-13.59	-7.42
Mean	2.75	2.53	0.10	-1.14	-0.18	4.99	-6.66	-1.95
± SEM	± 4.44	± 2.02	± 4.04	± 2.20	± 4.92	± 5.26	± 5.17	± 2.61

A 100-g sample of grapefruit juice contains 36–40 mg of vitamin C,[11] which is known to increase the collagen fibers in the dermis.[35-39] With an increase in collagen, conditions for hydration are improved.[40] In addition, vitamin C improves the barrier function of the stratum corneum (SC), in turn improving moisture in the skin.[41]

In both formulations tested, glycerin was incorporated in the internal aqueous phase to enhance the skin moisture level. Glycerin is a humectant with excellent sensorial properties that moisturizes the full thickness of the SC while creating an apparent "reservoir" of moisture in the skin. This makes the skin more resistant to dry conditions.[24]

In the present study, a slight increase in moisture was found[c] from the first to third week after application of the control, and a slight decrease was observed at the fourth week; however, after the application of the test formulation, the skin moisture content was more pronounced from the first to the fourth week.

ANOVA testing found that the control showed an insignificant change with respect to the basic values, at 0 hr before application of creams, whereas the test formulation showed a significant variation throughout the study period of 28 days.

By applying an LSD test, the change in moisture content was found to be statistically significant after application of the test formulation. A paired sample t-test confirmed a significant difference in the moisture values was produced at the fourth week when comparing the control to the test formulation (see **Table 5**).

Table 5. Percent change in skin moisture content after application of control (Ctrl) and test (Test) formulas

Volunteer #	First week		Second week		Third week		Fourth week	
	Ctrl	Test	Ctrl	Test	Ctrl	Test	Ctrl	Test
1	27.83	34.62	16.10	41.00	-11.93	46.92	-13.52	59.00
2	56.04	17.38	39.61	22.80	-8.21	29.35	-41.30	33.41
3	14.11	42.29	3.60	28.08	20.87	39.86	-5.71	53.03
4	-1.09	4.63	-3.27	8.30	-26.73	17.76	-5.82	21.24
5	-3.20	6.26	-16.16	11.18	-13.39	14.31	-21.40	15.20
6	9.78	1.47	8.26	-4.26	8.94	0.29	26.81	11.91
7	-1.12	37.41	-3.54	35.37	23.84	41.50	19.37	54.20
8	10.59	26.90	-2.97	36.55	-2.97	42.98	-10.41	47.66
9	7.94	3.74	11.56	9.07	30.61	-6.05	45.58	7.12
Mean	13.43	19.41	5.91	20.90	2.34	25.21	-0.71	33.64
± SEM	± 6.21	± 5.40	± 5.30	± 5.19	± 6.54	± 6.52	± 8.89	± 6.78

Sebum Content

Sebaceous glands, located in each hair follicle, produce sebum to lubricate and protect the skin.[33] Sebum production is measured using a special opalescent plastic film[d] that becomes transparent when it comes in contact with sebum lipids.[42]

A probe is used to press a piece of the film onto the skin for a measured length of time and sebum is adsorbed onto the film, similarly to ink on blotting paper, thus turning the film transparent.

The probe is then placed into a device that radiates a light beam onto the film. A metal mirror behind the film reflects the beam back again through the film and into an instrument called a *photomultiplier*, which measures the amount of light in the beam. The more sebum on the skin, the more transparent the film and the greater the amount of light reflected.

In the present study, the effects of the control and test formulations on sebum content in human facial cheeks were investigated. Sebum was measured weekly in all test subjects using the control and test formulations; both samples were found to increase sebum content from the first to fourth week of the study period.

An ANOVA test confirmed a statistically significant effect of the control and test formulation on skin sebum throughout the study period. By applying an LSD test, it was evident that significant changes in sebum content were observed at different time intervals after application of both formulations (see **Table 6**).

With a paired sample t-test it was found that the control and test formulations showed insignificant variations regarding the skin sebum content. Thus, researchers attributed the increase in sebum content to the oily nature of the w/o emulsions, since they contained paraffin oil.[14]

Table 6. Percent change in sebum after application of control (Ctrl) and test (Test) formulas

Volunteer #	First week		Second week		Third week		Fourth week	
	Ctrl	Test	Ctrl	Test	Ctrl	Test	Ctrl	Test
1	34.43	180.33	139.34	17.24	183.61	25.00	180.33	96.55
2	47.19	205.62	84.27	49.52	115.73	56.19	205.62	147.62
3	42.11	205.26	173.68	409.09	350.00	581.82	205.26	754.55
4	58.06	464.52	103.23	192.31	170.97	276.92	464.52	976.92
5	271.43	771.43	309.52	81.25	771.43	140.00	771.43	196.25
6	10.42	206.25	64.58	82.35	108.33	105.88	206.25	402.94
7	-31.71	145.12	14.63	15.33	93.90	21.33	145.12	25.33
8	165.52	513.79	637.93	12.70	627.59	23.81	513.79	34.13
9	-40.65	-37.40	2.44	83.75	43.09	130.00	-37.40	196.25
Mean	61.86	294.99	169.96	104.84	273.85	151.22	294.99	314.50
± SEM	± 32.90	± 81.10	± 66.09	± 42.32	± 86.22	± 60.31	± 81.10	± 112.16

pH Values

The pH of skin ranges between 5 and 6; 5.5 is considered to be the average pH of skin. Therefore, formulations intended for application on skin should have a pH level close to this range.[28]

pH values in the volunteers' skin were measured at different time intervals before and after the application of the control and test formulation for a period of four weeks (see **Table 7**).

Table 7. Percent change in skin pH values after application of control (Ctrl) and test (Test) formulas

Volunteer #	First week		Second week		Third week		Fourth week	
	Ctrl	Test	Ctrl	Test	Ctrl	Test	Ctrl	Test
1	-20.86	-8.60	-17.65	-33.84	-3.80	-24.20	-3.63	-27.33
2	3.57	-4.38	1.07	-11.17	4.63	-7.82	-1.52	1.46
3	90.59	10.89	122.32	7.46	98.91	7.46	-1.31	-7.46
4	45.86	0.60	73.83	3.41	112.75	-15.23	154.81	114.83
5	16.00	-2.04	15.34	-5.92	23.29	-1.63	39.51	156.33
6	-10.46	-36.10	-4.77	-27.80	-4.59	-15.95	125.87	-42.86
7	87.35	6.64	7.96	15.35	8.78	92.53	148.16	-7.26
8	94.02	17.67	-5.25	13.36	53.08	120.47	131.70	142.24
9	-7.43	-54.13	-49.17	-47.26	-8.21	-57.51	-21.11	-53.63
Mean	33.18	-7.72	15.96	-9.60	31.65	10.90	63.61	30.70
± SEM	± 15.70	± 7.70	± 17.16	± 7.42	± 15.38	± 19.19	± 24.92	± 27.62

After application of the control, pH values of the skin was increased throughout the study period, whereas application of the test formulation decreased pH values during the first and second week, and increased during the third and fourth week.

ANOVA testing found a significant effect on skin pH values produced by the control, whereas an insignificant effect was observed by the test formulation. A paired sample t-test concluded that the change in skin pH in volunteers by both the test and control formulation was significant in the first and fourth week.

The absence of change in the pH of skin from the test formulation could be attributed to the presence of potent natural antioxidants in the grapefruit extract,[32] which can prevent the oxidative degradation of skin by scavenging free radicals, thus maintaining the natural integrity of human skin.

TEWL

Body loses water by constant evaporation through the skin, also known as trans epidermal water loss (TEWL).[42] TEWL changes are related to SC water-binding capacity.[42] Water makes up 70–75% of the basal layer weight but only 10–15% of the SC. If the water content of the SC falls below 10%, it becomes dry, less flexible and prone to damage, breakdown and infections.[43]

In the present study, a decrease in TEWL values was noted after the application of the control and test formulation throughout the 28-day study (see **Table 8**).

Table 8. Percent change in TEWL values after application of control (Ctrl) and test (Test) formulas

Volunteer #	First week Ctrl	First week Test	Second week Ctrl	Second week Test	Third week Ctrl	Third week Test	Fourth week Ctrl	Fourth week Test
1	21.36	-16.88	-10.91	-30.52	17.27	-21.10	-28.64	-48.05
2	-6.91	-4.50	-16.59	-8.00	-27.19	-19.50	-32.72	-24.50
3	16.23	13.44	1.05	6.45	5.76	3.76	-12.57	-2.69
4	-4.68	-17.76	-24.26	-23.03	-28.51	-32.57	-14.04	-37.50
5	-8.56	-13.10	-28.02	-13.54	-33.85	-11.35	-30.35	-32.31
6	-21.68	-9.84	-32.87	-12.99	-46.50	-40.55	-14.69	-28.74
7	-15.27	-21.85	-27.27	-23.33	-26.55	-28.15	-36.36	-36.67
8	-9.84	-39.11	-12.30	-14.92	-42.21	-37.50	-45.90	-34.27
9	5.16	-0.25	-13.10	-53.44	-27.78	-51.65	-19.05	-58.78
Mean	-2.69	-12.21	-18.25	-19.26	-23.28	-26.51	-26.03	-33.72
± SEM	± 4.75	± 4.91	± 3.57	± 5.53	± 7.04	± 5.54	± 3.86	± 5.18

ANOVA testing confirmed that changes in TEWL produced by both formulations were statistically significant during the four-week study. By applying an LSD test, the change in TEWL values became significant for both formulations after the first week of application. With a paired sample t-test, insignificant variation in TEWL was found with respect to the control and test formulation throughout the study.

Researchers concluded that both formulations prevented TEWL probably due to a number of factors including their glycerin and paraffin oil content. Glycerin moisturizes the full thickness of the SC[24] and paraffin oil, as mentioned previously, forms an occlusive covering on skin thus preventing TEWL. Therefore, due to moisture-retaining properties, both formulations enhanced the SC's ability to attract, hold and redistribute water, in turn reducing TEWL.[24, 34, 44]

Panel Test

A questionnaire was given to each volunteer for sensory evaluation of each of the two creams. Average points were calculated for both the control and test formulations (see **Figure 1**).

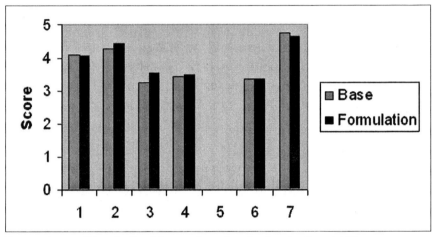

Figure 1. Average Values for Panel Test: 1= Ease of application; 2 = Spreadability; 3 = Sense just after application; 4 = Sense in long term (28 days); 5 = Irritation; 6 = Shine on skin; and 7= Sense of softness

The average points for ease of application were 4.12 and 4.08 for the control and test formulation, respectively, indicating ease of application on the skin. Points for spreadability rated the test formulation higher—4.29 for the control and 4.42 for the test formulation. Feel upon application was rated as 3.25 points for the control and 3.54 for the test formulation, an indication the test formulation felt better upon application to skin.

Average points for the 28-day application period were 3.43 and 3.5 for the control and test formulation, respectively. The numbers indicated the test formulation produced a more pleasant feeling; there also was no irritation on the skin in both formulations thus they were assigned 0.0 points for irritation by all volunteers.

Shine on skin was rated 3.35 for the control and 3.36 for the test formulation. This was expected since the two formulations contained the same quantity of paraffin oil. Similarly, the control produced a higher rating for softness of the skin; the average points was 4.74 for the base and 4.63 for the test formulation.

From a paired sample t-test, an insignificant difference was noted between the average points of sensitivity for both formulations. Thus, researchers concluded that little variation existed between the control and test formulation in regards to sensory evaluation. Both creams behaved similarly, from a sensory point of view.

Conclusion

Antioxidant-rich grapefruit extract, when used at a concentration of 1% in topical creams, was not found to realize its full skin benefit potential in a 28-period of application. It is therefore suggested, to maximize the cosmetic benefits, that the grapefruit extract be used in higher concentrations and for longer period of time.

Published January 2008 *Cosmetics and Toiletries* magazine

References

1. JPF Macedo et al, Micro-emultocrit technique: A valuable tool for determination of critical HLB value of emulsions, *AAPS Pharm Sci Tech* 7(1) (2006)
2. K Welin-Berger, Formulations, release and skin penetration of topical anesthetics, Dissertation for the Degree of Doctor of Philosophy (Faculty of Pharmacy), Uppsala University (2001) pp 17–18
3. F Nielloud, G Marti-Mestres and MM Gilberte, *Pharmaceutical Emulsions and Suspensions*, New York: Marcel Dekker (2007)
4. G Kutz, P Biehl, M Waldmann-Laue and B Jackwerth, On the choice of oil-in-water emulsifiers for use in skin care products for sensitive skin, *SOFW J*, 123 145–150 (1997)
5. TO Ngai, SH Behrens and H Auweter, Novel emulsions stabilized by pH and temperature sensitive microgels, *The Roy Soci of Chem* (2004)
6. US Pat 7,138,128, Preparations of the W/O emulsion type with an increased water content, and comprising cationic polymers, B Andreas, K Rainer and Schneider Gu, assigned to Beiersdorf AG (Hamburg, Germany) (Nov 21, 2006)
7. NV Yanishlieva, E Marinova and J Pokorny, Natural antioxidants from herbs and spices, *Eu J of Lip Sci and Tech* 108 (9)776–793 (2006)
8. D Roberts, Antioxidant values in fruits and vegetables, Macular Degeneration Support Web site; *www.mdsupport.org* (Accessed Feb 27, 2007)
9. L Curtis, *Juice Up*, Northbrook, IL USA: Virgo Publishing (1997)
10. FP Mary et al, A furanocoumarin-free grapefruit juice establishes furanocoumarins as the mediators of the grapefruit juice–felodipine interaction, *Ameri J of Clinic Nutr*, 83(5) 1097–1105 (2006)
11. *Grapefruit*, Wikipedia, the free encyclopedia Web site; *www.en.wikipedia.org/wiki/grapefruit#column-one*; Wikimedia Foundation Inc. 15(59) (Accessed Mar 28, 2007)
12. British Pharmacopoeia 2 (2004) pp 1132–1134
13. Code of Federal Regulations, U.S. Food and Drug Administration, Sec.146.132, *Grapefruit juice*, Department of Health and Human Services, U.S. Government Printing Office 2 (2002) pp 439–440

14. RC Rowe, PJ Sheskey and PJ Weller, Dimethicone, mineral oil, wax white; wax yellow, *Handbook of Pharmaceutical Excipients*, 4th ed, Chicago: The PhP London, and Washington, D.C.: the APhA Washington (2003) pp 213–214, 395–396, 687–690

15. J Swarbrick, JT Rubino and OP Rubino, Coarse dispersions, in *Remington: The science and practice of pharmacy*, 21st edn, Philadelphia: Lippincot Williams and Wilkins (2006) pp 316–334

16. NM Mostefa, AH Sadok, N Sabri, A Hadji, Determination of optimal cream formulation from long-term stability investigation using a surface response modelling, *Int J of Cosmet Sci*, 28 (3) 211–218 (2006).

17. M Muehlbach, R Brummer and R Eggers, Study on the transferability of the time temperature superposition principle to emulsion, *Int J of Cosmet Sci*, 28(2) 109–116 (2006)

18. HA Lieberman, MM Rieger and GS Banker, Pharmaceutical Emulsions, in *Pharmaceutical Dosage Forms: Disperse Systems*, New York and Basel: Marcel Dekker 1 (1988) pp 199–240, 285–288

19. L Song, X Ge, M Wang and Z Zhang, Direct preparation of silica hollow spheres in a water in oil emulsion system: The effect of pH and viscosity, *J of Non-Cry Sol* 352(21–22) 2230–2235 (2006)

20. L Lachman, HA Lieberman and JL Kanig, in *Emulsions, The Theory and Practice of Industrial Pharmacy*, 3rd edn, Bombay: Varghese Publishing House (1990) p 502

21. A Abdelbary and SA Nour, Correlation between spermicidal activity and haemolytic index of certain plant saponins, *Pharmazie* 34(9) 560–561 (1979)

22. K Tauer, Emulsions, in *MPI Colloids and Interfaces*, D-14476 Golm, Germany: Am Mühlenberg (2006)

23. ST Mabrouk, The preparation and testing of a common emulsion and personal care product: Lotion, *J of Chem Edu* 81(1) 83–86 (2004)

24. TL Diepgen, Professional care for dry and sensitive skin, Medical and economic costs of skin disease, in *White Book of Dermatology*, Heidenberg, Germany: European Dermatology Forum, University of Heidenberg (2005)

25. Grapefruit, International Cyber Business Services Inc; *www.holisticonline.com* (2000)

26. TE Wallis, *Text book of Pharmacognosy,* 5th edn, New Delhi: CBS publishers, (2004) p 194

27. A Prakash, Antioxidant activity, What are antioxidants? *Medallion Laboratories* 19(2) (2001)

28. N Akhtar, Formulation and evaluation of a cosmetic multiple emulsion system containing macademia nut oil and two antiaging agents, Dissertation for the Degree of Doctor of Philosophy, the Department of Pharmaceutical Technology, Anadolu University (2001) pp 104,107

29. P Shoukat et al, Survey and mechanism of skin depigmenting and lightening agents, *Wily Int Sci J* 20(11) 921–934 (2006)

30. DG Meyers and PA Maloley, Safety of antioxidant vitamins, *Arch of Int Med* 156(9) 925–935 (1996)

31. CD Villarama and HI Maibach, Glutathione as a depigmenting agent: An overview, *Int J of Cosmet Sci* 27(3) 147–153 (2005)

32. D Roberts, Antioxidant Values in Fruits and Vegetables, Macular Degeneration Support Web site; *www.mdsupport.org* (Accessed Feb 15, 2007)

33. G Mateljan, Grapefruit, The World's Healthiest Foods, Honolulu, Hawaii: McGraw Hill Professional, Science and Technology Encyclopedia, *www.healthline.com* (2007)

34. JN Kraft and CW Lynde, Moisturizers: What They Are and a Practical Approach to Product Selection, Skin therapy letter, indexed by the U.S. National Library of Medicine 10 (2005)

35. R Hata and H Senoo, L-ascorbic acid 2-phosphate stimulates collagen accumulation, cell proliferation and formation of a three dimensional tissue like substance by skin fibroblasts, *J Cell Physiol*, 138(1) 8–16 (1989)

36. S Murad, D Grove, KA Lindberg, G Reynolds, A Sivaraja and SR Pinnel, Regulation of collagen synthesis by ascorbic acid, *Proc Natl Acad Sci USA* 78 2879–2882 (1981)

37. JC Geesin, D Darr, R Kaufmann, S Murad and SR Pinnel, Ascorbic acid especially increases type 1 and type III procollagen messenger RNA levels in human skin fibroblast, *J Invest Derma* 90(4) 420–424 (1988)

38. SR Pinnel, S Murad and D Darr, Induction of collagen synthesis by ascorbic acid: A possible mechanism, *Arch Derma* 123(12) 1684–1686 (1987)

39. K Scharffetter-Kochanek et al, Photoaging of the skin from phenotype mechanisms, *Exp Gerontol* 35(3) 307–316 (2000)

40. SJ Padayatty and M Levine, New insights into the physiology and morphology of vitamin C, *Canad Med Assoc J* 164(3) 353–355 (2001)

41. M Ponec et al, The formation of competent barrier lipids in reconstructed human epidermis requires the presence of vitamin C, *J Invest Derm* 109(3) 348–355 (1997)

42. J Gray, The world of skin care, ed 1, London: Macmillan Press (2000) p 7

43. D Mitsushiro, Influence of drug environment on epidermal functions, *J Derm Sci* 24(1) 22–28 (2000)

44. HK Biesalski and JUC Obermueller, UV light β-carotene and human skin beneficial and potentially harmful effect, *Arch Biochem Biophys* 389(1) 1–6 (2001)

CHAPTER 21

Tetrapeptide Targets Epidermal Cohesion

G. Pauly, MD; P. Moussou, PhD; J.-L. Contet-Audonneau, MD; C. Jeanmaire, PhD; O. Freis, PhD; M. Sabadotto; L. Danoux; V. Bardey, PhD; I. Benoit; and A. Rathjens, PhD

Cognis France, Division de Laboratoires Sérobiologiques, Pulnoy, France

KEY WORDS: *glycosaminoglycans, proteoglycans, syndecan-1, aging, type XVII collagen*

ABSTRACT: *Most antiaging products claim to act on the dermis; however, the epidermis, a key element of cutaneous aging, is often forgotten. In the present study, researchers selected an acetylated tetrapeptide for its effect on epidermis cohesion, triggered by activity on syndecan-1 and collagen XVII; these effects are confirmed in vivo.*

Actives proposed for skin care generally are focused on wrinkle prevention—but another sign of aging is fragile skin. During aging, the epidermis becomes thinner, the cohesion of the epidermal cells diminishes and the epidermis loses its resistance to environmental aggressors. The skin becomes dry and slack and consequently is easily damaged even with the lightest friction or shock.

To enhance epidermal cohesion, Laboratoires Sérobiologiques has developed an antiaging active designed to target two proteins that affect epidermis cohesion: syndecan-1 and type XVII collagen.

Syndecan-1

In the skin, proteoglycans (PG) and glycosaminoglycans (GAG) are present not only in the extracellular matrix of the dermis, but also in the epidermis. Syndecans represent the major form of PG synthesized by the epidermis with syndecan-1, a small PG with a MW <60,000 da, located in supra-basal layers of the epidermis. Syndecan-1 plays an important role in keratinocyte activation during wound healing.[1] In addition, it has diverse functions including the regulation of cell signaling such as by fibroblast growth factors, participation in cell-to-cell and cell-to-laminin adhesion,[2] and in the organization of cell matrix adhesion. According to Carey,[3] syndecan-1 may link the intracellular cytoskeleton to the interstitial matrix.

Much data exists on the alteration of the synthesis and the structure of GAG and some PGs during skin aging,[4] but little information is available concerning small PGs in the epidermis, in particular syndecan-1. One recent study on cell cultures from donors of different ages showed a reduced synthesis of syndecan-1 by keratinocytes during aging.[5] This data has been confirmed by immunohistochemistry (IHC) on skin biopsies from donors of different ages (**Figure 1**).

In **Figure 1a**, syndecan-1, revealed in yellow-green in the epidermis (E), is not very visible in skin from a 3-year-old donor. It is more strongly visible in skin from a 41-year-old donor (+222%, p<0.01), yet greatly reduced in skin from a 55-year-old donor (-88%, p<0.05) (**Figure 1b**). This type of level evolution, according to aging, is usually observed for proteoglycan skin components.[6]

Type XVII Collagen

Type XVII collagen is a component of hemidesmosomes, participating in the adhesion of basal keratinocytes to the extracellular matrix of the dermo-epidermal junction (**Figure 2**).

Hemidesmosomes are composed from different proteins such as plakin BP230, a6 b4 integrins, tetraspanin/CD151, plectin and type XVII collagen, also called BP180 (**Figure 3**).

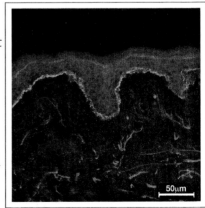

Figure 2. Visualization, in green, of type XVII collagen on human skin by immunohistochemistry and confocal microscopy

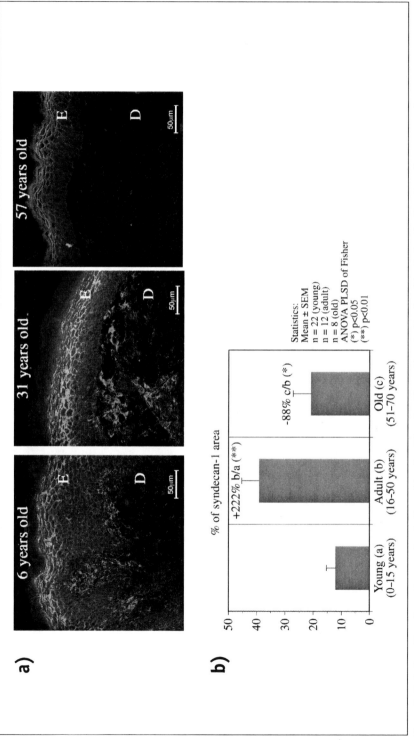

Figure 1. Variation of syndecan-1 expression in the epidermis with aging (E = epidermis, D = dermis); a) visualization, in yellow-green, of skin sections; b) quantification

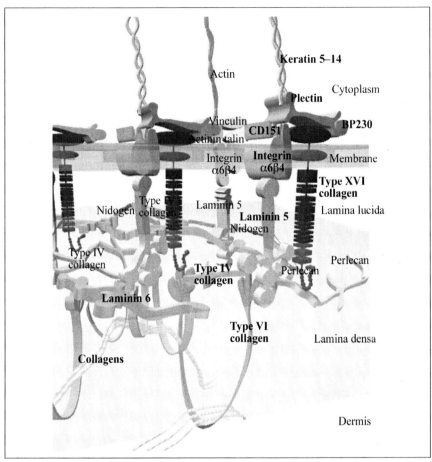

Figure 3. Schematic representation of the hemidesmosome structure between basal keratinocytes and the extracellular matrix; type XVII collagen is represented in green.

Mutations in the type XVII collagen encoding gene (COL17A1) led to a decrease in epidermal adhesion, as well as skin blistering in response to minimum mechanical deformation.[7] This underlines the fundamental importance of stabilizing interactions between type XVII collagen and laminin-5 and integrins to maintain the correct cohesion between different skin layers.

During the aging process, skin becomes more fragile and presents an increased blistering response to weak physical constraints such as external shock.[8] Because type XVII collagen plays a role in anchoring and cohesion, any alteration of this protein may at least be partly responsible for skin weakness.

N-Acteyl-tetrapeptide-11

With the aim of reducing consequences of the aging process and maintaining the level of syndecan-1 and type XVII collagen in the epidermis, an active ingredient was developed based on an acetylated tetrapeptide N-acetyl-Pro-Pro-Tyr-Leu (AcTP11) (**Figure 4**)[a].

The peptide sequence corresponds to four amino acids of an antimicrobial polypeptide, cathelicidin PR-39, that is expressed during wound healing and induces syndecan-1 expression.[9]

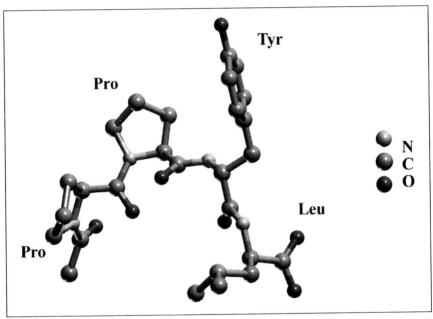

Figure 4. Chemical structure of AcTP11 (N-acetyl-Pro-Pro-Tyr-Leu)

In vitro Efficacy

Keratinocyte cultures: Human keratinocyte suspensions were prepared by trypsinization of human skin biopsies from adult donors. Keratinocytes were cultured at 37°C, CO_2 5%, within medium containing fetal calf serum (FCS) at 5%.

- *Keratinocyte culture for syndecan-1:* After incubation for two days, the growth medium was changed for medium (DMEM without FCS) but containing AcTP11 (at 0.87 and 2.6mg/mL) or KGF as reference substance at 0.01mg/mL.[10] The

---

[a] SYNiorage (INCI: Glycerin (and) acetyl tetrapeptide-11) is a product of Cognis.

cultured cells were processed five days later for visualization of syndecan-1 by immunocytochemistry (ICC)[b] and quantification by image analysis.

- *Keratinocyte culture for type XVII collagen:* After incubation for three to five days, the growth medium was changed for medium (DMEM without FCS) containing AcTP11. The cultured cells were processed three days later for visualization of type XVII collagen by ICC[c] and quantification by image analysis.

Reconstructed full thickness skin models: Reconstructed full-thickness skin models[d] contain growing keratinocytes overlaying a pseudo-dermis that is formed by viable fibroblasts dispersed in collagen matrix. The skin models were treated by AcTP11 or KGF at the beginning of the differentiation. After nine days of incubation, models were analyzed by IHC.

DNA-array analysis: DNA-array analyses were performed on human keratinocyte cultures treated or untreated with AcTP11. Four strains taken from different donors were mixed to take into account inter-individual variabilities.

After incubation for 3 hr or 24 hr, to identify shorter and moderate time-lapse effects, total RNAs were extracted from cell cultures[e]. During the reverse transcription step, complementary DNAs (cDNAs) were synthesized and labeled either with cyanine-3 (Cya3) for total RNA extracted from nontreated cultures, or with cyanine-5 (Cya5) for AcTP11 treated cultures. Competitive hybridizations of the two labeled cDNAs were performed on the same specific DNA-array[f].

After washing with stringent buffer to eliminate nonspecifically bound cDNA, the red and green fluorescence of Cya3 and Cya5 were measured to evaluate the gene expression rates in the two tested conditions—control and AcTP11 treatment. Each gene was analyzed four times in the slide and statistical analyses were elaborated to identify significant gene expression modifications.

---

[b] Primary polyclonal rabbit antibody antihuman syndecan-1, SC-5632, was obtained from Tebu, France; also, secondary sheep antibody anti-rabbit—FITC, was obtained from BIO-RAD, France.
[c] Primary polyclonal rabbit antibody antihuman collagen XVII, Ab28440, was obtained from Abcam, Cambridge, UK; and secondary monoclonal goat antibody anti-rabbit, 4010-2, was obtained from Southern Biotechnology Associates, Birmingham, USA.
[d] Epiderm FT Kit EFT 200 was obtained from MatTek, USA.
[e] The Nucleospin RNA II kit from Macherey-Nagel, France, was used for this test.
[f] 1300 genes PIQOR Skin by Memorec Biotec GmbH, Germany, was used to perform this test.

qRT-PCR: A quantitative reverse transcription-polymerase chain reaction (qRT-PCR) for type XVII collagen encoding gene (COL17A1) was realized on total RNAs extracted from keratinocytes cultured for two days with or without AcTP11.

Microscopy and image analysis: After staining by ICC or IHC, cell cultures and tissue sections were observed by a confocal laser scanning microscope[g] and images were quantified by an image analyzer[h].

For skin sections, the percentage of stained PG area was quantified (% of stained epidermis). For cell cultures, the results were expressed as: expression index 1 = number of stained pixels x fluorescence intensity in green channel in arbitrary unit. For the full-thickness skin model sections, the result was expressed as: expression index 2 = number of stained pixels x fluorescence intensity in green channel/epidermal thickness in arbitrary unit.

Results

Global effect of AcTP11 on DNA array: The expression of two strategic genes was potentially modified by AcTP11 treatment: the expression of the Discoidin Domain Receptor 1 (DDR1) gene was down-regulated, and the type XVII collagen encoding gene expression was increased.

The DDR1 gene codes for a cellular receptor, which is activated by numerous extracellular collagens.[11] Signals transduced from this receptor induce a cell growth decrease[12] and a repression of the expression of some genes of the extracellular matrix (ECM), including the syndecan-1.[13] Since AcTP11 seemed to decrease DDR1 expression, it could also induce a keratinocyte growth stimulation and thus limit syndecan-1 gene repression.

The collagen XVII or BP180 protein is implicated in the hemidesmosome structure that forms a bridge between cytoskeleton of basal epidermal keratinocytes and the extracellular matrix of the dermo-epidermal junction. This collagen is strongly implicated in the cohesion of the different skin layers.

---

[g] The CLSM 310 is a device of Zeiss, France.
[h] The TCS-SP2 is a device of Leica, France.

AcTP11 on syndecan-1, keratinocytes, full-thickness models: The stimulation of keratinocyte cell growth by AcTP11 was confirmed on in vitro cell cultures (+13%, p<0.05), and the decrease of syndecan-1 gene repression by AcTP11 was confirmed by in vitro tests. On keratinocyte cultures, AcTP11 significantly increased the rate of syndecan-1 in keratinocyte cultures (**Figure 5a**), with a dose dependent and significant effect, comparatively to the control (**Figure 5b**).

On the full-thickness skin model, AcTP11, introduced in the culture medium at 2.60 µg/mL, significantly increased the rate of syndecan-1 (**Figure 6a**), comparatively to the control (+38%, p<0.02) (**Figure 6b**).

AcTP11 on type XVII collagen, keratinocyte cultures: The increase of type XVII collagen encoding gene expression also has been confirmed by in vitro tests. AcTP11 at 2.60 µg/mL significantly increased the COL17A1 gene expression by human epidermal keratinocytes in culture (+18%, p<0.05) (**Figure 7**).

This result has been confirmed by visualizing the production of type XVII collagen protein (shown in green) on cell culture (**Figure 8**).

In vivo Efficacy

A clinical study was conducted on 19 healthy female volunteers aged 60 to 70 years who were experiencing loss of elasticity on the face. This study evaluated the antiaging effects of a cream incorporating 3% (13.5 ppm) of the active ingredient based on AcTP11 at 60mg/cm^2 (see **Formula 1**), after 56 days of twice-daily use, versus a placebo cream.

The antiaging activity in the skin was evaluated by biomechanical measurements since some biomechanical parameters such as firmness and elasticity decrease with skin aging.[14]

The biomechanical properties of the skin were measured on the upper cheek by a torquemeter before treatment (D0) and after 28 (D28) and 56 (D56) days of treatment. Macrophotographs of the temples were taken at the same time.

The torquemeter is designed to measure the angular displacement of skin in response to torsional forces applied by the torque motor incorporated into the probe. The gap between the central rotating disk and the external stationary ring of the probe determines the

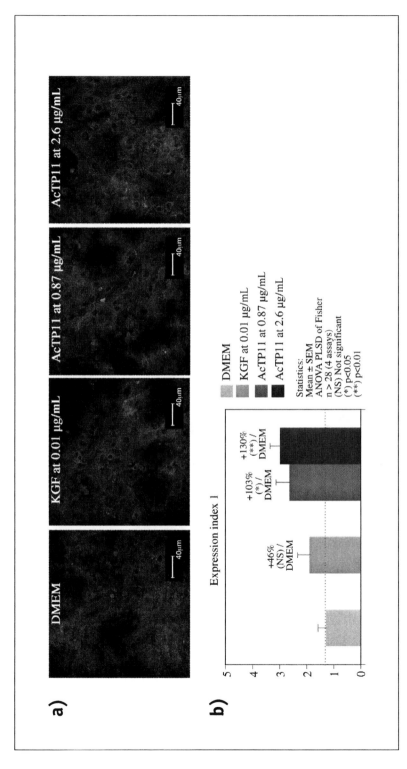

Figure 5. Effect of AcTP11 on the syndecan-1 synthesis by human keratinocytes in primary cell culture; a) visualization of the cells, in green; b) quantification

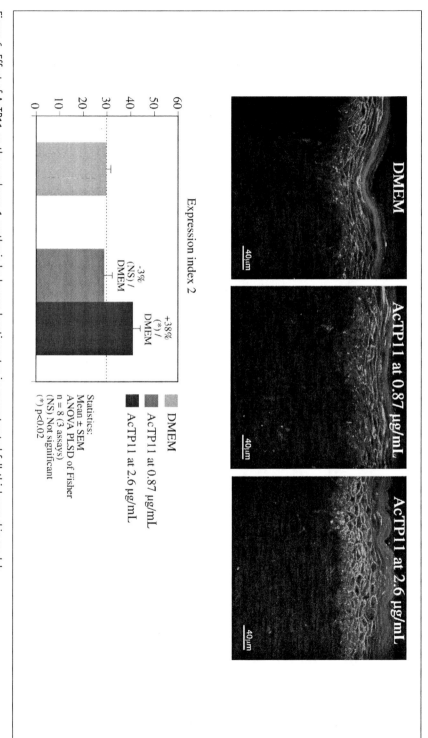

Figure 6. Effect of AcTP11 on the syndecan-1 synthesis by human keratinocytes in reconstructed full-thickness skin model; a) visualization of the sections, in green; b) quantification

depth of the skin solicitation. A gap of 1 mm was used for the characterization of the biomechanical behavior of the superficial layers of epidermis.[15] The parameters measured are shown in **Figure 9**.

After 56 days of treatment, a significant increase was observed in the biomechanical properties of firmness and elasticity in the superficial layers of the epidermis. Skin texture was improved, skin relief was smoothed and skin radiance was increased (**Figure 10a**).

A sample cream with 3% AI based on AcTP11 had a 5–10% greater effect than the placebo cream (**Figure 10b**).

The significant increase in firmness and elasticity reflects an improvement of epidermal cohesion and consequently an antiaging effect.

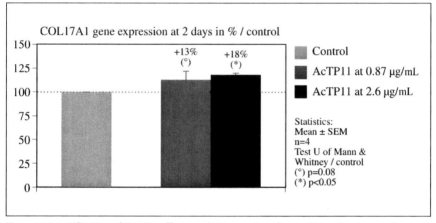

Figure 7. Quantification of AcTP11 effect on the expression of type XVII collagen encoding gene (COL17A1) in human epidermal keratinocytes by qRT-PCR

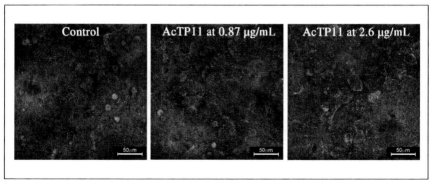

Figure 8. Visualization of AcTP11 effect on type XVII collagen, shown in green, in human epidermal keratinocytes by ICC

Formula 1. Antiaging test cream incorporating AcTP11 active

A. Lauryl glucoside (and) polyglyceryl-2 dipolyhydroxystearate
    (and) glycerin   4.00% w/w

   Behenyl alcohol   2.00

   Ethylhexyl stearate   4.00

   Hexyldecanol (and) hexyldecyl laurate   4.00

   Dicaprylyl ether   2.00

   Dimethicone   1.00

   Sodium polyacrylate   1.00

B. Water (*aqua*)   qs to 100.00

   Propylene glycol (and) phenoxyethanol (and) chlorophenesin

      (and) methylparaben (Elestab 388, Laboratoires

      Sérobiologiques)   2.50

   Xanthan gum   0.25

   Glycerin   3.00

   Sodium cocoyl glutamate   0.80

C. Glycerin (and) acetyl tetrapeptide-11 (SYNiorage LS 9748, Cognis)   3.00

                                                          100.00

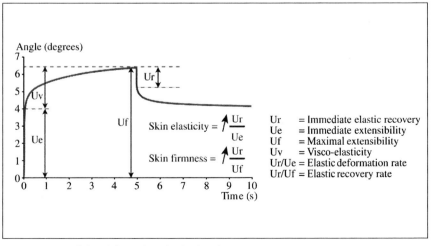

Figure 9. Curve of skin deformation obtained with a torquemeter

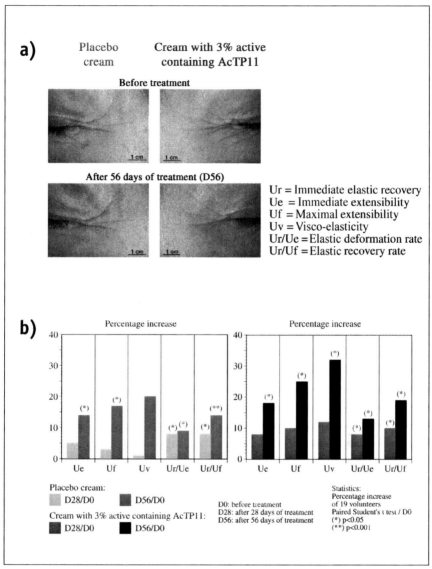

Figure 10. Evolution of cutaneous relief in vivo after treatment (D56); a) with 3% AI cream with AcTP11, versus placebo cream (macrophotography); and b) effect on biomechanical properties of the skin (torquemeter)

Conclusions

The newly developed tetrapeptide AcTP11 was shown to have an in vitro stimulating effect on keratinocyte growth via a DNA array and growth test, and on syndecan-1 synthesis by keratinocytes via a DNA array, ICC and IHC. This increase of syndecan-1 level may induce a better homeostasis of the epidermis due to its multiple functions on skin organization, regulation and intercellular adhesion. By stimulating the synthesis of type XVII collagen, shown by DNA array, q-RT PCR and ICC, AcTP11 also allowed for the improvement of cohesion between epidermis and dermis.

There is a discrepancy between the spirit of seniors and the appearance of their skin. Whereas they acquire strength and serenity with age, their skin on the contrary becomes more fragile and blemished as a consequence of epidermis weakening. By targeting two specific constituents of the epidermis responsible for its cohesion, syndecan-1 and type XVII collagen, an AI-based AcTP11 can help the skin to recover resistance, a refined texture and consequently better radiance, a growing market request in an aging society.

Published January 2008 *Cosmetics and Toiletries* magazine

Acknowledgements: This work was supported by the contribution of imagery laboratories, D. Gauché and M.D. Vazquez-Duchene; technicians in histology, C. Naudin, C. Tedeschi and P. Sthrudel; in cell culture, L. Martin and E. Charrois; in molecular biology, N. Bari; and A. Courtois from the scientific department.

References

1. MA Stepp et al, Defects in keratinocyte activation during wound healing in the syndecan-1-deficient mouse, *J Cell Sci* 115 4517–31 (2002)
2. O Okamoto et al, Normal human keratinocytes bind to the 3LG4/5 domain of unprocessed laminin-5 through the receptor syndecan-1, *J Biol Chem* 278(45) 44168–11477 (2003)
3. DJ Carey, Syndecans: Multifunctional cell-surface co-receptors, *Biochem J* 327 1–16 (1997)
4. B Vuillermoz, Y Wegrowski, JL Contet-Audonneau, L Danoux, G Pauly and FX Maquart, Influence of *aging on glycosaminoglycans and small leucine-rich proteoglycans production by skin fibroblasts, Mol Cell* Biochem 277 63–72 (2005)
5. Y Wegrowski, L Danoux, JL Contet-Audonneau, G Pauly and FX Maquart, Decreased syndecan-1 expression by human keratinocytes during skin aging, *J Invest Dermatol* 125(5), Abstracts 029 (2005)
6. L. Robert, Tissue conjonctif I Introduction, in *Précis de physiologie cutanée,* France La porte verte Eds, (1980) pp131–136
7. AM Powell, Y Sakuma-Oyama, N Oyama and MM Black, Collagen XVII/BP180: A collagenous transmembrane protein and component of the dermoepidermal anchoring complex, *Experimental Dermatol* 30 682–687 (2005)
8. NA Fenske and CW Lober, Structural and functional changes of normal aging skin, *J Am Acad Dermatol* 15 571–585 (1986)
9. RL Gallo et al, Syndecans, cell surface heparan sulfate proteoglycans, are induced by a proline-rich antimicrobial peptide from wounds, *Proc Natl Acad Sci* USA 91 11035–9 (1994)

10. P Jaakkola and M Jalkanen, Transcriptional regulation of Syndecan-1 expression by growth factors, *Progress in Nucleic Acid Research & Molecular Biology*, 63 109–138 (1999)

11. W Vogel, Discoidin domain receptors: Structural relations and functional implications, *FASEB J* 13(Suppl.) S77–S82 (1999)

12. CA Curat and WF Vogel, Discoidin Domain Receptor 1 Controls Growth and Adhesion of Mesangial Cells, *J Am Soc Nephrol* 13 2648–2656 (2002)

13. E Faraci, M Eck, B Gerstmayer, A Bosio and WF Vogel, An extracellular matrix-specific microarray allowed the identification of target genes downstream of discoidin domain receptors, *Matrix Biol* 22 373–381 (2003)

14. C Escoffier, J De Rigal, A Rochefort, R Vasselet, PG Agache and JL Leveque, Age-related mechanical properties of human skin: An in vivo study, *J Invest Dermatol* 93(3) 353–357 (1989)

15. PG Agache, Twistometry measurement of skin elasticity, in *Noninvasive Methods & Skin*, J Serup eds, Denmark: GBE Jemec (1995) pp 319–328

CHAPTER 22

From the Sea: Algal Extracts for Skin Homeostasis

Diane Bilodeau and Isabelle Lacasse
Atrium Innovations Inc., Quebec City, Quebec, Canada

KEY WORDS: *algal extracts, skin barrier improvement, free radical protection, antiaging benefits, anti-inflammatory action*

ABSTRACT: *The authors discuss the abilities of marine-derived active ingredients to protect the skin from barrier disruption, aging, free radicals and inflammation. Four marine species are examined that provide such benefits via various sulfated polysaccharides and polyphenols.*

Homeostasis refers to the ability that all living organisms possess to achieve and maintain physiological stability while facing constant environmental changes. Being at the frontier of the internal and external milieus, the skin certainly is one of the most challenged organs. Desiccants, free radicals, inflammatory mediators or even the simple passage of time are major insults capable of disrupting skin homeostasis.

Supporting Homeostasis with Marine Extracts

A global strategy for skin care must protect the skin on multiple fronts. Therein, the marine biomass has various solutions to offer. For example, the brown seaweed, *Ascophyllum nodosum*, which typically is found in the cold marine waters of the Northern Hemisphere, can easily tolerate desiccation, temperature variations and high saline water. Desiccation tolerance in algae has been linked to its capacity to increase cell wall thickness with emersion to air. As cell wall thickness increases, more polysaccharides become available for retaining water, thus decreasing the rate of dessication.[1]

Also of interest is the robust brown seaweed *Fucus serratus* that grows well on slow-draining shores where it has to protect itself from heavy wave action and sand abrasion. Not to be forgotten is the red seaweed *Palmaria palmata* found on moderately exposed rocky shores where it grows under the shade of other types of algae. *P. palmata* has developed pigments with antioxidant activity to better absorb light.[2]

Yet another promising biomass is *Enteromorpha compressa,* the marine green alga that grows abundantly in rock pools and sandy rocks. Being exposed to a high oxygen concentration in rock pools, *E. compressa* also has developed potent antioxidant mechanisms that may be linked to polycaccharides and polyphenol fractions.[3]

Each of these algae is rich in various and specific sulphated polysaccharides such as fucoidans and alginates (*A. nodosum* and *F. serratus*), carrageenans and galactans (*P. palmata*), and ulvans (*E. compressa*), that have found applications in the cosmetic industry. They also contain various polyphenols that may add to their benefits. To better characterize the cosmetic potential of these algal sources, a profile of their modulation of gene expression in skin fibroblasts and keratinocytes was established using cDNA microarray technology, as this paper describes, and the results were validated with corresponding in vitro functional assays performed on skin cells. The concurrent benefits of these ingredients were then assessed through consumer testing. Results shown here reveal that alone or in combination, these marine actives could be an answer for a global strategy to preserve skin homeostasis.

DNA Microarray: The Technique

DNA (gene) arrays are commonly used for monitoring expression levels of numerous genes simultaneously. The technique is particularly useful to decipher how cells react to a particular treatment and may give important clues as to the molecular mechanism of action of active ingredients in the cosmetic field. The protocol is fairly complex and is based on the specificity of DNA-RNA interactions.

In cells, messenger RNAs (mRNA) are molecules produced in the nucleus through transcription, as a reflection of gene activation. These mRNAs are then exported into the cytoplasm where they serve as blueprints to guide protein synthesis. The level of mRNA for a given protein varies with cellular activity.

To measure the effect of an active on the gene expression of skin cells, the mRNA content of treated cells is extracted and tagged with red fluorescence, then mixed with the mRNA content of control cells previously labeled with green fluorescence. Samples of this mixture of RNA transcripts are gently placed over an array of pre-identified microscopic DNA spots attached to a solid surface such as glass. These various DNA fragments are complementary (cDNAs) and can therefore bind, as Velcro bands[a], to their unique corresponding messenger mRNA. The end result fluorescence for each cDNA spot will obviously depend upon the ratio between red and green mRNA.

If a gene has been more activated in treated cells, the corresponding mRNA will be more abundant than in control cells, resulting in red fluorescence of the complementary cDNA spot on the array. On the opposite, gene silencing following treatment will result in green fluorescence. Should treatment have no impact on a specific gene, the corresponding spot on the array would appear as yellow, reflecting an equal amount of red and green mRNA transcripts.

In vitro Tests

To characterize the skin's response to selected marine water extracts, a fibroblast suspension was prepared and integrated into a reconstructed epidermis model. Following incubation of the co-cultures for 24 hr at 37°C, in medium containing the extract in water only or without the test compound as the control, total RNA was extracted for each culture, purified and fluorescently labeled. Microarray hybridization was assayed using a confocal laser scanner to measure fluorescence intensities, allowing simultaneous determination of the relative expression levels of all the genes represented in the array. A selection of up to 164 genes pertinent to skin physiology was grouped by clusters of physiological interest on the mini chips.

---

[a] Velcro is a product of Velcro Industries B.V.

F. serratus: The DNA array-based profiling of *F. serratus* extract points toward its role as a modulator of keratinocyte differentiation. In the presence of the extract[b] alone, gene expression of cell cytokeratins 14 and 16 was up-regulated while that of cytokeratins 1 and 10 was down-regulated (see **Table 1**). This activity is in line with the stimulation of a pro-differentiation pathway.[4]

Table 1. Results obtained with *F. serratus* extract in the reconstructed epidermis cDNA microarray experiment

Gene	Up-regulation	Down-regulation	No effect
		Effect of *F. serratus* extract	
Antigen KI-67			X
Aquaporin 3	X		
β-defensin 4	X		
Corneodesmosin	X		
Cornulin	X		
Cytokeratin 1		X	
Cytokeratin 10		X	
Cytokeratin 14	X		
Cytokeratin 16	X		
Involucrin	X		
NICE-1	X		
RNAse 7	X		
Transglutaminase K	X		

Other markers of differentiation, including corneodesmosin, cornulin, involucrin, NICE-1 and especially transglutaminase K (TGK/TGase1), were also up-regulated. TGK is an enzyme that plays an important role in the formation of the cornified layer during the differentiation of epithelial keratinocytes.[5] The lack of influence of the extract on the expression of the Ki-67 antigen, a proliferation marker, supports a rather selective effect in modulating epidermal differentiation for improved barrier function.[6] In addition, β-defensin-4 and RNAase 7 expressions were also up-regulated, indicative of *F. serratus*' potential to provide antimicrobial resistance for additional skin protection.[7]

[b] Homeo-Shield (INCI: F. serratus extract (and) glycerol) is a registered trademark of Atrium Innovations, Quebec City, Quebec, Canada.

The up-regulating effect of *F. serratus* extract on transglutaminase (TGK) gene expression has been validated at the protein level through a measure of TGK activity. Normal Human Epidermal Keratinocytes (NHEK) were incubated at 37°C for 72 hr with or without (control) the extract alone, at a concentration of 0.33%. The enzyme TGK was then extracted from cells and assayed by measuring the covalent addition of 3H-putrescin to casein. The casein was precipitated with trichloroacetic acid (TCA), the precipitates collected on filters, and the radioactivity measured by liquid scintillation.

Following *F. serratus* extract treatment, transglutaminase activity was significantly induced—5 x over control cells, p < 0.01 (see **Figure 1**). This result supports the cDNA microarray observations and demonstrates that *F. serratus* extract modulates the epithelial differentiation process.

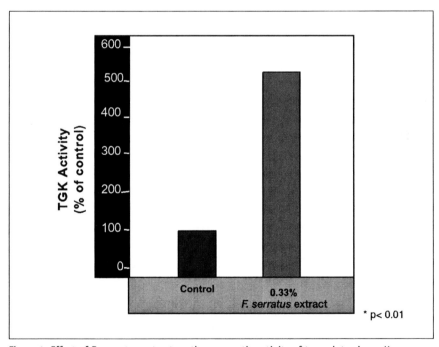

Figure 1. Effect of **F. serratus** extract on the enzymatic activity of transglutaminase K

An increase in transglutaminase activity by promoting maturation of the cornified envelope should improve skin barrier function.[5,8] This suggests *F. serratus* extract would be beneficial in skin care formulas aimed at protecting from adverse environmental influences and transepidermal water loss (TEWL).

E. compressa **and** *P. palmata:* A DNA array-based profile obtained on combined *E. compressa* and *P. palmate* water extracts[c] demonstrated that this combination synergizes to switch on gene coding for various antioxidant enzymes in aged fibroblasts and reconstructed epidermis (see **Table 2**).

Both the green *E. compressa* and the red *P. palmata* are known to develop antioxidant strategies when challenged by higher level of stress, an activity that has been associated with the presence of polysaccharides and some phenolic compounds that may also be responsible for their remarkable color.[2,3]

The gene expression of catalase, SOD 1 (cytosolic form), SOD 2 (mitochondrial form) and glutathione peroxidase was augmented in the presence of the combination of water extracts from *E. compressa* and *P. palmata*. Such a stimulation of the cellular antioxidant machinery would be expected to limit the destructive effects of reactive oxygen species (ROS).[9] The reduced expression of oxidative stress-responsive 1 (OXSR1), a stress marker whose expression normally correlates with a high concentration of ROS, further validates the free radical scavenging ability of the ingredient.

The combination of *E. compressa* and *P. palmata* extracts acts at other levels of antioxidant protection as well by increasing the gene expression of heme-oxygenase 1 (HO-1) without affecting the constitutively expressed heme-oxygenase 2. HO-1 is part of an inducible protection system that primes skin defenses against UV-induced oxidative stress.[10] Finally, the mixture's ability to induce thioredoxin could assist in protecting skin cells from UV-induced lipid peroxidation.[11] This effect on lipid peroxidation was further documented using fluorescence cytometry analysis.

Young and aged fibroblasts were both studied. It is known that cellular aging causes an increase in the endogenous formation of metabolically generated ROS, leading to significant lipid peroxidation.[12] Accordingly, the mixture[c] was tested for its efficacy in reducing the level of lipid peroxidation occurring in aged fibroblasts.

---

[c] Homeoxy (INCI: Sorbitol (and) E. compressa extract (and) P. palmata extract (and) water (aqua)) is a registered trademark of Atrium Innovations, Quebec City, Quebec, Canada.

Table 2. Results obtained with *E. compressa* and *P. palmata* extracts on the expression of antioxidant enzymes in different skin cell systems analyzed in the described cDNA microarray experiment

Gene	Aged fibroblasts			Reconstructed epidermis*
	Up-regulation	Down-regulation	No effect	Up-regulation
Catalase	X			
Glutaredoxin	X			
Glutathione peroxidase	X			
Glutathione reductase	X			
Heme oxygenase 1	X			X
Heme oxygenase 2			X	
Metal-regulatory transcription factor		X		
Oxidative stress response 1		X		
Peroxiredoxin 1	X			
SOD 1 (cytosolic)			X	X
SOD 2 (mitochondrial)	X			X
Thioredoxin		X		X
Thioredoxin reductase 1			X	

*Note: On reconstituted epidermis, up-regulation was the only observed effect

Aged cells were incubated at 37°C for 24 hr with or without (control) the test product at a concentration of 1% in water only. A probe specific for lipid peroxides was added to the culture media for 45 min and washed away. The test mixture was then reintroduced or not (control) in the culture media.

Following an additional incubation, cells were trypsinized and fluorescence measured by flow cytomety. The presence of oxidation is reflected by a decrease in the fluorescence of the probe. Results showed that the presence of the extracts significantly reduced lipid peroxidation in aged cells to a level similar to that of young cells; 41%, $p < 0.01$.

UV exposure also is known to trigger lipid peroxidation. Thus, using a similar protocol, researchers also investigated the action of the ingredient on aged fibroblasts exposed to UVA and UVB irradiation at 180 mJ/cm^2. While UV exposure caused a further increase in the level of lipid peroxidation in aged fibroblasts, a protective effect was observed in the presence of the extracts; 32%, $p < 0.01$ (see **Figure 2**).

The *E. compressa* and *P. palmata* blend allowed aged skin cells to restore their innate free radical scavenging capacity to that of younger cells, therefore limiting membrane lipid peroxidation. These activities could reduce and prevent the signs of chronological as well as actinic aging in the skin.

A. nodosum on aging: cDNA array-based profiles differ between young and aged skin fibroblasts and this fact provides information on the effects of aging in skin cell biology. Not surprisingly, genes responsible for the synthesis of structural proteins such as α-smooth muscle actin, collagen 1 and 3, cytoplasmic β-actin, decorin and lamin A, as well as genes involved in cell adhesion such as integrin beta-1 and laminin beta-1, displayed reduced expression in aged cells in the microarray experiment.

On the other hand, expression of MMP3 gene was up-regulated in these cells. MMP3 activation has been associated with the breakdown of extracellular matrix components such as collagen fibers and fibronectin during the processes of chronological and actinic aging.[13] Interestingly, incubating these aged cells in the presence of a depolymerized fucan fraction derived from *A. nodosum*[d] reverses these deleterious effects of aging, re-establishing a younger pattern of gene expression (see **Table 3**).

[d] Homeo-Age (INCI: A. nodosum extract (and) sorbitol (and) water (aqua)) is a registered trademark of Atrium Innovations, Quebec City, Quebec, Canada.

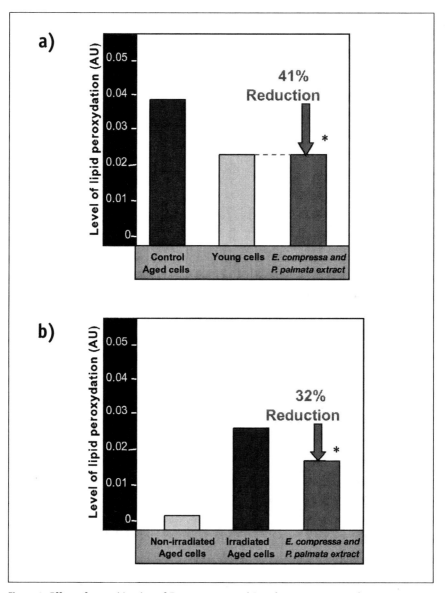

Figure 2. Effect of a combination of **E. compressa** and **P. palmata** extract on a) metabolically- and b) UV-induced lipid peroxidation

Table 3. Results obtained with A. nodosum fraction, enriched in depolymerized fucans, in an aged-cell cDNA microarray experiment

Gene	Effect of cellular aging[1]			Reversal effect of extract[2]	
	Up-regulation	Down-regulation	No Effect	Up-regulation	Down-regulation
α-smooth muscle actin		X		X	
Collagen 1 α-1		X		X	
Collagen 3 α-1		X		X	
Cytoplasmic β-actin		X		X	
Decorin		X		X	
Glutathione reductase		X		X	
HSP 27		X		X	
Integrin β-1		X		X	
Lamin A		X		X	
Laminin β-1		X		X	
MMP3	X				X
Plasminogen activator inhibitor 1			X		X

[1] Effect of aging on gene expression: Aging mainly translates into a down-regulation of mRNA transcript levels of genes coding for important functional and structural proteins
[2] Effect of A. nodosum fraction, enriched in depolymerized fucans, on the reversion of aging-induced modulation of gene expression

The rejuvenating potential of the *A. nodosum* fraction was confirmed when aged cells were found to recover their lost responsiveness to growth factors such as epidermal growth factor (EGF) while grown in the presence of the extract. EGF is naturally produced in the body where, among other things, it stimulates skin cell production, an effect that is diminished with aging.[14] In a proliferation assay, EGF was used to stimulate cell turnover in young and aged fibroblasts.

Aged and young cells were seeded at low density and incubated for 72 hr in the presence or not (control) of EGF, with and without (control) the tested 0.1% in water extract. Supernatants were removed, cells were rinsed and cell nuclei were stained by incubating with Hoechst dye solution. After extensive washing, analysis of the labeling by nuclei count was performed with a cell analyzer.

As expected, and contrary to young cells, aged cells initially did not respond to the presence of the growth factor; however, addition of an extract derived from *A. nodosum* restored the responsiveness of aged cells to EGF, as revealed by an increase in proliferation capacity (see **Figure 3**).

The proliferation assay results obtained with *A. nodosum* are in line with the cDNA profiling and support a rejuvenating potential for this active; it may help to restore the integrity of the extracellular matrix, especially at the dermal-epidermal junction, and it may also promote optimal cell turnover and increase the rate of skin renewal to a level normally associated with younger age.

A. nodosum on inflammation: A different fraction[e] of *A nodosum*, this time enriched in nondepolymerized fucans, was shown to reduce inflammatory activity.

To reproduce inflammatory conditions, keratinocytes were stimulated with phorbol 12-myristate 13-acetate (PMA). In response to such stress, cells normally release prostaglandin E2 (PGE2), a lipid involved in inflammatory reactions.[11] However, when keratinocytes were stressed with PMA ($0.1\mu g/mL$) in the presence of the active water extract at 0.6%, PGE_2 production was reduced by 60%, $p < 0.01$ (see **Figure 4**). PGE_2 production was measured from the culture supernatant using an ELISA detection system.

---

[e] Homeo-Soothe (INCI: A. nodosum extract (and) sorbitol (and) water (aqua)) is a registered trademark of Atrium Innovations, Quebec City, Quebec, Canada.

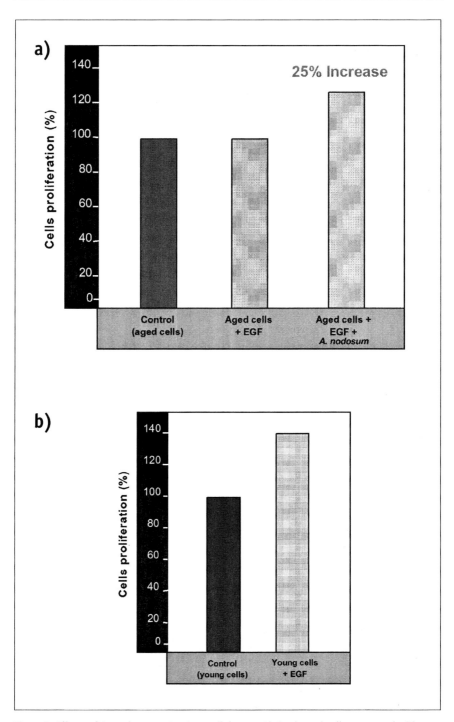

Figure 3. Effects of **A. nodosum** extract on cellular growth in a) aged cells, compared with b) a young cell control and young cells treated with only EGF

In accordance with this result, the active derived from a fraction of *A. nodosum* enriched in nondepolymerized fucans could be used to protect the skin from harmful inflammatory responses that may result from environmental insults such as chemical or UV exposure.

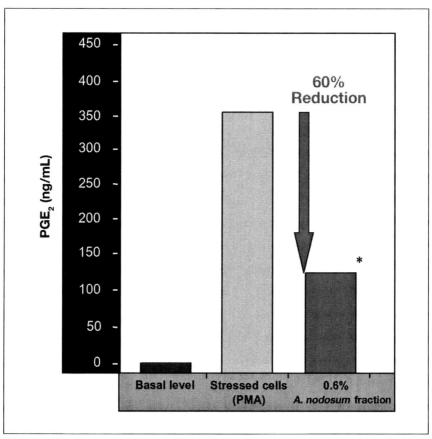

Figure 4. Effect of **A. nodosum** fraction, enriched in nondepolymerized fucans, on stress-induced production of PGE2.

In vivo Tests

The compatibility and complementarity of the described ingredients in combination[f] were evaluated using consumer assessments. Such tests make it possible to directly identify and evaluate the benefits generated to the end users.

[f] The Homeosta-SEA line of ingredients is a registered trademark of Atrium Innovations, Quebec City, Quebec, Canada.

For the first consumer test, a panel of 105 women aged 40–75 years was asked to apply a daily regimen consisting of two different cosmetic formulations for a period of 28 days. The tested day cream contained 0.5% nondepolymerized *A. nodosum* plus 0.5% of the combined *E. compressa* and *P. palmata* extract (**Formula 1**), while the night cream contained 0.5% depolymerized *A. nodosum* plus 1% *F. serratus* extract (**Formula 2**).

Formula 1. Antiaging day cream

A. Cetearyl glucoside (and) cetearyl alcohol	1.5% w/w
Glyceryl stearate	1.0
Sodium cetearyl sulfate	0.3
Squalene	1.0
Dicaprylyl carbonate	2.0
Dicaprylyl ether	2.0
Paraffinum liquidum (mineral) oil	5.0
Dimethicone	1.0
Sodium polyacrylate	1.0
B. Glycerin	3.0
Water (*aqua*)	qs to 100.00
Preservative	0.7
C. *A. nodosum* extract (and) sorbitol (and) water (*aqua*) (Homeo-Soothe, Atrium)	0.5
Sorbitol (and) *E. compressa* extract (and) *P. palmata* extract (and) water (*aqua*) (Homeoxy, Atrium)	0.5

Procedure: Heat A and B to 80°C. Add B to A and slowly cool to 60°C. Homogenize until sodium polyacrylate is dispersed and begin cooling to ambient temperature. Add C and mix until homogeneous. Viscosity: 41,000cps; Brookfield RVF#6–10 rpm 25°C.

Formula 2. Antiaging night cream

A. Cetearyl glucoside (and) cetearyl alcohol		1.5% w/w
Glyceryl stearate		1.0
Sodium cetearyl sulfate		0.3
Squalene		1.0
Dicaprylyl carbonate		2.0
Dicaprylyl ether		2.0
Paraffinum liquidum (mineral) oil		5.0
Dimethicone		1.0
Sodium polyacrylate		1.0
B. Glycerin		3.0
Water (*aqua*)		qs to 100.00
Preservative		0.7
C. *A. nodosum* extract (and) sorbitol (and) water (*aqua*) (Homeo-Age, Atrium)		0.5
F. serratus extract (and) glycerol (Homeo-Shield, Atrium)		0.5

Procedure: Heat A and B to 80°C. Add B to A and slowly cool to 60°C. Homogenize until sodium polyacrylate is dispersed and begin cooling to ambient temperature. Add C and mix until homogeneous. Viscosity: 44,500cps; Brookfield RVF#6–10 rpm 25°C.

Subjects were asked to evaluate the benefits of the cream formulations with respect to defined criteria linked to the appearance of signs of aging such as wrinkles, skin tone and skin firmness. The rationale supporting potential antiaging effects for these specific cream formulations relied on the presence of ingredients with anti-irritant and antioxidant activities—i.e., *F. serratus* extract plus *E. compressa* and *P. palmata* extract, respectively—in the day cream, and ingredients with metabolic-enhancing and skin barrier replenishing activities—depolymerized *A. nodosum* and *F. serratus* extract, respectively—in the night cream. The regimen performance is summarized in **Figure 5**. An overall satisfaction of 84% was reported after 28 days and this particular regimen was reported to reduce the appearance of wrinkles, improve skin texture and complexion, and to protect the skin from dehydration.

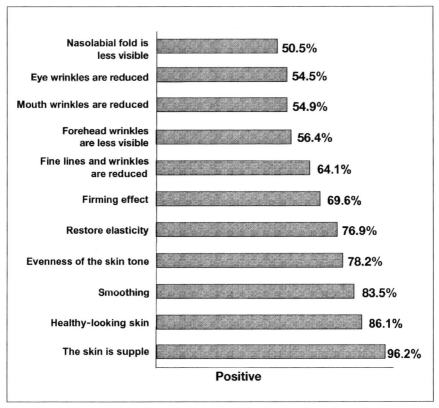

Figure 5. Self-appreciation of a twice daily application of the described algae extract regimen cream formulations on the appearance of signs of aging

In a second consumer test, the soothing effect of a different regimen was self-assessed by subjects presenting a general sensitive skin as evaluated by a dermatologist. This test cream incorporated 0.5% nonde-polymerized *A. nodosum* extract, and 0.5% of the combined *E. compressa* and *P. palmata* extract plus 0.5% *F. serratus* extract (**Formula 3**).

The rationale behind testing this formulation was that sensitive skin expresses pro-irritant, pro-oxidant and defective barrier compo-nents.[16] A panel of 102 women with sensitive skin, aged 18–50 years, used the test cream formulation twice daily for a period of 28 days. Results were reported as a self-assessment of the formulation's efficacy toward signs of skin sensitivity such as tingling sensations being reduced, soothing and calming effects (see **Figure 6**). Results showed that 85% of the consumers were satisfied with the soothing cream after 28 days of use, with reports that skin better resisted aggressions and protected sensitive skin from inflammatory reactions.

Formula 3. Soothing cream

A. Cetearyl glucoside (and) cetearyl alcohol	1.5% w/w
Glyceryl stearate	1.0
Sodium cetearyl sulfate	0.3
Squalene	1.0
Dicaprylyl carbonate	2.0
Dicaprylyl ether	2.0
Paraffinum liquidum (mineral) oil	5.0
Dimethicone	1.0
Sodium polyacrylate	1.0
B. Glycerin	3.0
Water (*aqua*)	qs to 100.00
Preservative	0.7
C. *A. nodosum* extract (and) sorbitol (and) water (*aqua*) (Homeo-Sooth, Atrium)	0.5
F. serratus extract (and) glycerol (Homeo-Shield, Atrium)	0.25
Sorbitol (and) *E. compressa* extract (and) *P. palmata* extract (and) water (*aqua*) (Homeoxy, Atrium)	0.5

Procedure: Heat A and B to 80°C. Add B to A and slowly cool to 60° C. Homogenize until sodium polyacrylate is dispersed and begin cooling to ambient temperature. Add C and mix until homogeneous. Viscosity: 36,500cps; Brookfield RVF#6–10 rpm 25°C.

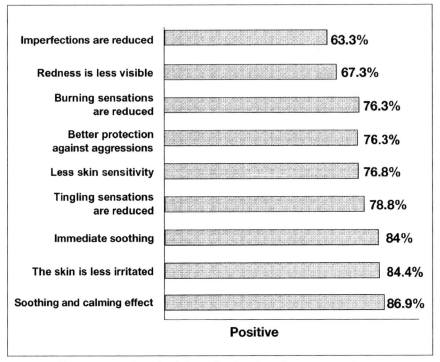

Figure 6. Self-appreciation of a twice daily application of an algae extract regimen cream formulation on sensitive skin parameters

Conclusion

Each ingredient from the discussed line of algal extracts shows a biological activity profile addressing at least one major threat to skin homeostasis. *F. serratus* extract, for example, could be used to protect the epidermal barrier; *E. compressa* and *P. palmata* extracts exhibited free radical scavenging affects; and the profiles of a depolymerized fucan fraction of *A. nodosum*, as well as a different fraction of *A. nodosum*, are indicative of reversing the signs of aging and controlling pro-inflammatory mediators in the skin, respectively. The specificity and complementarity of these ingredients suggest their use alone or in combination to aid skin health and appearance. The proposed line of algal extracts represents an armamentarium for the formulation chemist wishing to develop finished products endowed with defined biological mechanisms of action while respecting the delicate skin homeostasis.

Published April 2008 *Cosmetics and Toiletries* magazine

References

1. AD Boney, Biology of marine algae, *Hutchinson Educational Ltd*, London (1969)
2. YV Yuan, MF Carrington and NA Walsh, Extracts from dulse (*P. palmata*) are effective antioxidants and inhibitors of cell proliferation in vitro, *Food Chem Toxicol* 43(7) 1073–81 (2005)
3. AD Ansell, RN Gibson and M Barnes, Oceanography and marine biology, an annual review, *UCL Press,* London (1998)
4. C Jacques, AM de Aquino and M Ramos-e-Silva, Cytokeratins and dermatology, *Skinmed* 4(6) 354–60 (2005)
5. K Hitomi, Transglutaminases in skin epidermis, *Eur J Dermatol* 15(5) 313–9 (2005)
6. T Scholzen and J Gerdes, The Ki-67 protein: From the known and the unknown, *J Cell Physiol* 182(3) 311–22 (2000)
7. F Niyonsaba and H Ogawa, Protective roles of the skin against infection: Implication of naturally occurring human antimicrobial agents beta-defensins, cathelicidin LL-37 and lysozyme, *J Dermatol Sci* 40(3) 157–68 (2005)
8. T Hirao, A novel non-invasive evaluation method of cornified envelope maturation in the stratum corneum provides a new insight for skin care cosmetics, *IFSCC Magazine* 6(2) 103–109 (2003)
9. DR Bickers and M Athar, Oxidative stress in the pathogenesis of skin disease, *J Invest Dermatol* 126(12) 2565–75 (2006)
10. M Allanson and VE Reeve, Immunoprotective UVA (320–400 nm) irradiation up-regulates heme oxygenase-1 in the dermis and epidermis of hairless mouse skin, *J Invest Dermatol* 122 1030–1036 (2004)
11. Y Nishinaka, H Nakamura, H Masutani and J Yodoi, Redox control of cellular function by thioredoxin: A new therapeutic direction in host defense, *Arch Immunol Ther Exp (Warsz)* 49(4) 285–92 (2001)
12. J Vinson and S Anamandla, Comparative topical absorption and antioxidant effectiveness of two forms of coenzyme q10 after a single dose and after long-term supplementation in the skin of young and middle-aged subjects, *IFSCC Magazine* 8(4) 287–92 (2005)
13. P Brenneisen, H Sies and K Scharffetter-Kochanek, UVB irradiation and matrix metalloproteinases: From induction via signaling to initial events, *Ann N Y Acad Sci* 973:31–43 (2002)
14. KT Tran, SD Rusu, L Satish and A Wells, Aging-related attenuation of EGF receptor signaling is mediated in part by increased protein tyrosine phosphatase activity, *Exp Cell Res* 289(2) 359–67 (2003)
15. JN Lawrence, JJP Dally and DJ Benford, Measurement of eicosanoid release in keratinocyte cultures to investigate skin irritation and tumour promoting activity, *Toxicol in vitro* 9(3) 285–290 (1995)
16. M Lebwohl and LG Herrmann, Impaired skin barrier function in dermatologic disease and repair with moisturization, *Cutis* 76(6 Suppl) 7–12 (2005)

CHAPTER 23

A DNA Repair Complex to Decrease Erythema and UV-induced CPD Formation

Giorgio Dell'Acqua
Dellacqua Consulting, Vevey, Switzerland

Kuno Schweikert
Induchem AG, Volketswil, Switzerland

KEY WORDS: *UV, DNA repair, cyclobutane pyrimidine dimer, proline, tyrosine, erythema*

ABSTRACT: *The authors describe how a DNA-repair complex based on amino acids decreases UV-induced DNA damage in reconstituted human skin and reduces related skin inflammation in human volunteers.*

Solar radiation such as UVA and UVB induces physiological damage in the skin. Photoaging is a classic example of UV-induced wrinkle formation and thinning of the skin. This phenotype change reflects a deeper impact at the molecular level, in particular on the DNA double helix present in each cell nucleus. The cumulative effect of repeated damage strongly contributes to the development of DNA mutations and down-regulates proteins essential to maintain normal skin turnover.

Prominent among UV-induced lesions on DNA are cyclobutane pyrimidine dimers (CPDs) formed between adjacent pyrimidines on the same DNA strand exposed to UVB (280–320 nm) irradiation[1]

(**Figure 1**). Pyrimidine dimers alter the biological function of DNA and are a major cause of lethal,[2] transformational[3] and tumorigenic[4] events induced by UV exposure. UV-induced CPDs may be repaired by enzymatic processes, or by a light-dependent reaction mediated by electron transfer.[5] Importantly, the repairing mechanism decreases with aging, contributing to increased mutational risk.[6,7]

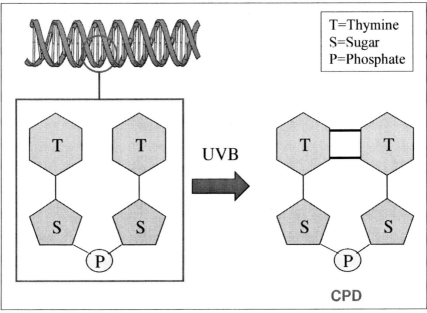

Figure 1. Environmental aggressions such as UVB lead to formation in the DNA filament of cross-linked dimers between adjacent thymines, such as cyclobutane pyrimidine dimers (CPDs)

Furthermore, studies in cell lines and in animals have demonstrated a link between DNA damage and erythema formation.[8,9] Mediators of inflammation such as NF-kB, IL-6, IL-10 and TNF-α were induced by CPDs,[10,11] and the reduction of these inflammatory mediators was stimulated by mechanisms that increase CPD repair.[10–12] In vivo studies on animals such as knockout and transgenic mice further proved that when enzymes essential to DNA repair were over-expressed or deleted, a clear correlation with the onset of UV-induced skin erythema was evidenced.[13,14] Studies on the kinetics of CPD removal in humans revealed that the number of CPDs in the epidermis is significantly decreased three days after UV exposure, and CPDs were almost entirely removed 10 days after UV irradiation.[15]

In order to increase the natural repairing mechanism of the skin, Induchem has previously formulated a DNA-repairing bioactive complex[a] to boost the natural repairing mechanism of the skin. The repair activity of the complex is due to the presence of a high amount of amino acids such as acetyl tyrosine and proline (see **Figure 2**).[16] Acetyl tyrosine has shown interesting redox properties[17] and is a target for phosphorylation of many kinases involved in the DNA repairing mechanism.[18] Proline has been shown to be a survival factor in plants and fungi[19,20] and also to have redox properties.[17] Proline is also a target for protein kinases in the repairing pathway, especially for the so-called proline-directed protein kinases.[18] The combination of acetyl tyrosine and proline promotes an increase of the natural repairing mechanism.

The study presented here shows that treatment of reconstituted human skin with the repair complex[a] (TRC) decreases the formation of UVB-induced CPDs and dramatically reduces UV light-induced erythema in the skin of human volunteers.

Materials and Methods

Ruling out a UV absorbance effect: In order to rule out a possible sunscreen-like effect of TRC, given the aromatic nature of some of the active ingredients, a UV absorbance test was performed; TRC at different concentrations was compared to a UV filter. No UV absorbance on the whole spectrum was observed, while the sunscreen filter fully absorbed the UV light as expected (data not shown). The authors therefore excluded a possible protection effect due to UV absorbance capacity.

Reconstituted human skin model study: The reconstituted human skin model[b] was chosen to test the effect of UVB on CPD formation,[21] and the influence of treatment with TRC on DNA repair efficacy. Readout was performed by immunohistological staining for CPD-positive cell nuclei and the results were documented by microscopic photography.

---

[a] Unirepair T-43 (INCI: Acetyl tyrosine (and) proline (and) hydrolyzed vegetable protein (and) adenosine triphosphate) is a product of Induchem.

[b] 0.5 cm2, aged day 17, Skinethic, France

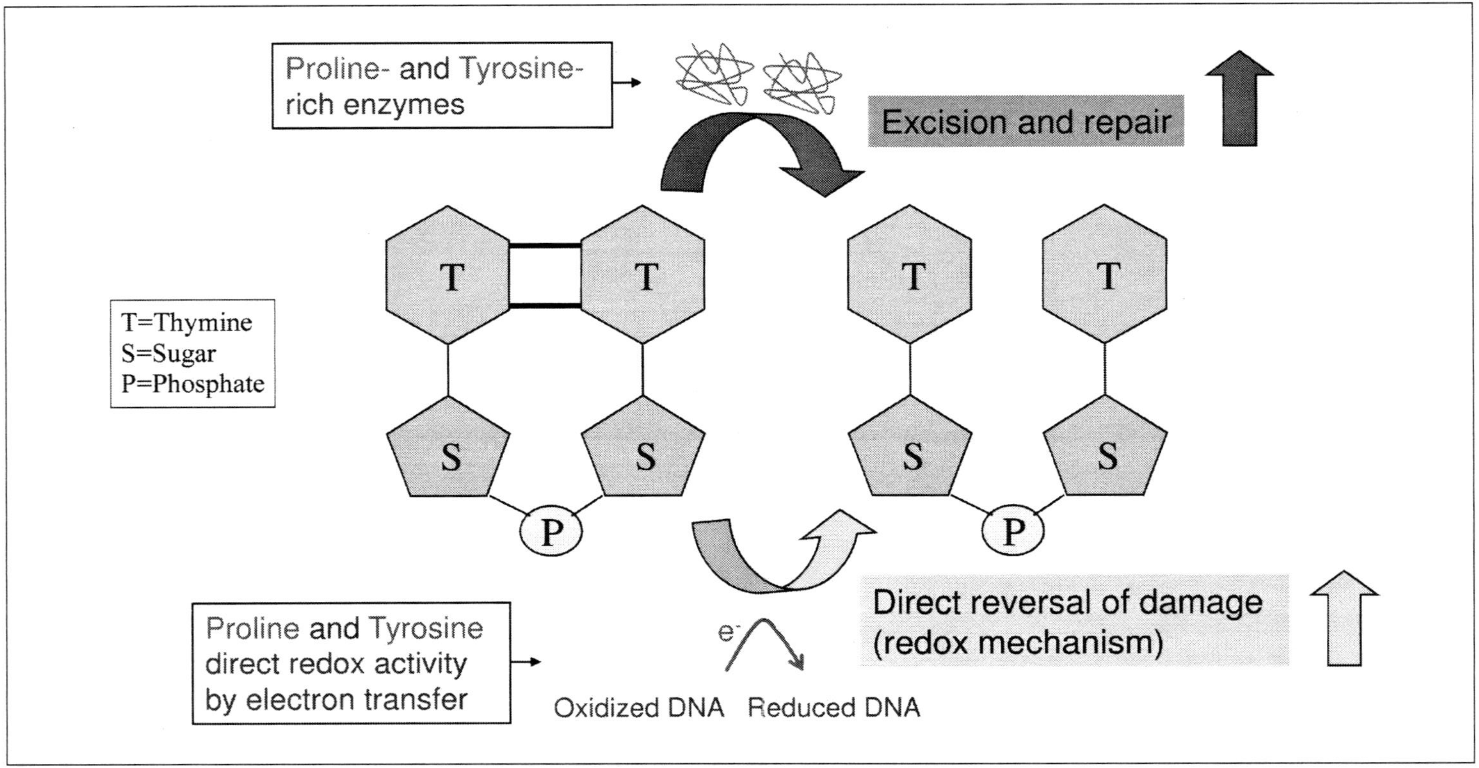

Figure 2. Amino acids such as tyrosine and proline have direct and indirect action in DNA repairing steps. Directly, both amino acids have shown electron transfer capacity to decrease oxidative damage. Indirectly, they are precursors of enzymes, such as proline-directed protein kinases, that are phosphorylated during the repairing mechanism.

TRC was applied on the skin 20 min before UVB irradiation (300 mJ/cm^2) in two different concentrations (1% or 3%, diluted in medium). After irradiation the skin models were fixed in 10% formalin solution (0.3 hr later) or incubated with 1% or 3% of TRC for further 5 hr and then fixed. Irradiated but untreated controls were performed in parallel. TRC was present on the skin for the whole experiment to simulate the in vivo condition. The timeline of the experiment on reconstituted human skin is given in **Figure 3**.

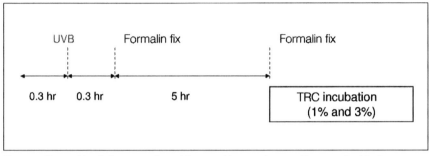

Figure 3. Time table of the reconstituted human skin experiment; skin treated with the repair complex (TRC) was compared to untreated skin.

The skin models were fixed in 10% formalin solution at 4°C for at least 24 hr and subsequently embedded in paraffin. Sections of each prepared skin model were cut 4 μm thick and subjected to immunohistochemical detection of CPDs in the epidermal cell nuclei.

Sections were extracted from paraffin by incubation at 65°C for 30 min and immersion in xylene followed by rehydration (immersion in 100%, 90%, 70% ethanol for 2 min each).

After a mild alkaline hydrolysis, sections were dehydrated and incubated with proteinase K at 37°C for 15 min. Incubation with the primary monoclonal antibody[c] was performed at 4°C overnight. The primary antibody was washed off with tris-buffered saline (TBS) and sections were treated with the secondary antibody goat antimouse IgG conjugated with a signal enhancer polymer labeled with alkaline phosphatase (AP) molecules[d].

---

[c] 1:400, Anti-Thymine Dimer, clone KTM53, mouse IgG, Kamiya Biomedical Company, Seattle, Washington, USA

[d] DAKO Diagnostika GmbH, Hamburg, Germany. DAKO is a registered trade name

Sections were then incubated in a fuchsin substrate/chromogen solution[e] for 8 min; color reaction was stopped by rinsing with aqua bidest. AP-fuchsin substrate/chromogen yields a fuchsin red-colored reaction product at the site of the target antigen.

After staining, the sections were microscopically photographed and evaluated by quantitative and qualitative analysis.

Quantification (score) of cyclobutane pyrimidine dimers: The number of stained CPD-positive cells in the cut sections was determined microscopically. For each model, CPDs were counted in five different locations on the section using a 40x objective[f]. In addition, the signal intensity of each positive nucleus was rated as strong (score value 3), middle (score value 2) or weak (score value 1), and then the CPDs with each of the score values were counted. Representative areas were also documented by photography with 220x and 880x magnification[g].

Both the number and intensity of the stained nuclei were used to calculate the Total CPD Score of each skin model according to the following expression:

$$\text{Total CPD Score} = 3N_S + 2N_M + N_W$$

where N_S is the number of strong stained nuclei, N_M is the number of middle stained nuclei, and N_W is the number of weak stained nuclei.

The Total CPD Score of irradiated but untreated skin models directly after irradiation (t0) was set as maximal damage or 100% (all nuclei stained positive, intensive signals).

Because there were two models per treatment (1% and 3% TRC) per time point (0.3 hr and 5 hr), mean values were calculated and standard deviations were given.

Human volunteers study: Twenty-five volunteers were selected and informed about the importance and meaning of the study. Written informed consent was obtained from all the subjects prior to entry into the trial.

---

[e] DAKO Diagnostika GmbH, Hamburg, Germany
[f] Olympus CK40 microscope, 400x magnification.
[g] Microscope: DXC-950 OP, Olympus; Video documentation: Sony Deutschland GmbH

The following criteria were used for subject inclusion in the study: clinically healthy and older than 18 years. Criteria for exclusion included skin diseases, pregnancy, uneven skin tone, sunburn, scars or lesions in the test area and Fitzpatrick skin phototype greater than III. The subjects of this study were between 27 and 58 years of age (average: 39.8). They could withdraw from the study at any time without giving any reason. Subjects were instructed not to use any topical preparations on the inner forearms starting from seven days prior to testing and until the end of the test. For cleansing, only water or a mild syndet[h] was allowed during the entire study, including the run-in phase.

Each volunteer's inherent reactivity to UV radiation was assessed by a series of UV exposures of varied time intervals given at six spots on the forearm one day prior to the test. Each spot had a diameter of 0.8 cm. The time intervals selected were a geometric series, in which each exposure was 25% greater than the previous exposure. The irradiated sites were assessed 16–24 hr after irradiation and the provisional MED for unprotected skin was determined. The provisional MED was used as indicator from which to determine the exposure times required in the main test.

When this step was complete, the provisional MED (adaptation time: 30 min, room temperature: 21±1°C, relative humidity: 50±5%) had been determined and the required irradiation times had been calculated to achieve a centered final MED.

The next step was induction of erythema and measurement of redness. Three test areas (untreated, placebo, test product) on one of the forearms of each volunteer were delineated with a skin marker. Subsequently, a staff member applied the test cream (**Formula 1A**) with 3% TRC to one test area and a placebo cream (**Formula 1B**) to the second test area, while leaving the third area untreated. Each dose was approximately 2 mg/cm^2; it was checked for loss by weighing and spread for 40 sec with a presaturated finger cot.

After a waiting period of 20 min, all tested areas were irradiated with UV light[k], adjusted to 125% of MED. Skin redness (representing erythema) was measured 24 and 48 hr after UV irradiation (adaptation time: 30 min; room temperature: 21±1°C; relative

---

[h] Eubos flüssig – blau, manufactured by Dr. Hobein, Meckenheim-Merl, Germany. Eubos is a registered trade name.
[k] Solar Light Model 601-300 Multiport

humidity: 50± 5%) with a color meter[m] as a positive change on the green-red (a*) axis of a three-dimensional color coordinate system.

Before each measuring series, the instrument was calibrated against the standard white tile. Measurements were performed according to the guidelines of the Standardization Group of the European Society of Contact Dermatitis.[22]

Data were analyzed using the Student's t-test. The timeline of the experiment on human volunteers is given in **Figure 4**.

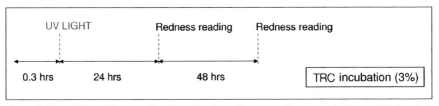

Figure 4. Time table of the experiment on the inner forearms of human volunteers. Skin treated with the repair complex (TRC) cream was compared to skin treated with a placebo cream or to untreated skin.

[m] Chromameter CR 400, Minolta, Japan

Formula 1. Cream used in the test of erythema reduction

	A Test (% w/w)	B Placebo (% w/w)
Water (aqua)	85.20	88.20
Octyldodecyl neopentanoate	4.00	4.00
Octyldodecanol	3.00	3.00
Butylene glycol* (and) acetyl tyrosine (and) proline (and) hydrolyzed vegetable protein (and) adenosine triphosphate (Unirepair T-43, Induchem)	3.00	0.00
Butylene glycol	2.00	2.00
Myristyl myristate	1.00	1.00
Acrylates/C10-30 alkyl acrylate crosspolymer	0.58	0.58
Phenoxyethanol (and) methylparaben (and) ethylparaben (and) propylparaben (and) butylparaben (and) isobutylparaben (Uniphen P-23, Induchem)	1.00	1.00
Sodium hydroxide	0.07	0.07
Fragrance (parfum)	0.15	0.15
	100.00	100.00

* This butylene glycol is the solvent for the Unirepair T-43 actives. It represents 17.5% of the complex, or approximately 0.5% of Formula 1A.

Results

As shown in **Figure 5**, pretreatment of reconstituted human skin for 20 min with TRC at 3% before UVB irradiation followed by 5 hr of further incubation with TRC significantly reduces both the number and intensity of CPDs. This is particularly evident in the skin's basal layer (see arrows). CPD quantitative scoring (**Figure 6**) shows that at all time points from UVB irradiation the skin treated with TRC at 1% and 3% has significantly less DNA damage, and therefore a better repair rate, when compared to irradiated but untreated control. This difference reached 50% at 5 hr with 3% TRC treatment and was statistically significant ($p < 0.05$, Student's t-test). These results confirm previously published effects of TRC on the same model when applied after UVB irradiation.[16]

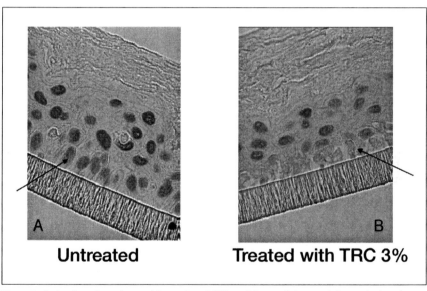

Untreated   **Treated with TRC 3%**

Figure 5. Reduction of number and intensity of CPD positive nuclei, especially at the basal layer (see arrow), in reconstituted human skin treated with the repair complex (TRC) versus an untreated equivalent. Red staining indicates CPD positive nuclei after UVB irradiation at 300 mJ/cm².

In human volunteers, pretreatment of inner forearm skin for 20 min with a cream containing TRC at 3% significantly ($p < 0.001$, Student's t-test) reduced the parameter a* (erythema index), measured quantitatively by color meter (**Figure 7**). This decrease was observed after 24 hr and 48 hr from UV light irradiation and was −36.8%

and –51.6%, respectively, when compared to the treatment with the placebo cream. The data represented an average from 25 volunteers.

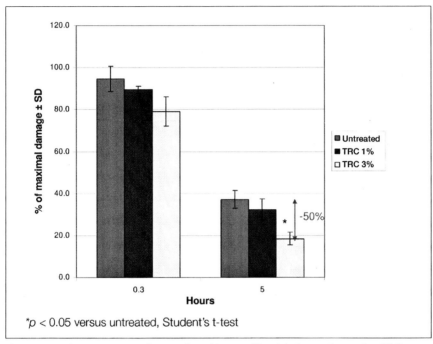

Figure 6. 20 min pretreatment of reconstituted human skin with the repair complex (TRC) followed by UVB radiation decreases maximal damage by 50% when compared withuntreated skin.

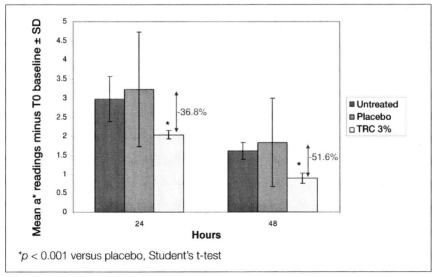

Figure 7. Skin redness in human volunteers after treatment with a placebo cream or a cream containing the repair complex (TRC) at 3% followed by UV irradiation. * indicates green-red color

Discussion and Conclusion

The repair complex[a] (TRC) discussed in this article has been shown to decrease the damaging effect of UV solar radiation both in a reconstituted skin model and in vivo on the inner side of the arm of human volunteers. It accelerated the removal of CPDs in the reconstituted skin model and it drastically reduced erythema formation on the arm of human volunteers.

Although this set of experiments did not prove a direct link between CPDs formation and erythema development, several published papers[10–14] suggest a strong association between DNA damage repair and erythema formation, concluding that protection or repair from UV-induced DNA damage would inhibit or reduce skin erythema development. Based on these observations the current authors believe that the erythema reduction that occurred on human volunteers after pretreatment with TRC followed by UV irradiation is due to the capacity of TRC to accelerate repair of CPDs and therefore to reduce DNA damage and the consequent triggering of the inflammation reaction. Further study of CPDs in vivo would be needed to fully demonstrate this hypothesis.

The repairing nature of TRC is also supported by previous studies in human reconstituted skin where the complex was applied 5 hr after UVB exposure and showed the same pattern of efficacy, i.e., an increased removal of CPDs when compared to control.[16]

Skin pretreatment of human volunteers with TRC before UV exposure was chosen instead of an aftertreatment. This decision was based on the longest time of compound absorbance by the skin in vivo compared to the human reconstituted skin model where the absorbance is faster.[23] Therefore, the compound was allowed more time in vivo to penetrate the skin in order to fully perform its repairing function.

Based on these results, one can conclude that TRC is strongly suggested when developing products that fight UV-induced DNA damage and products formulated to reduce or prevent erythema (sunburn) after sun exposure.

The usefulness of TRC is further highlighted by recent interest in products that would help the skin respond to the deleterious effect of UV light by increasing the mechanisms that help to repair damage at the molecular level, such as oxidation of DNA, protein and lipids. The combination of TRC with sunscreen filters in a formulation would assure a better protection from the effect of UV-induced oxidation.

It is possible, in fact, that sunscreen products would not assure a complete screening of UV, especially when final SPF is not elevated, typically in day creams. The authors have recently demonstrated that an SPF 20 cream is not able to avoid UV-induced down regulation of oxidation repairing enzymes (data not published yet), demonstrating a "leaking" of protection by UV sunscreens.

In these situations, products like TRC would help the skin to react to UV light not screened by the filter. In the future, further products to help repair or protect oxidized protein and lipids would ideally complement TRC to ensure a better skin reaction to UV light. Some of these products are in current development at Induchem and will be presented shortly.

Finally TRC has proven to be compatible and easy to formulate in various cosmetics forms, being water-soluble and stable at pH values ranging from 4 to 8. Moreover, skin patch tests (TRC 10%) and repeated insult patch tests (RIPT) in human volunteers have proved the safety profile of TRC (data not shown).

The authors conclude that TRC could be used as a pretreatment or an aftertreatment in day products to act immediately against UV-induced skin oxidation and in night products to help recovery and repair.

Published May 2008 *Cosmetics and Toiletries* magazine

References

1. RB Setlow, Cyclobutane-type pyrimidine dimers in polynucleotides, *Science* 153(734) 379–386 (1966)

2. H Harm, Repair of UV-irradiated biological systems: photoreactivation, In *Photochemistry and Photobiology of Nucleic Acids,* vol 2, SY Yang, ed, New York, NY: Academic Press 219–262 (1976)

3. BM Sutherland, NC Delihas, RP Oliver and JC Sutherland, Action spectra for ultraviolet light-induced transformation of human cells to anchorage-independent growth, *Cancer Res* 41(6) 2211–2214 (1981)

4. R Hart, RB Setlow and AD Woodhead, Evidence that pyrimidine dimers in DNA can give rise to tumors, *Proc Natl Acad Sci USA* 74(12) 5574–5578 (1977)

5. L Roza L, FR de Gruijl, JB Bergen Henegouwen, K Guikers, H van Weelden, GP van der Schans and RA Baan, Detection of photorepair of UV-induced thymine dimers in human epidermis by immunofluorescence microscopy, *J Invest Dermatol* 96(6) 903–907 (1991)

6. Y Takahashi, S Moriwaki, Y Sugiyama, Y Endo, K Yamazaki, T Mori, M Takigawa and S Inoue, Decreased gene expression responsible for post-ultraviolet DNA repair synthesis in aging: a possible mechanism of age-related reduction in DNA repair capacity, *J Invest Dermatol* 124(2) 435–442 (2005)

7. M Yamada, MU Udono, M Hori, R Hirose, S Sato, T Mori and O Nikaido, Aged human skin removes UVB-induced pyrimidine dimers from the epidermis more slowly than younger adult skin in vivo, *Arch Dermatol Res* 297(7) 294–302 (2006)

8. AA Vink and L Roza, Biological consequences of cyclobutane pyrimidine dimers, *J Photochem Photobiol B* 65(2–3) 101–104 (2001)

9. DB Yarosh, DNA repair, immunosuppression and skin cancer, *Cutis* 74(5 Suppl) 10–13 (2004)

10. C Petit-Frère, PH Clingen, M Grewe, J Krutmann, L Roza, CF Arlett and MHL Green, Induction of interleukin-6 production by ultraviolet radiation in normal human epidermal keratinocytes and in a human keratinocyte cell line is mediated by DNA damage, *J Invest Dermatol* 111(3) 354–359 (1998)

11. P Wolf, H Maier, RR Mullegger, CA Chadwick, R Hofmann-Wellenhof, HP Soyer, A Hofer, J Smolle, M Horn, L Cerroni, D Yarosh, J Klein, C Bucana, K Dunner Jr, CS Potten, H Honigsmann, H Kerl and ML Kripke, Topical treatment with liposomes containing T4 endonuclease V protects human skin in vivo from ultraviolet-induced upregulation of interleukin-10 and tumor necrosis factor-α, *J Invest Dermatol* 114(1) 149–156 (2000)

12. H Stege, L Roza, AA Vink, M Grewe, T Ruzicka, S Grether-Beck and J Krutmann, Enzyme plus light therapy to repair DNA damage in ultraviolet-B-irradiated human skin, *Proc Natl Acad Sci USA* 97(4) 1790–1795 (2000)

13. W Schul, J Jans, YMA Rijksen, KHM Klemann, APM Eker, Jan de Wit, O Nikaido, S Nakajima, A Yasui, JHJ Hoeijmakers and GTJ van der Horst, Enhanced repair of cyclobutane pyrimidine dimers and improved UV resistance in photolyase transgenic mice, *Embo J* 21(17) 4719–4729 (2002)

14. RJW Berg, HJT Ruven, AT Sands, FR de Gruijl and LHF Mullenders, Defective global genome repair in XPC mice is associated to skin cancer susceptibility but not with sensitivity to UVB induced erythema and edema, *J Invest Dermatol* 110(4) 405–409 (1998)

15. SK Katiyar, MS Matsui, and H Mukhtar, Kinetics of UV light-induced cyclobutane pyrimidine dimers in human skin in vivo: an immunohistochemical analysis of both epidermis and dermis, *Photochem Photobiol* 72(6) 788–793 (2000)

16. K Schweikert, W McGregor, C Klein and G Dell'Acqua, Amino acids to increase DNA repair after UVB irradiation of reconstituted human skin, *SOFW J* 132(11) 22–26 (2006)

17. JR Milligan, JA Aguilera, A Ly, NQ Tran, O Hoang and JF Ward, Repair of oxidative DNA damage by amino acids, *Nucleic Acids Res* 31(21) 6258–6263 (2003)

18. K Bender, C Blattner, A Knebel, M Iordanov, P Herrlich and HJ Rahmsdorf, UV-induced signal transduction, *J Photochem Photobiol B* 37(1–2) 1–17 (1997)

19. C Chen and MB Dickman, Proline suppresses apoptosis in the fungal pathogen *Colletotrichum trifolii, Proc Natl Acad Sci USA* 102(9) 3459–3464 (2005)

20. PP Saradhi, S Alia Arora and KVSK Prasad, Proline accumulates in plants exposed to UV radiation and protects them against UV induced peroxidation, *Biochem Biophys Res Commun* 209(1) 1–5 (1995)

21. JP Therrien, M Rouabhia, EA Drobetsky and R Drouin, The multilayered organization of engineered human skin does not influence the formation of sunlight-induced cyclobutane pyrimidine dimers in cellular DNA, *Cancer Res* 59(2) 285–289 (1999)

22. A Fullerton, T Fisher, A Lahti, KP Wilhelm, H Takiwaki and J Serup, Guidelines for measurement of skin colour and erythema. A report from the standardization group of the European Society of Contact Dermatitis, *Contact Derm* 35(1) 1–10 (1996)

23. FP Schmook, JG Meingassner and A Billich, Comparison of human skin or epidermis models with human and animal skin in in vitro percutaneous absorption, *Int J Pharm* 215(1–2) 51–56 (2001)

CHAPTER 24

Macroalgae in Nutricosmetics

J.H. Fitton, PhD, and M. Irhimeh, PhD
Marinova, Hobart, Tasmania

KEY WORDS: *nutricosmetic, macro- and microalgae, anti-inflammatory, anti-glycation, tyrosinase inhibition*

ABSTRACT: *Ingested macroalgae and its extracts can provide antiaging benefits such as inhibition of matrix enzymes, glycation, inflammatory activity and elastin calcification. Here, the authors investigated macroalgal extracts on insulin levels of test subjects to determine whether they could control glucose levels.*

Nutricosmetics are specific macro- and micronutrients that are orally delivered to help provide positive changes in the quality of the skin and general appearance. Dietary intake has clear connections with skin health and can even limit UV-induced damage.[1]

Macroalgae contains a number of components including micronutrients, carotenoids, fucoidan, vitamin K and omega-3 lipids that are known to provide inhibitory effects on skin damage.[2]

There is a well-known disparity between skin aging in Japanese women who include macroalgae in their diet compared with Causcasian women of the same age who generally do not ingest macroalgae.[3] Environmental factors responsible for these differences include sun exposure and diet.

In general, fucoidan and fucoxanthin products derived from seaweed are appearing more often on the market. As whole macroalgae and its extracts gain an increased presence in the nutraceutical sector, its untapped potential for the antiaging market as a detoxifying ingredient and micronutrient provider is being realized, in addition to its use in topical cosmetic preparations.

In a previous article, the authors described the historical use and current applications of macroalgae and a bioactive extract, fucoidan, as ingredients in skin care and spa products.[4] In addition to its cosmetic role, macroalgae has long provided mankind with sources of food and medicine and offered certain specific benefits as nutricosmetics. This article outlines the nutricosmetic benefits of macroalgae and discusses the potential for these natural ingredients to be utilized in the development of novel formulations.

Iodine: Essential Bioactive for Health, Beauty

Macroalgae and its extracts are commonly found in food products. The Asian diet is especially rich in macroalgae based products such as the red macroalga *Porphyra* or nori, the brown alga *Undaria* or wakame, and another brown macroalga *Laminaria sp.* or kombu. All of these macroalgae make excellent food supplements, being nutrient and micronutrient dense, with protein yields exceeding 30% in some cases.

Iodine and other trace elements tend to be more concentrated in perennial kelps,[5] for example, and protein contents are highest in edible species such as *Porphyra* and *Ulva*.[2] Macroalgae also contain all the essential amino acids, omega-3 lipids and soluble fiber,[2] as well as a wide variety of bioactives including lipid-modulating, blood pressure-lowering and glucose metabolism-modifying compounds.[4] For instance, small peptides found in the brown macroalga *Undaria pinnatifida* have angiotensin-converting enzyme (ACE)-inhibitory activity, which lowers blood pressure.[6]

Micronutrient supplementation is essential to supporting normal healthy skin. Key micronutrients in this area include zinc, selenium and iodine. Macroalgae is a particularly rich source of iodine, and also contributes to selenium and zinc intake. Iodine is a trace element essential for synthesis of the thyroid hormones triiodothyronine and thyroxine, which affect processes and pathways mediating the intermediary metabolism of carbohydrates, lipids and proteins in almost all tissues, including skin.[7]

Selenium is also necessary for the formation of these important hormones. Individuals suffering from thyroid hormone deficiencies also often experience dry skin and thinning hair. Recent research has demonstrated a marked effect of topically applied thyroid hormone on hair density and epidermal proliferation in a mouse model.[8]

Most studies conducted on thyroid hormone tissue effects tend to concentrate on lipid metabolism. The use of iodine supplements for weight loss has been popular in both Western and Asian cultures for centuries. Eating seaweed was a popular Victorian remedy for weight loss, according to the popular Mrs. Grieves.[9] In addition, there are several traditional Chinese medicines that include macroalgae, such as "concoction of the Jade flask," which includes the brown macroalgae species *Ecklonia* and *Sargassum* and is used to treat goiter, a condition in which the thyroid gland is enlarged due to iodine deficiency.[10]

Today in the Western market, generally the most common use of whole macroalgae in nutraceuticals is as iodine supplements. It is important for manufacturers to consider the iodine levels in products since concentrations vary widely in the different species, from relatively low levels in *Porphyra* and *Undaria* (up to 50 micrograms/g), to extremely high levels (thousands of micrograms/g) in some kelps.[5]

The upper limit for intake is 300 micrograms/day and the upper limit for toxicity is 1,000 micrograms/day.[11] In some countries such as Australia, iodine intake is low or marginal due to its paucity in the soil, and supplementation is probably wise.[12] It is important to note that iodine-containing supplements should not be taken by persons already diagnosed with thyroid deficiencies except on the advice of their medical practitioner.

Vitamin K for Youthful Skin

Macroalgae also contains vitamins and other bioactive components. Brown, red and green macroalgae can provide vitamins A, B and C in modest dietary amounts.[2] These vitamins are essential for healthy skin—for example, vitamin C is necessary for collagen production[1] while the vitamin B group controls homocysteine levels.[13]

Vitamin K or phylloquinone is often overlooked as an essential vitamin for maintenance of elasticity and capillary integrity in skin, and recent studies have emphasized its critical role for the inhibition of elastin degradation. Vitamin K is a required coenzyme for the carboxylation of the amino acid glutamic acid in a small protein called matrix Gla protein or MGP.[14]

This carboxylated protein is essential in inhibiting the calcification and subsequent degradation of elastin fibers. Elastin is an elastic matrix component of vascular tissues and skin. The integrity of elastin is an important feature of youthful and healthy tissues. Degradation of elastin by proteases may also lead to the induction of inflammatory processes or so called *inflamm-aging*.[15]

Dried seaweeds have very high vitamin K content; for example, dried wakame contains 1,293 µg/100 g, as compared with broccoli, at 305 µg/100 g.[16] This fat-soluble vitamin is best taken orally where the entire benefit can be realized. Thus, orally delivered dried macroalgae could make good nutricosmetic elastin support ingredients.

Carotenoids to Inhibit UV-induced Damage

The active components of macro-algae include pigments such as polyphloroglucinols and carotenoids such as fucoxanthin. Many of these have antioxidant qualities and contribute to the antioxidant nature of aqueous and nonaqueous extracts. Additionally, they are antimutagenic and protect against environmental damage.[17]

It has been found that UV-induced skin damage can be ameliorated by dietary means. Components that confer some protection include carotenoids, tocopherols, ascorbate, flavanoids and omega-3 fatty acids.[1] Beta-carotene, lycopene, phytotene, phytofluene and lutein have all been identified in epidermal and dermal layers. They provide some protection from UV-induced skin damage, especially in combination with other antioxidants and immunoprotectives.[1] Carotene, phytotene, phytofluene and lutein are all found in edible macroalgae such as *Porphya*, wakame and kombu. Indeed, excess intake of beta-carotene derived from the red alga *Porphyra* is expressed as carotenodermia, an orange color in the skin.[16]

However, the main antioxidant found in brown macroalgae is fucoxanthin.[18] Fucoxanthin and its derivative, fucoxanthinol, have marked protective effects against inflammation in vitro, and also a profound antiobesity effect in animal models and in vitro.[19, 20] This component offers significant promise as a nutricosmetic ingredient.

Glutathione, an antioxidant that is sometimes used as an orally delivered skin whitening agent, is a constituent of all macroalgae, with some species containing as much as 3,082 µg/100g.[21] Additionally, omega-3 fatty acids such as stearidonic acid and hexadecatetraenoic acid are found in edible marine algae such as *Undaria pinnatifida* and *Ulva*, contributing up to 40% of the plants' total fatty acid content.[22]

Enzyme Inhibition to Reduce Skin Aging

One of the major effects of UV-induced damage is increased elastase activity in the skin. Thus the inhibition of this enzyme could increase the overall elasticity of the skin when combined with the elastin-sparing activity of vitamin K. Macroalgae can provide ample activity in both these areas.

Fucoidan fractions, alginates and phloroglucinols isolated from marine algae have enzyme inhibitory properties against hyaluronidase, heparanases, phospholipase A2, tyrosine kinase and collagenase expression.[23–27] Profound antiviral activity against coated viruses such as herpes and HIV is exhibited by the sulphated polysaccharides found in macroalgae.[28, 29]

Fucoidans are known to have substantial activity on dermal elements within in vitro models. For example, fucoidan acts to enhance dermal fibroblast proliferation and deposition of collagen and other matrix factors.[30] Matrix metalloproteases that modulate connective tissue breakdown are inhibited by low molecular weight fucoidan due to increased association with its inhibitors. In addition, the serine protease leukocyte elastase was inhibited, thus protecting the elastic fiber network in human skin cultures.[31] Tyrosinase is also inhibited by fucoidan fractions, indicating its potential for inclusion as whitening agents,[32] an effect additional to that of glutathione.

Current Fucoidan Research

Marinova has developed a solvent-free coldwater process to extract fucoidan and is currently developing purified, organically certified extracts from a range of brown macroalgae species sourced from Tasmania, Nova Scotia, Tonga and Patagonia.

Over the last six years, the company has funded research into fucoidan, including work by Irhimeh et al., that has demonstrated a low but significant serum uptake of a high molecular weight *Undaria* derived fucoidan using a novel antibody technique.[33] This finding was important since it confirmed that systemic effects can be attributed to serum uptake, even from a high molecular weight fucoidan.

Irhimeh et al. also demonstrated a profound increase in the sticky receptor CXCR4 on blood stem cells, attributed to the fucoidan extract. This increase was accompanied by healthy changes in cholesterol levels and an increase in the immune regulating cytokine interferon gamma.[34] The significant effects of orally ingested fucoidan suggest potential for rejuvenation nutraceuticals, designed to give the body a boost of immune function.

The company is now carrying out a long term project to determine the effects of macrolgal fractions on matrix enzyme (elastase) activity and glycation, with a particular focus on cosmetics and nutricosmetics.

Glycation is one of the determinants of skin aging. High or irregular blood glucose levels and high insulin levels all correlate with higher levels of glycation. Matrix and serum protein components are gradually glycated in a nonenzymatic process—similar to the browning process that takes place during cooking. The end products of the glycation process are known as advanced glycation end products or AGEs.

In a previous report,[4] data was discussed on fucoidan extracts with alpha-glucosidase activity. The action of alpha-glucosidase inhibitors is to delay carbohydrate absorption, reducing the post-prandial increase in blood glucose.[35] *Undaria* and *Fucus vesiculosus* fucoidans were found to be particularly efficacious since they inhibited the activity of alpha-glucosidase by 50% at a concentration of less than 20 µg/mL, in comparison with luteolin that inhibited alpha-glucosidase activity at approximately 18 µg/mL.

In the previous report,[4] researchers hypothesized that this inhibitory action on alpha-glucosidase would be reflected in reduced insulin levels in serum. In data reported here, the authors investigated insulin levels as a determinant of glucose control and thus potential for glycation.

Methodology

Insulin levels in volunteer blood samples were quantitatively measured using insulin kits and an insulin analyzer[a]. The sole restriction was that volunteers were not to have ingested seafood.

This method is a solid-phase, two-site chemiluminescent immunometric assay. The reference fasting range used for the study is 6-27 μIU/L. The insulin levels were tested in a group of volunteers (n = 10) after receiving the active treatment of 75% *Undaria fucoidan*, 3 g/day, divided into three one-gram doses, for a total of 12 days. The insulin was tested only at two points: baseline and 12 days from receiving the active treatment. Another group of volunteers (n = 3) who received the placebo-control treatment was also tested for insulin levels at the same test points (see **Figure 1**).

[a] Immulite 2500 insulin kits and the Immulite 2500 analyzer are products of Diagnostic Products Corp., A Siemens Company, Calif. USA.

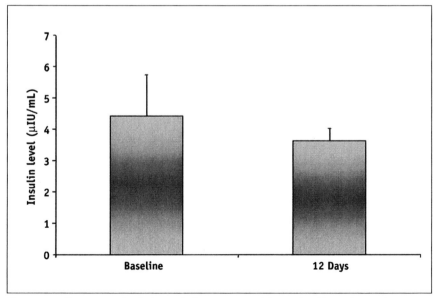

Figure 1. Insulin concentration before and after treatment with 75% fucoidan active; each point represents the average of 10 different individuals (5 male and 5 female) ± MSE

Results

No change in the average insulin level was found in the placebo group and only a slight decrease was found in the average insulin level of the active treatment group. The slight decrease in insulin levels, however, does suggest that fucoidan extract could act as an inhibitor of glycosidase and reduced glucose loads; yet, this trial was not sufficiently powered to achieve a statistically significant result in healthy adults.

The nutricosmetic area is still modest and relatively underdeveloped. While various fish collagen-based preparations including some vitamin blends have been around for a while, overall there is a much smaller market presence. Further research is definitely warranted.

Anti-inflammatory Fucoidans

Fucoidan is a well-known anti-inflammatory agent with potential for inclusion in nutricosmetics with an antiaging or sunscreen focus. Marinova is currently in clinical trials in this area to investigate the immunomodulatory and anti-inflammatory properties of fucoidans of interest for nutriceutical and nutricosmetic developers. These trials aim to underline the relevance of fucoidans as anti-inflammatory and antiaging ingredients. The trials are being managed and designed by professor Stephen Myers, founding director of the Australian Centre for Complimentary Medicine Education and Research and one of Australia's leading alternative medicine researchers and practitioners.

As explained in the previous article,[6] fucoidans can be considered to be a dietary fiber and are nontoxic in cell culture. No toxicological changes were observed in rats administered up to 300 mg/kg of fucoidan from *Laminaria japonica* orally. Anticoagulant effects were observed at doses of 900 to 2,500 mg/kg, but no other signs of toxicity were observed.[36] Marinova has also undertaken a safety trial in cancer patients in Australia and demonstrated that ingestion of up to 6 g per day of fucoidan has no observable side effects. This study is currently unpublished.

Conclusion

Macroalgae and its extracts are novel nutricosmetic ingredients that can provide cosmetic antiaging benefits such as inhibition of matrix enzymes, glycation inhibition and anti-inflammatory activity, in addition to inhibition of elastin calcification. While macroalgae remain a staple of the spa industry, fucoidan-rich macroalgal extracts have strong potential for commercial success in cosmetics. Key components include fucoidan, vitamin K, minerals and trace elements and carotenoids.

From a consumer's point of view, it tends to take longer to generate beneficial effects on skin through oral supplements, although the effects may be longer-lasting. It is more difficult to market a product that requires persistence and this may account for limited research currently in the nutricosmetics area. Combination products offering two levels of effect—topical, more immediate effects, plus orally administered, longer-term effects—may make more of an impact on consumers.

The nutraceutical world generally does not focus on taking skin measurements as part of clinical studies on supplements, although some supplements likely generate benefits for the skin. As the market matures, the industry may see more of a focus on the health of skin via nutrition.

Published May 2008 *Cosmetics and Toiletries* magazine

References

1. H Sies and W Stahl, Nutritional protection against skin damage from sunlight, *Annu Rev Nutr* 173–200 (2004)
2. S Aaronson, Algae, in *The Cambridge World History of Food*, K Kiple and KC Ornelas, eds, Cambridge University Press, Cambridge, UK, Vol I, Ch. II.C.I 231–249 (2000)
3. K Tsukahara et al, Comparison of age-related changes in wrinkling and sagging of the skin in Caucasian females and in Japanese females, *J Cosmet Sci* 55(4) 351–71 (Jul/Aug 2004)
4. JH Fitton, M Irhimeh and N Falk, Macroalgal fucoidan extracts: A new opportunity for marine cosmetics, *Cosm & Toil* 122, 55–64 (2007)
5. J Teas, S Pino, A Critchley and LE Braverman, Variability of iodine content in common commercially available edible seaweeds, *Thyroid* 14, 836 (2004)
6. K Suetsuna and T Nakano, Identification of an antihypertensive peptide from peptic digest of wakame (*Undaria pinnatifida*), *J Nutr Biochem* 11(9) 450–4 (Sep 2000)
7. M Moreno, P de Lange, A Lombardi, E Silvestri, A Lanni and F Goglia, Metabolic effects of thyroid hormone derivatives, *Thyroid* 18(2) 239–53 (Feb 2008)
8. JD Safer et al, Thyroid hormone action on skin: Diverging effects of topical versus intraperitoneal administration, *Thyroid* 13(2) 159–65 (Feb 2003)

9. M Grieve, *A Modern Herbal*, Dover Publications Inc., New York (1971)

10. C Tseng, Algal biotechnology industries and research activities in China, *J Appl Phycol* 13, 375 (2001)

11. European Commission Web site, Safe upper intake levels for vitamins and minerals, available at: *http://ec.europa.eu/food/food/labellingnutrition/supplements/documents/denmark_annex2.pdf* (Accessed Mar 28, 2008)

12. M Li et al, Are Australian children iodine deficient? Results of the Australian National Iodine Nutrition Study, *Med J Aust* 184(4) 165–9 (Feb 20, 2006)

13. P Gisondi, F Fantuzzi, M Malerba and G Girolomoni, Folic acid in general medicine and dermatology, *J Dermatolog Treat* 18(3) 138–46 (2007)

14. D Gheduzzi et al, Matrix Gla protein is involved in elastic fiber calcification in the dermis of *Pseudoxanthoma elasticum* patients, *Lab Invest* 87(10) 998–1008 (Oct 2007)

15. F Antonicelli, G Bellon, L Debelle and W Hornebeck, Elastin-elastases and inflamm-aging, *Curr Top Dev Biol* 79 99–155 (2007)

16. M Kamao et al, Vitamin K content of foods and dietary vitamin K intake in Japanese young women, *J Nutr Sci Vitaminol* (Tokyo) 53(6) 464–70 (Dec 2008)

17. Y Okai, K Higashi-Okai, Y Yano and S Otani, Identification of antimutagenic substances in an extract of edible red alga, *Porphyra tenera* (Asakusa-nori), *Cancer Lett* 100(1-2) 235–40 (Feb 27, 1996)

18. Y Nishimura, N Ishii, Y Sugita and H Nakajima, A case of carotenodermia caused by a diet of the dried seaweed called Nori, *J Dermatol* 25(10) 685–7 (Oct 1998)

19. X Yan et al, Fucoxanthin as the major antioxidant in *Hijikia fusiformis*, a common edible seaweed, *Biosci Biotechnol Biochem* 63(3) 605–607 (1999)

20. H Maeda et al, Fucoxanthin from edible seaweed, *Undaria pinnatifida*, shows antiobesity effect through UCP1 expression in white adipose tissues, *Biochemical and Biophysical Research Communications* 332, 392–397 (2005)

21. H Maeda, M Hosokawa, T Sashima, N Takahashi, T Kawada and K Miyashita, Fucoxanthin and its metabolite, fucoxanthinol, suppress adipocyte differentiation in 3T3-L1 cells, *Int J Mol Med* 18(1)147–52 (Jul 2006)

22. M Kakinuma, CS Park and H Amano, Distribution of free L cysteine and glutathione in seaweeds, *Fisheries Science* 67, 194 (2001)

23. T Katsube, Y Yamasaki, M Iwamoto and S Oka, Hyaluronidase-inhibiting polysaccharide isolated and purified from hot water extract of *Sporophyll of Undaria pinnatifida*, *Food Sci Technol Res* 9, 25 (2003)

24. CR Parish, DR Coombe, KB Jakobsen, FA Bennett and PA Underwood, Evidence that sulphated polysaccharides inhibit tumour metastasis by blocking tumour cell derived heparanases, *Int J Cancer* 40, 511 (1987)

25. T Shibata, K Nagayama, R Tanaka, K Yamaguchi and T Nakamura, Inhibitory effects of brown algal phlorotannins on secretory phospholipase A_2s, lipoxygenases and cyclooxygenases, *J Appl Phycol* 15, 61 (2003)

26. M Wessels, G Konig and A Wright, A new tyrosine kinase inhibitor from the marine brown alga *Stypopodim zonale*, *J Nat Prod* 62, 927 (1999)

27. MJ Joe et al, The inhibitory effects of eckol and dieckol from *Ecklonia stolonifera* on the expression of matrix metalloproteinase-1 in human dermal fibroblasts, *Biol Pharm Bull* 29(8) 1735–9 (Aug 2006)

28. DJ Schaeffer and VS Krylov, Anti-HIV activity of extracts and compounds from algae and cyanobacteria, *Ecotoxicology and Environmental Safety* 45, 208 (2000)

29. KD Thompson and C Dragar, Antiviral activity of *Undaria pinnatifida* against herpes simplex virus, *Phytother Res* 18, 551 (2004)

30. R O'Leary et al, Fucoidan modulates the effect of transforming growth factor (TGF) - β1 on fibroblast proliferation and wound repopulation in in vitro models of dermal wound repair, *Biol Pharm Bull* 27(2) 266–270 (2004)

31. K Senni et al, Fucoidan, a sulfated polysaccharide from brown algae, is a potent modulator of connective tissue proteolysis, *Arch Biochem Biophys* 1 445(1) 56–64 (Jan 2006)

32. XJ Kang, FX Wang, CM Sheng and Y Zhu, *Undaria pinnatifida* stem fucoidan biological activity of the composition and bioactivity, *Chinese Pharmaceutical Journal* 41(22) 1748-1750 (2006)

33. MR Irhimeh, JH Fitton, RM Lowenthal and P Kongtawelert, A quantitative method to detect fucoidan in human plasma using a novel antibody, *Methods Find Exp Clin Pharmacol* 27(10) 705–710 (Dec 2005)

34. MR Irhimeh, JH Fitton and RM Lowenthal, Fucoidan ingestion increases the expression of CXCR4 on human CD34+cells, *Exp Hematol* (2007) (in press)

35. HP Rang, MM Dale and JM Ritter, *Pharmacology*, 3rd edn. Churchill Livingstone, New York (1995)

36. N Li, Q Zhang and J Song, Toxicological evaluation of fucoidan extracted from *Laminaria japonica* in Wistar rats, *Food Chem Toxicol*, 43 421 (2005)

CHAPTER 25

Lightening, Boosting and Protecting with Colorless Carotenoids

Liki von Oppen-Bezalel

IBR Ltd., Ramat Gan, Israel

KEY WORDS: *phytoene, phytofluene, colorless carotenoids, antiaging, SPF booster, anti-inflammatory, brightening, whitening*

ABSTRACT : *Phytoene and phytofluene (P&P) are carotenoids that are precursors in the biosynthetic pathway of other carotenoids. These materials occur naturally in microorganisms, algae and other plants and exhibit benefits for skin care including skin lightening, anti-inflammatory activity and protection against UV and oxidative damage, as is shown here.*

Biologically, carotenoids are a significant group of organic pigments with more than 700 members. They are found widely throughout nature but are synthesized only by plants, algae, fungi and bacteria, where they aid in the absorption of light and capture excessive energy, neutralizing tissue-damaging free radicals.[1] Chemically, carotenoids are isoprenoid, C-40 molecules that are either linear or cyclized at one or both ends of the molecule. The chemical structure determines their physico-chemical properties and biological activity.

Carotenoids, specifically β-carotene and lycopene, were used as a treatment against photosensitization as early as 1964.[2] Since then, a vast number of studies have shown that carotenoids act as antioxidants, anti-inflammatories and antimutagenic agents. These materials also are believed to potentially inhibit certain cardiovascular diseases and cancers. In addition, many carotenoids show beneficial immunological effects. Thus, these molecules are of interest for protective applications against premature aging and age-related disorders resulting from oxidative damage and stress.

Unfortunately, most carotenoids are sensitive to light, a property that considerably limits their use and shortens the shelf life of products that contain them.[3] In addition, most carotenoids have a distinctive visible color that is undesirable in most cosmetic and some food applications. In contrast to other carotenoids, however, phytoene and phytofluene (P&P) lack visible color and absorb light in the ultraviolet (UV) range. They are also precursors in the biosynthetic pathway of other carotenoids (see **Figure 1**).

Phytoene has been shown to act as an anticarcinogen in mouse skin cancer models[4] and may play a role in cell-to-cell communication, as some studies with phytoene-producing transgenic mice have suggested.[5] In addition, dietary P&P accumulate in human skin,[6] offering protection by acting as UV absorbers, antioxidants and anti-inflammatory agents, suggesting they could play a protective role in beauty and skin applications.

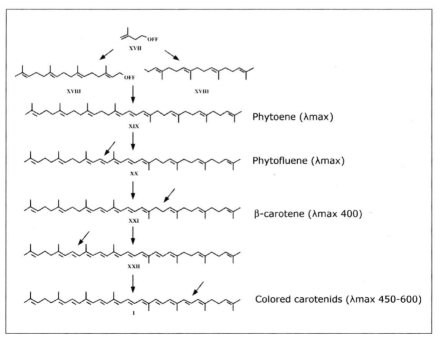

Figure 1. The biosynthetic pathway of carotenoids, where phytoene and phytofluene are the first precursors

Bioavailability and Tissue Distribution

Dietary carotenoids are found in most human tissues including the blood and skin.[1, 7-11] The distribution of carotenoids throughout the human body is not uniform; for example, higher concentrations are found in the skin, compared with the lungs, plasma or lymphocytes. In addition, P&P accumulate in greater amounts than other carotenoids.[9] Interestingly, the carotenoid content found within the human body also is notably greater than the content found in foods containing the molecule.[12]

UV Protection

UV radiation generates reactive oxygen species (ROS) and free radicals, which lead to DNA damage, lipid peroxidation, inflammation, collagen degradation and more, resulting in premature skin aging and potential skin cancer. UV irradiation causes DNA damage in two primary ways:

1. UVB damages DNA directly. Energy from sunlight causes an alteration in the chemical composition of the nucleotide bases, altering the molecular structure and disrupting DNA transcription; and

2. UVA causes damage indirectly. Here, the sunlight itself does not change the physical structure of DNA but rather triggers an array of molecules in the cell to break down in turn producing free radicals and ROS. These mutagenic agents can cause alterations in the physical structure of DNA.

P&P[a] carotenoids can be employed to protect skin from UVA and UVB damage since phytoene has been shown to absorb UVB, while phytofluene absorbs UVA (see **Figure 2**). Together, they reduce UV transmission through partial absorption by reflecting or emitting light (see **Figure 3)**. Mathews-Roth has demonstrated that carotenoids and phytoene specifically have photo-protective capabilities and can prevent UV-induced skin cancer.[4, 13-15]

---

[a] Phytoene and phytofluene are nutraceutical beauty supplements in the product Phytofloral TP and topical active ingredients in IBR-TCLC and IBR-CLC.

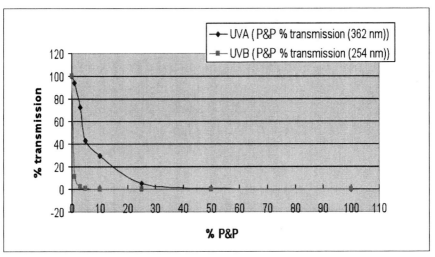

Figure 2. Transmission of UVB and UVA by P&P

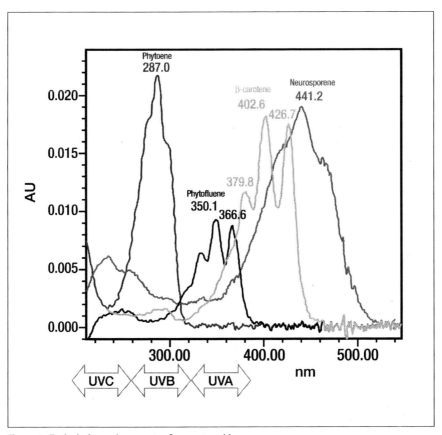

Figure 3. Typical absorption spectra for carotenoids

Hydroxyl Radical Quenching

Hydroxyl radicals play a significant role in UV damage and are several levels of magnitude more reactive toward cellular constituents than superoxide radicals and hydrogen peroxide. This type of free radical can be formed from $\cdot O_2^-$ and H_2O_2 via the Harber Weiss reaction, which generates hydroxyl radicals from hydrogen peroxide and superoxide. The interaction of copper or iron with H_2O_2 also produces $\cdot OH$, as first observed by Fenton.

These reactions are significant, because the constituents ($\cdot O_2^-$, H_2O_2 and H_2O) are found within the body and on the skin, and can easily interact to generate damaging free radicals.[16] Sunlight is a source for topical generation of hydroxyl radicals, as was demonstrated by Taira et al.[17] This group suggested that skin exposed to sunlight may lead to hydroxyl radical generation and simultaneous lipid peroxidation.

P&P are some of the few antioxidants that show efficacy in quenching hydroxyl radicals ($\cdot OH$) by trapping and neutralizing them, as the DPPH assay in **Figure 4** shows; however, they are more then antioxidants, as their comparison with BHT shows in **Figure 5**.[18–20]

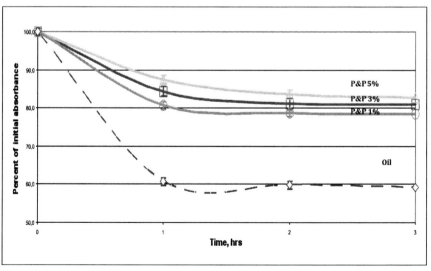

Figure 4. Hydroxyl radical scavenging activity of colorless carotenoids as shown by quenching of 1,1-diphenyl-2-picrylhydrazyl (DPPH)

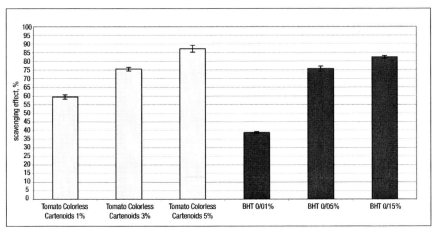

Figure 5. DPPH Scavenging activity comparing colorless carotenoids with BHT (courtesy of IBR Ltd.)

Anti-inflammation and DNA Damage

UVB light induces erythema formation. However, colorless carotenoids have been shown to significantly reduce the expression of inflammatory markers interleukin-6 and interleukin-12 in activated lymphocytes[18] as well as reduce inflammation and potentially sun-damaged cells.[18-22] Specifically, a 46% reduction in PGE-2 expression in interleukin-1-induced normal human fibroblasts has been observed.[21] The anti-inflammatory activity of P&P carotenoids could thus reduce erythema formation.

Other studies have show a reduction of UV-induced erythema with a dietary intake of a combination containing the colorless carotenoids P&P.[7, 23, 24] In most of these studies, researchers noted that added protection was likely due to the ability of P&P to absorb UV light, providing additional protection against UV-generated free radicals.[3, 7, 24-27]

Another detrimental effect of free radicals formed by UVA/UVB is collagen degradation, which leads to the premature skin aging expressed by wrinkles and loss of skin elasticity and shine. In vitro studies have shown that P&P are able to inhibit MMP-1 expression—which is involved in the breakdown of the extracellular matrix—at the low concentration of 15 µg/mL by 14%, a mild but significant effect. Therefore, P&P carotenoids could reduce the downstream collagen degradation effect of UV light.[21]

P&P also have demonstrated protective effects against DNA damage caused by hydroxyl radicals formed in vitro. This was measured by a reduction in fluorescence derived from biotinylated base pairs introduced to a reaction system following free radical damage to plasmid DNA. The DNA was protected by P&P, as shown by the change in fluorescence level indicated in **Table 1,** as well as following repair (not shown).

Table 1. P&P protection against damage to plasmid DNA caused by free radicals[13]

Compound	Conc. µg/mL	% inhibition in the presence of hydroxyl radicals	% non-specific inhibition	% specific inhibition	Concentration giving 50% of activity
Phytoene	140	86	24	62	
and	14	74	19	55	11.2 µg/mL
phytofluene	1.4	6	7	1	
	0.14	1	1	0	
Postive	1000	88	9	79	
control	100	69	11	58	80 µg/mL
	10	5	0	5	
	1	4	0	4	

These findings are in accord with an intervention study conducted by Porinni et al.[9] with carotenoids from natural tomato extract containing mostly lycopene, phytoene, phytofluene and β-carotene. This study showed modification of plasma and lymphocyte levels and improved antioxidant protection against DNA damage to lymphocytes with increasing values of plasma and lymphocyte carotenoid levels, especially in the case of phytoene.

Skin Brightening with P&P

Human skin tone varies between fair to dark brown. Skin type, according to the Fitzpatrick scale, ranges from I to VI with the higher numerals indicating darker, ethnic skin tones. Although these darker types are more resistant to sun irradiation, they are also at risk for skin cancer.

Differences in skin color are primarily determined by the amount of melanin present in melanocytes. Melanin production is stimulated by UVA light, leading to a tanning effect in skin. Aging, exposure to sun, hormonal abnormalities and various skin disorders increase the deposition of melanin pigment in skin, resulting in dark spots and freckles. These pigmented spots are undesired in many cultures and also considered unhealthy.

To eliminate pigmentation on skin or achieve a lighter skin tone, whitening or bleaching compositions are useful. Typical lightening agents in cosmetic formulations include kojic acid, arbutin, licorice extract and vitamin C. These are effective tyrosinase inhibitors and antioxidants but tend to be unstable since they are easily oxidized and degraded. Moreover, these compounds carry a higher risk for potential skin irritation and inflammation.

A combination of P&P has demonstrated efficacy on skin pigmentation by reducing the melanin content in skin cells.[20] In addition, these natural carotenoids have not been shown to cause adverse effects when applied to skin or taken orally. An example of a skin-lightening formulation incorporating P&P carotenoids is shown in **Formula 1**.

P&P carotenoids in concentrations lower than known skin-lightening ingredients such as arbutin have in fact shown greater effects on melanin synthesis than such ingredients. For instance, P&P

carotenoids have shown a 22% reduction in melanin content in B16 murine melanocytes at a concentration of 7.5 µM with no effect on cell viability, whereas arbutin, a known skin-lightening agent, has shown an effect on melanin synthesis without an inhibitory effect on cell growth at maximum concentrations of 50 µM.[28] Although the lightening effect of P&P carotenoids has not been tested on ethnic skin, they have been formulated into ethnic products in Asia. These materials could in theory be used on ethnic skin to lighten, protect against UV damage and reduce inflammation.

Formula 1. Lightening o/w day cream

A. Potassium cetyl phosphate	3.00% w/w
Glyceryl stearate	0.50
Triethylhexanoin	6.00
Isopropyl isostearate	6.00
Cyclopentasiloxane	6.00
Phenyl trimethicone	2.00
B. Water (*aqua*)	qs to 100
Carbomer	0.40
C. Squalane (and) *Solanum lycopersicum* (tomato) fruit extract (IBR-TCLC, IBR)	0.50
Water (*aqua*) (and) *Narcissus tazetta* bulb extract (IBR Dormin, IBR)	1.50
D. Titanium dioxide (and) boron nitride (and) acrylates/ ammonium methacrylate copolymer (WhiteCap2, Tagra)	1.00
E. Aluminum oxide	0.50
Glycerin	4.00
F. Propylene glycol (and) diazolidinyl urea (and) methylparaben (and) propylparaben (Sharomix DMP, Sharon Laboratories)	1.00

Procedure: Combine B with stirring. Separately combine A. Heat A and B at 80°C. Add A to B while stirring moderately (approx. 300 rpm). Homogenize AB for 90 sec. Prepare E and add to AB in the homogenizer. Homogenize again for 90 sec. Cool to 40-45°C and add C and F to batch, stirring slowly. Add D to batch without homogenization. Cool to RT stirring slowly. Adjust final pH if necessary to 6.5.

Boosting Sunscreen SPF

Frequently, when sunscreens are exposed to sunlight, some of the light energy goes toward generating harmful free radicals and ROS. However, an active molecule that could quench or prevent free radical generation may stabilize the formulation and increase its safety and efficacy.

P&P carotenoids were tested in this capacity. Two sunscreen creams were prepared with 3.5% w/w octyl methoxycinnamate and 1% butyl methoxydibenzoylmethane. One sunscreen cream contained 5% P&P carotenoids from algae while the control did not contain the compounds. The in vitro SPF of both sunscreens was determined using a testing substrate that mimics the surface properties of human skin[b]. 2 mg/m^2 was applied to the substrate and irradiated. The reflected light was measured by transmittance analyzer[c]. The Minimum Protection Factor (MPF) was obtained and SPF was calculated.

The P&P carotenoids were shown to provide stabilization and to reduce the generation of free radicals and damage derived from irradiation of TiO$_2$ (see **Figure 6**); in addition, they boosted the SPF of a test sunscreen (see **Table 2**).

---

[b]Vitro-Skin is a product of IMS Inc.
[c]UV-1000F Ultraviolet Transmittance Analyzer is a product of Labsphere.

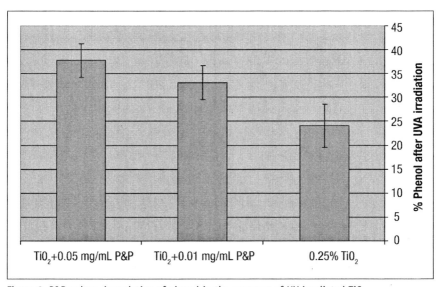

Figure 6. P&P reduce degradation of phenol in the presence of UV irradiated TiO$_2$

Table 2. SPF of sunscreen creams with and without P&P

Sunscreen	SPF in vitro (382 nm)
Sunscreen cream	18.7 ± 0.4
Sunscreen cream + 5% P&P	32.5 ± 0.1

Conclusion

The colorless carotenoids P&P have been shown to protect the skin via oral and topical application against UV and oxidative damage that leads to premature aging and other disorders. This article summarizes the protective activities of colorless carotenoids against UV irradiation, free radicals and DNA damage as well as anti-inflammatory benefits, collagen production promotion and reduction of skin pigmentation. Finally, P&P carotenoids can efficiently stabilize sunscreens and boosts their sun protection capabilities.

Published March 2009 *Cosmetics and Toiletries* magazine

References

1. A Bendich and JA Olson, Biological actions of carotenoids, *FASEB J* 3 1927–32 (1989)
2. MM Mathews, Protective effects of β-carotene lethal photosensitization by haematoporphyrin, *Nature* 203 1092 (1964)
3. NI Krinski, MM Mathews-Roth and RF Taylor (Eds), in: *Carotenoids, Chemistry and Biology*, New York, London: Platinum Press (1989)
4. MM Mathews-Roth, Antitumor activity of beta-carotene, canthaxanthin and phytoene, *Oncology* 39(1) 33–7 (1982)
5. Y Satomi, N Misawa, T Maoka and H Nishino, Production of phytoene, a carotenoid, and induction of connexin 26 in transgenic mice carrying the phytoene synthase gene crt, B. *Biocem Biophy Res Comm* 320 398–401 (2004)
6. F Khachik, L Carvalho, PS Bernstein, GJ Muire, DY Zhao and NB Katz. Chemistry, distribution, and metabolism of tomato carotenoids and their impact on human health, *Exp Biol Med* 227 845–851 (2002)
7. O Aust, W Stahl, H Sies, H Tronnier and U Heinrich, Supplementation with tomato-based products increases lycopene, phytofluene, and phytoene levels in human serum and protects against UV-light-induced erythema, *Int J Vitam Nutr Res* 75(1) 54–60 (2005)
8. IV Ermakov, MR Ermakova, W Gellermann and J Lademann, Noninvasive selective detection of lycopene and beta-carotene in human skin using Raman spectroscopy, *J Biomed Opt* 9(2) 332–8 (2004)
9. M Porrini, P Riso, A Brusamolino, C Berti, S Guarnieri and F Visioli, Daily intake of a formulated tomato drink affects carotenoid plasma and lymphocyte concentrations and improves cellular antioxidant protection, *Brit J of Nutrition*, 93(1) 93–99 (2005)
10. F Khachik, GR Beecher, MB Goli and WR Lusby, Separation, identification, and quantification of carotenoids in fruits, vegetables and human plasma by high performance liquid chromatography, *Pure App Chem*, 63(1) 71–80 (1991)
11. PD Fraser and PM Bramley, The biosynthesis and nutritional uses of carotenoids, *Progress in Lipid Research* 43 228–265 (2004)
12. TR Hata, TA Scholz, IV Ermakov, RW McClane, F Khachik, W Gellermann, LK Pershing, Non-invasive raman spectroscopic detection of carotenoids in human skin, *J Invest Dermatol*, 115(3) 441–8 (2000)

13. MM Mathews-Roth and NI Krinsky, Carotenoids affect development of UVB induced skin cancer, *Photochem Photobiol* 46(4) 507–9 (1987)

14. MM Mathews-Roth, Carotenoid functions in photoprotection and cancer prevention, *J Environ Pathol Toxicol Oncol*, 10(4–5) 181–92 (1990)

15. MM Mathews-Roth, Photoprotection by carotenoids, *Fed Proc* 46(5) 1890–3 (1987)

16. B Halliwell and JMC.Gutteridge, The chemistry of oxygen radicals and other oxygen-derived species. *Free Radicals in Biology and Medicine*, New York: Oxford University Press (1985) pp 20–64

17. J Taira, K Mimura, T Yoneya, A Hagi, A Murakami and K Makino, Hydroxyl radical formation by UV-irradiated epidermal cells, *J Biochem* 111(6) 693–5 (1992)

18. L Von Oppen-Bezalel, E Lerner, DG Kern, B Fuller, E Soudant and A Shaish, IBR-CLC, Colorless Carotenoids: Phytoene and Phytofluene from Unicellular Algae–Applications in Cosmetics, Wellness and Nutrition, *Fragrance J*, 34 48–53 (2006)

19. L Von Oppen-Bezalel, Colorless Carotenoids, phytoene and phytofluene for the skin: For prevention of aging/photo-aging from inside and out, *SÖFW*, 7 (2007)

20. L Von Oppen-Bezalel, UVA, A main concern in sun damage: Protection from the inside and outside with phytoene, phytofluene, the colorless carotenoids and more, *SÖFW*, 11 (2007)

21. BB Fuller, DR Smith, AJ Howerton, D Kern, Anti-inflammatory effects of CoQ10 and colorless carotenoids, *J Cos Derm* 5(1) 30–38 (2006)

22. MM Mathews-Roth and MA Pathak, Phytoene as a protective agent against sunburn (>280 nm) radiation in guinea pigs, *Photochem Photobiol*, 21(4) 261–26 (1975)

23. JP Cesarini, L Michel, JM Maurette, H Adhoute and M Bejot, Immediate effects of UV radiation on the skin: Modification by an antioxidant complex containing carotenoids, *Photodermatol Photoimmunol Photomed* 19(4) 182–9 (2003)

24. Y Sharoni, Lycopene, skin cancer and UV exposure, in *Conference notes: Examining the Health Benefits of Lycopene from Tomatoes*, Washington, DC, conference convened by the Center for Food and Nutrition Policy at Virginia Tech (Apr 1–2, 2003)

25. W Stahl, U Heinrich, S Wiseman, O Eichler, H Sies and H Tronnier, Dietary tomato paste protects against UV-induced erythema in humans, *J Nutr* 131 1449–1451 (2001)

26. J Lee, S Jiang, N Levine and RR Watson, Carotenoid supplementation reduces erythema in human skin after simulated solar radiation exposure, *Proc Soc Exp Biol Med* 223 170–174 (2000)

27. H Sies and W Stahl. Carotenoids and UV protection, *Photochem Photobiol Sci* 3(8) 749–52 (2004)

28. S Akiu, Y Suzuki, T Asahara, Y Fujinuma and M Fukuda, Inhibitory effect of arbutin on melanogenesis—Biochemical study using cultured B16 melanoma cells, *Nippon Hifuka Gakkai Zasshi*, 101(6) 609–13 (1999)

CHAPTER 26

A Medicinal Plant Blend for Soothing and Anti-inflammatory Effects

Jongsung Lee, Eunsun Jung, Kwangseon Jung and Deokhoon Park

Biospectrum Life Science Institute, Gunpo City, Korea

Anthony Ansaldi and Roy Heckl

DKSH North America Inc., Baltimore, USA

KEY WORDS: *atopic dermatitis, anti-inflammatory effect, pro-inflammatory cytokines, EASI*

ABSTRACT: *The use of steroids to treat atopic dermatitis (AD) often causes side effects; thus, the authors present a blend of plant-derived materials designed as an alternative treatment or an adjuvant therapeutic agent. Through in vitro and in vivo evaluations, the blend is shown to provide effective anti-inflammatory and AD-mitigating effects.*

Atopic dermatitis (AD) is a chronic inflammatory skin disease that most commonly occurs during early infancy and childhood and is characterized by a chronically relapsing course where symptoms of AD are ameliorated and aggravated repeatedly. Although the pathogenesis of AD is not fully understood, it has been reported that it is associated with multiple immunologic abnormalities.[1,2] The most prominent findings of immune dysfunction are the high level of immunoglobulin E (IgE) in peripheral blood and increased IgE production by B cells. In AD, T helper 2 (Th2) cells are mainly activated and then secrete interleukin-4 (IL-4), interleukin-5 (IL-5) and interleukin-10 (IL-10).[1,3,4]

Symptoms of AD induced by signal transduction pathways of IgE, IL-4, IL-5 or IL-10 are associated with inflamed skin damage as well as skin dryness. Accordingly, the generally accepted prescription includes moisturizers and topical steroids that maintain a level of moisture in the skin and suppress inflammatory reaction, respectively. However, treating AD over time with topical steroid hormones has been known to induce adverse side effects.[5] In addition, nonsteroid therapeutic treatments including cyclosporin A and tacrolimus have been reported to induce cutaneous T cell lymphoma, fever, extreme rises in serum alkaline phosphatase in children, enhanced irritation and relapsing Kaposi's varicelliform eruption.[6-10] Therefore, much recent work has focused on the development of therapeutic agents that maximize anti-inflammatory effects while minimizing side effects.

As a first step, the authors selected chemicals with known anti-inflammatory and antioxidant mechanisms to prepare a variety of formulations. Subsequently, candidate formulations exhibiting high anti-inflammatory effects using a nuclear factor kappa-B (NF-κB) luciferase reporter were screened. The results of the screening led to the development of a blend consisting of seven medicinal plant components[a]. These components included: carnosic acid from *Rosmarinus officinalis*; apigenin from *Matricaria recubita*; epigallocatechin-3-gallate from *Camellia sinensis*; glycyrrhetinic acid from *Glycyrrhiza glabra*; resveratrol from *Polygonum cuspidatum*; baicalin from *Scutellaria baicalensis*; and asiaticoside from *Centella asiatica* (see **Formula 1** and **Table 1**). In the present study, the authors investigated in vitro the anti-inflammatory effects of this preparation for its potential to treat AD.

Formula 1. Test blend[a]

Dimethyl sulfoxide, 99.9%	0.59% w/w
Carnosic acid, 98%	0.20
Apigenin, 98%	0.20
Epigallocetechin-3-gallate, 98%	0.20
Glyceryrrhetinic acid, 98%	0.30
Resveratrol, 98%	0.01
Scutellaria baicalensis root extract, 98%	0.20
Centella asiatica extract, 98%	0.30

Materials and Methods

To set up the test for anti-inflammatory effects of the plant blend,

Table 1. Compounds formulated in the test blend

Structure	Source	Activity	Reference(s)
Carnosic acid	*Rosemarinus officinalis*	• Antioxidant effect • Photoprotection effect	Masuda et al., 2001 Offord et al., 2002
Apigenin	*Matricaria recubita*	• Antioxidant effect • Prevention of carcinogenesis	Lin et al., 2002 Liang et al., 1999 and inflammation
EGCG	*Camellia sinensis*	• Antioxidant effect • Prevention of carcinogenesis and inflammation • Photoprotection effect	Surh et al., 2001 Katiyar et al., 2001 Hong et al., 2001
Glycyrrhetinic acid	*Glycyrrhiza glabra*	• Anti-inflammatory effect • Anti-tumor effect	Nishino et al., 1984 Akamatsu et al., 1991 Ohuchi et al., 1981

Table 1. Compounds formulated in the test blend (cont.)

Structure	Source	Activity	Reference(s)
Resveratrol	*Polygonum cuspidatum*	• Antioxidant effect • Anti-inflammatory effect • Chemoprevention	Jang et al., 1997 Jang et al., 1998
Baicalin	*Scutellaria biacalensis*	• Antioxidant effect • Anti-inflammatory effect	Gabrielska et al., 1997 Nakajima et al., 2001
Asiaticoside	*Centella asiatica*	• Elevation antioxidant level • Wound healing	Shukla et al., 1999 (*Phytother Res*) Shukla et al., 1999 (*J Ethnopharmacol*)

researchers first obtained the following materials: lipopolysaccharide[b] (LPS), phytohematoaglutinin[c], IL-2 luciferase reporter DNA,[11] IL-8 ELISA kit[d], TNF-α ELISA kit[e] and NF-κB DNA[f]. Three formulations containing the preparation were then prepared using dimethyl sulfoxide as the solvent;[12] these included a face/body wash containing 1% test blend (**Formula 2**), a liposome lotion containing 1.5% test blend (**Formula 3**), and a liposome serum containing 3% test blend (**Formula 4**). The liposome lotion and serum were manufactured in a liposome base using the one-step homogenization technique as described by Brandl et al.[13] The face/body wash was a general liquid soap with a low detergent level.

Cell lines and cell culture: THP-1 human monocyte cells and Jurkat human leukemia cells were cultured in a bicarbonate buffering

---

[a] MultiEx BSASM (INCI: Chamomilia Recutita (Matricaria) Flower Extract (and) Centella Asiatica Extract (and) Glycyrrhiza Glabra (Licorice) Root Extract (and) Camellia Sinensis Leaf Extract (and) Polygonum Cuspidatum Root Extract (and) Rosmarinus Officinalis (Rosemary) Leaf Extract (and) Scutellaria Baicalensis Root Extract (and) Butylene Glycol (and) Water (aqua)) is a product of BioSpectrum Inc., distributed by DKSH North America Inc.

[b] Lipopolysaccharide is a product of Sigma-Aldrich.

[c] Phytohematoaglutinin is a product of EMD Chemicals/Calbiochem.

[d] IL-8 ELISA kit is a product of R&D System.

[e] TNF-a Human ELISA kit is a product of Invitrogen.

[f] NF- B DNA is a product of Stratagene.

Formula 2. Face/body wash

Test blend preparation (see **Formula 1**)	1.00% w/w
Disodium cocoamphodiacetate	15.00
Coco-glucoside	8.00
Sodium lauroyl glutamate	5.00
Glycerin	2.00
Camellia japonica seed oil	0.50
Citric acid	0.15
Tocopherol	0.05
Preservative	qs
Fragrance (*parfum*)	qs
Water (*aqua*)	qs to 100.00%

system with variations in the amounts of amino acids and vitamins[g] including 10% fetal bovine serum and 1x antibiotic solution. HaCaT cells were cultured in Dulbecco's modified eagle's medium (DMEM) including 10% fetal bovine serum and 1x antibiotic solution. Cells were incubated at 37°C in a 5% CO_2 incubator.[14, 15]

Transient cell transfection and luciferase reporter gene assay: THP-1 cells were transiently transfected with 2 mg of the firefly luciferase reporter gene under the control of NF-κB responsible element and 0.2 mg of renilla luciferase expression vector driven by thymidine kinase promoter[h] by superfect reagent. The transfected cells were transferred to 6 well plates and incubated for 24 hr at a density of 8 X 10^5 cells per mL.

---

[g] RPMI-1640 is a product of Sigma-Aldrich.
[h] Thymidine kinase promoter is a product of Promega.

Formula 3. Liposome lotion

Test blend preparation (see **Formula 1**)	1.50% w/w
Lecithin	3.00
Caprylic/capric triglyceride	2.00
Camellia japonica seed oil	0.50
Phytosterol	1.50
Phytosqualane	1.00
Oenothera biennis (evening primrose) oil	0.50
Borago officinalis seed oil	0.50
Shea butter	1.00
Tocopherol	0.30
Ceramide 3	0.10
Xanthan gum	0.28
Sodium PCA (and) trehaolse (and) sorbitol (and) glycerin (and) panthenol (and) sodium hyaluronate (and) water (*aqua*) (MultiEx HumiD-Max, BioSpectrum)	2.00
Glycerin	0.50
Preservative	qs
Fragrance (*parfum*)	qs
Water (*aqua*)	qs to 100.00%

After 24 hr, the cells were further cultured in the presence or absence of LPS and the test blend for 5 hr. Luciferase activity was determined using the high-throughput analysis of mammalian cells containing genes for firefly and renilla luciferases[j] and a luminometer[k], and were expressed as a ratio of NF-κ B-dependent firefly luciferase activity divided by control thymidine kinase renilla luciferase activity (relative luciferase unit). Results were confirmed by three independent transfections. To assay for IL-2 promoter activity, Jurkat T cells were transfected with 2 µg of reporter plasmids using a transfection reagent[m]. After 24 hr, cells were activated by treatment with PHA (10 µg/mL) and harvested. Luciferase activity was determined in triplicate for each experiment with a lumino-meter[j].[16, 17]

[j] The Dual-Glo Luciferase Assay System used for this study is a product of Promega.
[k] The LB953 luminometer is a product of Berthold.
[m] SuperFect Transfection Reagent is a product of Qiagen.

Formula 4. Liposome serum

Test blend preparation (see **Formula 1**)	3.00% w/w
Lecithin	3.50
Caprylic/capric triglyceride	3.00
Camellia japonica seed oil	2.00
Phytosterol	2.00
Phytosqualane	2.00
Oenothera biennis (evening primrose) oil	0.50
Borago officinalis seed oil	0.50
Shea butter	0.50
Tocopherol	0.04
Ceramide 3	0.10
Xanthan gum	0.30
Sodium PCA (and) trehaolse (and) sorbitol (and) glycerin (and) panthenol (and) sodium hyaluronate (and) water (*aqua*) (MultiEx HumiD-Max, BioSpectrum)	2.00
Glycerin	0.20
Preservative	qs
Fragrance (*parfum*)	qs
Water (*aqua*)	qs to 100

Measurement of cytokine production: Cell supernatants were analyzed for IL-8 and TNF-α by using commercially available ELISA kits with sensitivities of 3 and 1 pg/mL, respectively.

Cytotoxicity assay: HaCaT cells were cultured in DMEM including 10% fetal bovine serum and 1x antibiotic solution. Cells were incubated at 37°C in a 5% CO_2 incubator. Cells were seeded on 24 well plates and drug treatment began 24 hr after seeding. General viability of cultured cells was determined by reduction of 3-(4,5-dimety-2-thiazoyl)-2,5-dipheny-2H-ltetrazolium bromide (MTT) to formazan. After incubation of HaCaT cells treated with various concentrations of the test blend for 24 hr at 37°C in 5% CO_2 atmosphere, an MTT assay was performed. MTT (1 mg/mL in PBS) was added to each well, 1/10 volume of media. Cells were incubated at 37°C for 3 hr and harvested by centrifugation, after which dimethyl sulfoxide was added to dissolve the formazan crystals. The absorbance was then measured at 570 nm with a spectrophotometer[n].

Statistical analysis: Non-parametric, one-way analysis of variance (Kruskal Wallis test) and the Mann-Whitney test were used for statistical analysis. Differences between groups were considered significant at $p < 0.05$ (*).

AD-mitigating Effects

Thirty children with mild AD, including 11 boys and 19 girls, ages 6–15, participated in an in vivo study. Written consent was obtained in each case and three variations of the test blend preparations were administered using the following instructions:

1. Face and body wash was to be used when taking a bath with lukewarm water for approximately 10 min each evening. Liposome lotion was then applied to the entire body immediately after removing excess water from bathing.

2. Liposome serum was additionally applied to severely dry skin or severely affected AD lesions twice daily—once in the morning and once in the afternoon—irrespective of the bathing. Topical or systemic uses of corticosteroids were strictly prohibited during the study period except oral antihistamines offered to control severe pruritus.

---

[n] Power Wave is a product of Bio-tek Inc.

Clinical evaluation was performed objectively on the symptoms and degree of AD using the Eczema Area Severity Index (EASI) as presented by J. M. Hanifin et al.[18] Pruritus was evaluated using a 10-point visual analog scale. Transepidermal water loss (TEWL) was measured before treatment, at two weeks of treatment, and at four weeks after treatment on the abdomen and right antecubital fossa. In addition, a patch test was performed on the back or forearm in 10 patients to check for any irritative or allergic effects.

For statistical analysis, Kruskal-Wallis one-way ANOVA was used to compare the changes of EASI, TEWL and pruritus according to the treatment period. A p value of less than 0.05 was considered to be statistically significant. In addition, a dimethyl sulfoxide-only group was used as a placebo (negative control).

LPS-induced NF-κB activation: NF-κB is a protein transcription factor that was first identified by Sen and Baltimore;[19] it enhances the transcription of a variety of genes including cytokines and growth factors, adhesion molecules, immunoreceptors and acute-phase proteins. NF-κB reportedly has been involved in maximal transcription of many cytokines, including TNF-α, IL-1, IL-6 and IL-8, which are considered to be important in the generation of acute inflammatory responses.

As a preliminary step to determine whether the test blend affects cytokine production, a NF-κB luciferase assay was performed. As shown in **Figure 1**, LPS increased NF-κB reporter activity fivefold,

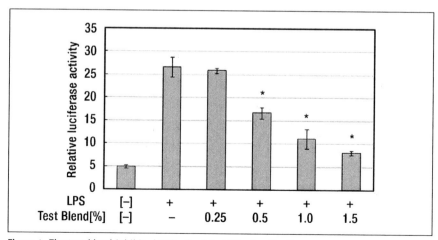

Figure 1. The test blend inhibited LPS-stimulated NF-κB activation.

whereas the test blend inhibited LPS-induced NF-κB reporter activity in a dose-dependent manner. In the experiment, THP-1 cells were transfected with NF-κB-luciferase using superfect. After incubation for 24 hr, cells were stimulated for 14 hr with LPS, harvested and lysed. Supernatants were assayed for luciferase activity.

Luciferase activity was determined three times in duplicate for each experiment. All values were significant (*p < 0.01) when compared with values for LPS alone. LPS-induced NF-κB reporter activity was diminished by one half when the test blend was treated at 1% concentration, indicating that IC_{50} of the blend is 1%. This result suggests the possibility that the test blend may be involved in blocking the production of proinflammatory cytokines.

LPS-induced production of IL-8 and TNF-α: The effect of the test blend on the production of IL-8 and TNF-α was also examined. Cells (10^6) were incubated with nothing, with LPS (100 ng/mL), or with LPS plus the test blend for 24 hr. Afterwards, supernatants were assessed for IL-8 by ELISA (**Figure 2**) or for TNF-α (**Figure 3**). Data is presented as the mean ± standard deviation of four separate experiments. All values were significant (*p < 0.01) compared with values for LPS alone. The test blend significantly reduced the production of IL-8 and TNF-α dose-dependently, confirming that the blend inhibits production of IL-8 and also suggesting the

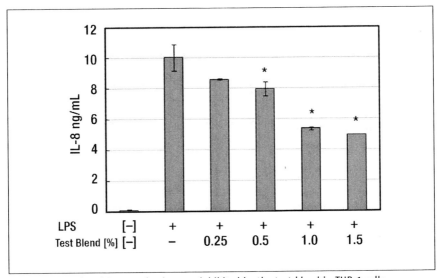

Figure 2. LPS-induced IL-8 production was inhibited by the test blend in THP-1 cells.

anti-inflammatory function of the test blend through inactivation of NF-κB promoter. These findings were similar to those found in **Figure 1**.

IL-2 production in Jurkat T cells: To explore the involvement of the test blend in T cell activation and proliferation, IL-2 luciferase reporter system was used. As shown in **Figure 4**, Jurkat T Cells were transfected with IL-2-luciferase using superfect. After incubation for 24 hr, cells were stimulated for 14 hr with PHA, harvested and lysed. Supernatants were assayed for luciferase activity. Luciferase activity

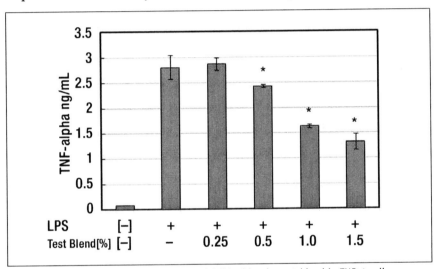

Figure 3. LPS-induced TNF-α production was inhibited by the test blend in THP-1 cells.

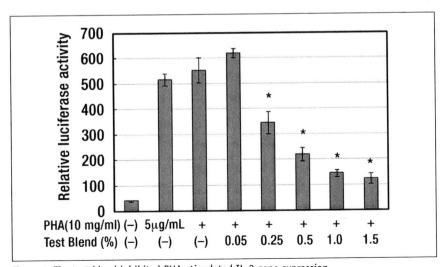

Figure 4. The test blend inhibited PHA-stimulated IL-2 gene expression.

was determined three times in duplicate for each experiment. All values were significant (p < 0.01), compared with values of PHA alone. PHA distinctly activated IL-2 reporter activity by tenfold. However, this increased reporter activity was inhibited by the test blend, indicating it has the potential to inhibit T cell activation and proliferation in Jurkat T cells.

Cytotoxic property in HaCaT cells: Next, the cytotoxic effects of the test blend were examined on HaCaT cells, human keratinocyte cell lines (see **Figure 5**). In this experiment, HaCaT cells were cultured for 24 hr in a medium with or without the test blend. The cellular cyto-toxicity was determined according to a rapid colorimetric MTT assay and expressed as the mean ± S.D. While the test blend at concentrations lower than 5% showed almost 100% cell viability, the tested blend at 10% showed a more than 80% cell viability of HaCaT cells. Thus, in HaCaT cells, the test blend did not show a significant cytotoxic effect (data not shown). This suggests the blend has low cytotoxic properties.

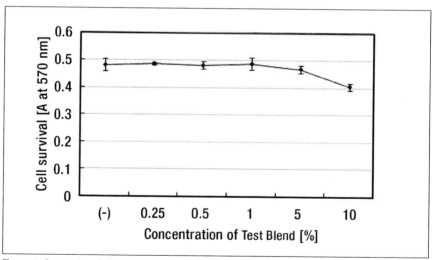

Figure 5. Cytotoxity of the test blend against HaCaT cells

Clinical Study

In a clinical study, a statistically significant reduction of EASI score was observed at 2 weeks (1.63 ± 00.60) and at 4 weeks (0.61 ± 0.48) after treatment with the test blend, compared with the EASI score prior to treatment (2.60 ± 0.57) (p = 0.001).

Pruritus also decreased significantly at 2 weeks (4.47 ± 0.53) and at 4 weeks (3.20 ± 0.49) after treatment (p = 0.022), compared with scores before treatment (5.13 ± 0.46). The effect of the test blend on TEWL also was studied on the antecubital fossa and on the abdomen. TEWL decreased after treatment, both on the antecubital fossa and abdomen, although only on the abdomen showed a statistically significant decrease (p = 0.01) 2 weeks (17.31 ± 1.85 $g/m^2/h$) and 4 weeks (13.46 ± 2.42 $g/m^2/h$) after treatment, when compared with scores prior to treatment (22.81 ± 2.18 $g/m^2/h$).

In regard to the patch testing, consistent with in vitro cytotoxic assays, no erythema, burning or pruritus reactions were observed in any patients based on the 2- and 4-day readings. Only one patient complained of pruritus immediately after application of liposome lotion and this patient dropped out of the study. The face/body wash containing the test blend and emollients was thus considered to be effective and safe for use in AD patients.

Discussion and Conclusions

As previously mentioned, despite the effectiveness of steroid hormones on AD, they have been known to induce side effects such as skin atrophy, dilation of blood vessels, depigmentation and so on.[5] Therefore, this study aimed to evaluate whether a blend of medicinal plant extracts could be used as an alternative or adjuvant therapeutic agent to treat AD. To this end, in vitro and in vivo experiments were performed.

In this report, the characterization of a test blend to act as an anti-inflammatory and AD-mitigating agent has been described and several benefits demonstrate its possibility as a therapeutic agent to treat AD. The blend inhibited LPS-induced NF-κB activation and reduced the LPS-induced production of IL-8 and TNF-α. In addition, it inhibited IL-2 production in Jurkat T cells, demonstrating anti-inflammatory effects and the involvement in blocking T cell-mediated immune responses.

In in vivo studies, after treatment with the test blend, a statistically significant reduction of EASI score was observed, as well as a decrease of pruritus and TEWL both on the antecubital fossa and abdomen. In addition, patch testing showed no reactions in any subjects, suggesting the test blend can safely be applied to human skin. Based on these results, the authors conclude that this medicinal plant blend can be safely applied to patients with AD. However, an understanding of the precise molecular mechanisms by which the blend improves AD remains incomplete. While cyclosporin A and tacrolimus, which inhibit IL-2 production in Jurkat T cells, are known to block PLC gamma-mediated Ca^{2+} signaling,[20-23] rosmarinic acid inhibits TCR-proximal $p56^{lck}$-mediated signaling.[24-26] In light of the IL-2 luciferase assay shown in **Figure 4**, the test blend may inhibit the Ca^{2+} signaling mediated by calcineurin or the $p56^{lck}$-mediated signaling that is known to play an important role in T cell activation and proliferation.[27-31]

Various agents that induce inflammation are known to activate NF-B.[32,33] In addition, several genes that are involved in inflammation are regulated by NF-κB.[34-36] Therefore, it was hypothesized that NF-κB promoter can be employed as a marker to screen anti-inflammatory candidates. The finding that the test blend inhibits LPS-induced NF-κB activation implicates its use in anti-inflammatory signaling and also suggests that its action mechanism may be mediated through suppression of the recruitment of signaling molecules involved in NF-κB activation.

Until now, a limited number of proteins involved in the NF-κB activation pathway have been identified, including TNFRSF1A-associated via death domain, NF-kB-inducing kinase (NIK), mammalian mitogen-activated protein kinase and Iκ B kinase.[37-40] The interaction between these molecules has previously been elucidated as critical in NF-κB activation signaling.[41,42] Therefore, it is likely that the test blend may block cross-talk among these signaling molecules.

As previously mentioned, the test preparation consists of seven compounds and their individual and/or combined effects are currently unknown. Studies to elucidate possible reciprocal interactions between them are in progress. Overall, however, the results procured thus far indicate this test blend can be used as an effective topical treatment for AD.

References

1. KD Cooper, Atopic dermatitis: Recent trends in pathogenesis and therapy, *J Invest Dermatol* 102 128–137 (1968)
2. JD Bos et al, Immune dysregulation in atopic eczema, *Archives of Dermatol* 128 1509–1512 (1992)
3. TR Mosmann et al, Two types of murine helper T cell clone. I. Definition according to profiles of lymphokine activities and secreted proteins, *J Immunol* 136 2348–2357 (1986)
4. L SH et al, Studies on serum IL-4 as a marker of symptom in patients with atopic dermatitis, *Korean J Dermatol* 36 95–102 (1998)
5. P Venge, Eosinophil and neutrophil granulocytes, *Allergy* 36 95–102 (1993)
6. B Kirby, Cutaneous T-cell lymphoma developing in a patient on cyclosporin therapy, *J Am Acad Dermatol* 47(2) S165–S167 (2002)
7. MD Thomas et al, Fever associated with cyclosporin for atopic dermatitis, *Br Med J* 317 1291 (1998)
8. T Van Meurs, Extreme rises in serum alkaline phosphatase in children with atopic dermatitis after intervention treatment with cyclosporin A, *Pediatric Dermatol* 15(6) 483 (1998)
9. M Ambo, Relapsing Kaposi's varicelliform eruption and herpes simplex following facial tacrolimus treatment for atopic dermatitis, *Acta Dermato-Venereologica* 82(3), 224–225 (2002)
10. M Fuchs et al, Tacrolimus enhances irritation in a 5-day human irritancy in vivo model, *Contact Dermatitis* 46(5) 290–294 (2002)
11. BC Young, KK Chan and Y Yungdae, An adapter protein interacting with the SH2 domain of p56lck, is required for T cell activation, *J Immunology* 163, 5242–5249 (1999)
12. L Jongsung et al, Evaluation of the anti-inflammatory and immunomodulatory effects of BSASM using in vitro experiments, *Korean J Pharmacognosy* 34(3) 228–232 (2003)
13. M Brandl et al, Three-dimensional liposome networks: Freeze fracture electron microscopical evaluation of their structure and in vitro analysis of release of hydrophilic markers, *Advanced Drug Delivery Reviews* 24 161–164 (1997)
14. H Nishino et al, Antitumor-promoting activity of glycyrrhetic acid in mouse skin tumor formation induced by 7,12-dimethylbenz[a]anthracene plus teleocidin, *Carcinogenesis* 5 1529–1530 (1984)
15. N Za et al, Jurkat cell proliferative activity is increased by luteinizing hormonereleasing hormone, *J Endocrinology* 153 241–249 (1997)
16. TM Williams et al, Advantages of firefly luciferase as a reporter gene: Application to the interleukin-2 gene promoter, *Analytical Biochem* 176 28–32 (1989)
17. PR Wenner et al, Detection and quantification of cyclosporine in body fluids using an interleukin-2 reporter-gene assay, *J Immunological Methods* 201 125–135 (1997)
18. JM Hanifin, M Thurston, M Omoto, R Cherill, SJ Tofte and M Graeber, The eczema area and severity index (EASI): Assessment of reliability in atopic dermatitis. EASI Evaluator Group, *Experimental Dermatol* 10 11–18 (2001)
19. R Sen and D Baltimore, Multiple nuclear factors interact with the immunoglobulin enhancer sequences, *Cell* 46 705–716 (1986)
20. GA Dos and EM Shevach, Effect of cyclo-sporin A on T cell function in vitro: The mechanism of suppression of T cell proliferation depends on the nature of the T cell stimulus as well as the differentiation state of the responding T cell, *J Immunology* 29 2360–2367 (1982)
21. M Eichhorn et al, IL-2 can enhance the cyclosporin A-mediated inhibition of Theileria parva-infected T cell proliferation, *J Immunology* 144 691–698 (1990)
22. MJ Tocci et al, The immunosuppressant FK506 selectively inhibits expression of early T cell activation genes, *J Immunology* 143 718–726 (1989)
23. SS Banerji et al, The immunosuppressant FK-506 specifically inhibits mitogen-induced activation of the interleukin-2 promoter and the isolated enhancer elements NFIL-2A and NF-AT1, *Mol Cellular Biol* 11 4074–4087 (1991)
24. J Won et al, Rosmarinic acid inhibits TCR-induced T cell activation and proliferation in an Lck-dependent manner, European, *J Immunology* 33 870–879 (2003)

25. MA Kang, Rosmarinic acid inhibits Ca2+-dependent pathways of T-cell antigen receptor-mediated signaling by inhibiting the PLC-gamma 1 and Itk activity, *Blood 101* 3534–3542 (2003)
26. SY Yun et al, Synergistic immunosuppressive effects of rosmarinic acid and rapamycin in vitro and in vivo, *Transplantation* 75 1758–1760 (2003)
27. SJ Anderson and RM Perlmutter, A signaling pathway governing early thymocyte maturation, *Immunology Today* 16 99–105 (1994)
28. TJ Molina et al, Profound block in thymocyte development in mice lacking p56lck, *Nature* 357 161–164 (1992)
29. M Hatakeyama et al and Taniguchi. Interaction of the IL-2 receptor with the src-family kinase p56lck: Identification of novel intermolecular association, *Science* 252 1523–1528 (1991)
30. Y Minami et al, Association of p56lck with IL-2 receptor beta chain is critical for the IL-2-induced activation of p56lck, *The EMBO Journal* 12 759–768 (1993)
31. JD Marth et al, Neoplastic transformation induced by an activated lymphocyte-specific protein tyrosine kinase (pp56lck), *Mol Cellular Biol* 8 540-550 (1988)
32. C Giuliani et al, NF-kappaB transcription factor: Role in the pathogenesis of inflammatory, autoimmune, and neoplastic diseases and therapy implications, *Clinical Therapeutics* 152 249-253 (2001)
33. R Donadelli et al, Protein traffic activates NF-kappaB gene signaling and promotes MCP-1-dependent interstitial inflammation, *Am J Kidney Disease* 36 1226-1241 (2000)
34. AV Miagkov et al, NF-kappaB activation provides the potential link between inflammation and hyperplasia in the arthritic joint, *Proceedings of the National Academy of Sciences of the United States of America* 95 13859-13864 (1998)
35. W Zheng-Ming et al, Chemokines are the main proinflammatory mediators in human monocytes activated by Staphylococcus aureus, peptidoglycan, and endotoxin, *J Biol Chem* 275(27) 20260–20267 (2000)
36. R Benjamin et al, Induction of proinflammatory cytokines by a soluble factor of *Propionibacterium acnes*: Implication for chronic inflammatory acne, *Infection and Immunity* 63(8) 3158–3165 (1995)
37. M Naofumi et al, Molecular mechanism of interleukin-8 gene expression, *J Leukocyte Biol* 56 554–558 (1994)
38. M Morgan et al, Nuclear and cytoplasmic shuttling of TRADD induces apoptosis via different mechanisms, *J Cell Biol* 157 975–984 (2002)
39. X Lin et al, Molecular determinants of NF-kappaB-inducing kinase action, *Mol Cellular Biol* 18 5899–5907 (1998)
40. AH Bild et al, MEKK1-induced apoptosis requires TRAIL death receptor activation and is inhibited by AKT/PKB through inhibition of MEKK1 cleavage, *Oncogene* 21 6649–6656 (2002)
41. D Krappmann et al, The I kappa B kinase (IKK) complex is tripartite and contains IKK gamma but not IKAP as a regular component, *J Biol Chem* 275 29779–29787 (2000)
42. G Takaesuet al, TAB2, a novel adaptor protein, mediates activation of TAK1 MAPKKK by linking TAK1 to TRAF6 in the IL-1 signal transduction pathway, *Mol Cell* 5 649–658 (2000)

CHAPTER 27

Orange Roughy Oil for Sensitive Skin and Other Topics: Literature Findings

Charles Fox
Independent Consultant

KEY WORDS: *skin, skin care, antioxidant, oily skin, gel, lotion, emulsion*

ABSTRACT: *Survey of recent patent and research literature describes moneymaking ideas for personal care product development including the influence of filaggrin on skin moisture, lotus extract for anticellulite and orange roughy oil for sensitive skin, among others.*

Skin and Skin Care

Filaggrin's role in skin moisture: Kezic et al. have reported that loss-of-function mutations in the filaggrin gene lead to a reduced level of natural moisturizing factor (NMF) in the stratum corneum (SC).[1] Since filaggrin (FLG) is the precursor protein for amino acid-derived components of the NMF, the researchers hypothesized that genetic carriers of FLG-null mutations would show reduced levels of NMF in the SC.

A reference spectrum of NMF was first constructed by super-imposing the spectra of pyrrolidone-5-carboxylic acid, ornithine, serine, proline, glycine, histidine and alanine. The researchers then screened 149 participants and 10 atopic dermatitis (AD) patients for four FLG mutations, including R501X, 2282del4, R2447X and S3247X. The study, including 16 carriers of an FLG mutation, was divided into one group of 12 female and four male participants, and another group of 23 individuals with wild type in respect to these mutations, broken into 15 female and eight male participants. Of the 16 mutation carriers, five were heterozygous for R5O1X, eight were heterozygous for 2282del4, and one was heterozygous for R2447X. The mean age of the carrier group was 33 years, comparable with that of non-carriers, with a mean age of 30.

The prevalence of AD history and active AD was found to be higher in carriers of an FLG mutation. Further, all carriers and 11 non-carriers reported dry skin. The study demonstrated that carriers of FLG-null mutations had significantly reduced levels of NMF in the SC and that FLG carriers with a history of AD had significantly lower NMF levels than non-carriers with a history of AD ($P < 0.0001$). In addition to reduced levels of NMF, carriers of FLG mutations showed higher transepidermal water loss than non-carriers.

Antioxidant compositions: The Lion Corp. has disclosed antioxidants containing carotenes, tocopherols or tocotrienol and coenzyme Q10 (CoQ10), in addition to compositions containing them.[2] The antioxidants, which inhibit the formation of lipid peroxides and prevent the formation of wrinkles, contain palm oil carotenes, lycopene and/or lutein; tocopherol and/or tocotrienol; and CoQ10 as active ingredients. A composition containing 39% w/w palm oil carotene, 8% tocotrienol, 32% tocopherol and 1% CoQ10 mmol/L showed 78% inhibition of lipid peroxide formation from linoleic acid in the presence of a radical generator in vitro. Soft capsules were formulated.

Proteoglycan photoaging inhibitors: Narisu Cosmetic Co., Ltd. introduced skin photoaging inhibitors containing proteoglycan-related substances, such as d-glucosamine-HCl, N-acetyl-d-glucosamine, d-xylose and sodium chondroitin sulfate, and cosmetics incorporating them.[3] A milky lotion containing 2.00% w/w N-acetyl-d-glucosamine significantly increased decorin and decreased the area of UVB-induced wrinkles in hairless mice.

Composition for oily skin: Kosei Co., Ltd. disclosed an oily skin composition that contains gamma-oryzanol and N-acyl glutamic acid diesters,[4] and wherein one compound contained is represented by the general formula: R1CONHCH(COOR2)CH2CH2COOR3 where R1 = C7-17 hydrocarbon; and R2 and R3 = C3-30 hydrocarbon; and wherein at least one compound is cholesteryl or phytosteryl. The composition showed improved storage stability of gamma-oryzanol and provided a fresh feeling on the skin without causing stickiness. An example is shown in **Formula 1**.

Formula 1. Oily skin care composition[4]

Gamma-oryzanol	2.00% w/w
N-lauroyl-L-glutamic acid di(cholesteryl/2-octyldodecyl)ester	18.00
Stearyl glycyrrhetinate	0.10
Macadamia nut oil	qs to 100.00

Improving stress with sweet orange oil: Shiseido Co., Ltd. used sweet orange oils, including orris oil and neroli oil, to improve stress response in cosmetics.[5] Formulation examples of creams, gels, shampoos, foods and cosmetic preparations were given.

Lotus extract for anticellulite activity: Lenaers et al. describe a three-pronged approach to reduce cellulite, including targeting fat storage, inflammation and adipose tissue degradation.[6] Silab has developed a lotus extract that provides anticellulite activity in these three areas. Research shows the extract reduces fat storage in mature adipocytes by activating lipolysis and inhibiting pre-adipocyte differentiation into mature adipocytes through the action of SIRT-1—a calorie restriction gene that limits the adipogenesis process. The extract also limits inflammation of adipose tissue by promoting the synthesis of adiponectin, an anti-inflammatory molecule; and finally, it preserves the adipose connective tissue by limiting its degradation.

Hair and Hair Care

Hair growth-promoting composition: Rath et al. disclose a composition and method for the promotion of hair growth on a mammal.[7] The composition—including lysine, proline, arginine, an ascorbic compound, polyphenols, calcium, magnesium, N-acetyl-cysteine, selenium, copper and manganese—was administered to a mammal and found to promote hair growth at certain levels.

Skin Pigmentation

The life cycle of melanocytes: Shinpou et al. have reviewed controlling the life cycle of human melanocytes by paracrine factors.[8] Hyperpigmentation and uneven pigmentation are cosmetic skin disorders that result from the aberrant proliferation and activation of melanocytes. To shed new light on the treatment of these disorders, an understanding of the life cycle of melanin-producing melanocytes would be of interest.

The life cycle of melanocytes includes several steps, beginning with the birth of undifferentiated precursor cells called *melanoblasts* followed by their maturation to fully differentiated melanocytes, their proliferation and activation, and their eventual death. This process is not fully understood in terms of identification of the precursor cells and the paracrine and intrinsic factors that regulate progress through the life cycle.

In order to identify such factors in vitro, the use of a completely defined culture medium has a major advantage. Researchers in the present study developed a normal melanocyte culture system based on a serum-free, chemically-defined medium to examine the in vitro effects of various paracrine factors on the life cycle of melanocytes with particular attention to their proliferation, activation and cell death.

Facultative skin pigmentation: Jimbow has reviewed aging and skin pigmentation including molecular targets for management.[9] Skin lightening for antiaging has recently become a large segment of the personal care industry, particularly for ethnic skin.

Skin pigmentation consists of two basic forms: a constitutive skin pigmentation, which reflects genetic skin color; and facultative skin pigmentation that is acquired from senescence and environmental exposure. Abnormal skin pigmentation associated with aging deals primarily with the facultative form, which reflects alterations of an epidermal melanin unit (EMU). The EMU defines the symbiotic interaction of a melanocyte and its associated pool of keratinocytes.

Thus, molecular targets for skin pigmentation associated with aging should be focused on mechanisms related to the EMU. There are three basic approaches. The first is the melanin/melanosome exfoliation process, which can be subdivided into exfoliation of horny-layered cells, accelerated growth of these cells, and their water and sebum content. The second is the transfer and degradation of melanin/melanosomes, which concerns molecules affecting the growth and differentiation of either melanocytes, keratinocytes or both. The third target are the molecules responsible for melanin and melanosome biosynthesis.

The step-by-step dissection of each of these processes should provide improved or novel management of aging-related facultative skin pigmentation.

Sunscreens

Photostable UV absorber: Shiseido Company Ltd. has disclosed sunscreens including dibenzoylmethane derivatives in combination with alkyl diphenylacrylate and benzalmalonate derivatives[10] that do not hinder the photostabilizing effect of the dibenzoylmethane derivatives. The composition is an effective UV absorber across a wide wavelength range, from UVA to UVB. Specifically, the composition contains a dibenzoylmethane derivative; an alkyl beta, beta-diphenylacrylate and/or an alpha-cyano-beta, beta-diphenylacrylate (for example, octocrylene); and a specific benzalmalonate derivative; for example, di-(2-ethylhexyl)-4-methoxybenzalmalonate.

Broad-spectrum UV filter: Herzog et al. review the development of broad-spectrum UV filters for cosmetic applications.[11] Modern sunscreens must protect against both UVB and UVA radiation. This requires UVB absorbers as well as photostable UVA or broad-spectrum UV filters. Bis-ethylhexyloxyphenol methoxyphenyltriazine (BEMT)[a] is a hydroxy-phenyl-triazine derivative that is designed for optimal spectral performance and solubility in cosmetic oils. Due to its molecular structure, the material exhibits a UV spectrum with two absorption peaks, indicating broad-spectrum protection even at the low concentration of 2%. It also exhibits efficacious photostability based on rapid photo-tautomerization, recognized by a change in molecular configuration brought about with exposure to UV.

The material can efficiently stabilize photo-labile UV filters such as T-butylmethoxydibenzoylmethane or ethylhexyl meth-

---

[a] Tinosorb S (INCI: Bis-ethylhexyloxyphenol Methoxyphenyltirazine) is a product of Ciba Specialty Chemicals.

[b] Tinosorb M (INCI: Methylene Bis-benzotriazolyl Tetramethylbutylphenol) is a product of Ciba.

oxycinnamate. Furthermore, it shows a synergistic effect on SPF with commonly used UVB filters as well as with bis-benzotriazolyl tetramethylbutylphenol.[b]

Makeup

Makeup remover stick: Kosei Co., Ltd. has developed a makeup remover stick containing solid fats of a melting point ≥ 70°C, di-C_{14-15} alkyl carbonates, and powders.[12] The remover is said to feel soft to the touch and leave no sticky residue after use. A combination of polyethylene wax[c], ethylene/propylene copolymer[d], C_{14-15} dialkyl carbonate[e], petrolatum[f], polymethyl methacrylate[g], silica[h], tocopherol acetate, propylparaben and polyglyceryl-2 triisostearate[j] showed effective removal of mascara.

Two-phase aqueous cosmetics: Kao Corp. has created two-phase aqueous cosmetics comprising powders coated with acrylic silicone graft copolymers, fluoro oils, water (*aqua*) and ethanol.[13] The cosmetics are said to have efficacious redispersibility after a long storage time, and remain in two separate phases of a transparent solution layer and a powder layer while standing. An example of such a makeup base is shown in **Formula 2**.

Formula 2. Two-phase makeup base[13]

Nylon powder treated with acrylate-dimethicone copolymer	3.00% w/w
Polyperfluoromethylisopropyl ether (Fomblin HC/04, Uniqema)	30.00
1,3-Butylene glycol	5.00
Ethanol	10.00
Fragrance (*parfum*)	qs
Water (*aqua*)	qs to 100.00

[c] Performalene 500 (INCI: Polyethylene Wax) is a product of New Phase Technologies.
[d] EPS Wax (INCI: Ethylene/Propylene Copolymer) is a product of Ina Trading.
[e] Lialcarb SR-1000/R (INCI: C_{14-15} Dialkyl Carbonate) is a product of EniChem.
[f] Vaseline is a registered trademark of Unilever.
[g] Microsphere M 101 (INCI: Polymethyl Methacrylate) is a product of Matsumoto Yushi Seiyaku Co., Ltd.
[h] Sylysia 770 (INCI: Silica) is a product of Fuji Silysia Chemical Co., Ltd.
[j] Cosmol 43V (INCI: Polyglyceryl-2 Triisostearate) is a product of Nisshin OilliO.

Interesting Raw Materials

Plant extracts as antioxidants: Shiseido Co., Ltd. has disclosed the use of plant extracts as antioxidants, DNA damage inhibitors, and topical drugs and cosmetics.[14] Plant extracts from *Sarcandra glabra*, *Saraca dives*, *Cudrania pubescens*, *Taxodium distichum*, *Ludwigia octovalis*, *Deutzianthus tonkinensis*, *Alchornea trewioides*, *Berchemia polyphylla*, *Glochidion puberum* and *Sassafras tzumu* are claimed to act as antioxidants, UV-induced DNA damage inhibitors, topical drugs and cosmetics. Formulation examples of creams, gels, cosmetic preparations and health drinks are presented.

Orange roughy oil for sensitive skin: Yamanouchi et al. review the properties of highly purified orange roughly oil, a marine-derived wax ester, for its physicochemical properties and effects on human skin, for application in cosmetics.[15] The oil posseses a fatty acid composition that is more like human skin than jojoba wax. The stability of the oil during storage was found to be similar to olive oil and jojoba wax. From a human study, the marine oil significantly improved skin condition and the moisture-maintaining ability of atopic and/or dry skin subjects. Researchers concluded that orange roughy oil is suitable for sensitive skin care.

Interesting Vehicles

Oily bases: Nippon Emulsion Co., Ltd. and Ajinomoto Co., Inc. disclose oily bases combining esters of amino acids with dimer diols and optional fatty acids, in addition to cosmetics or topical preparations containing them.[16] The bases are said to show good storage stability, pigment dispersibility and a good feel. Thus, titanium dioxide was mixed with N-myristoyl-N-methylalanine[k] for 3 min and allowed to stand for 3 days without resulting precipitation. A w/o cream foundation containing the aforementioned preparation and pigments showed effective covering properties and did not irritate skin.

Oily gel compositions: Asahi Kasei Chemicals Corp. has introduced oily gel compositions.[17] The described inventions contain a high amount of an oily component, a multichain polyhydrophilic compound having two or more long-chain hydrophobic groups and hydrophilic groups, a polyhydroxyl compound having two or more OH groups, a surfactant, water (*aqua*) and another oily component. A method to produce the oily gel composition and a method for mixing a water-containing composition to form an emulsion also are disclosed. For example, L-lysine hydrochloride was reacted with N-lauroyl-L-glutamic anhydride and neutralized with sodium hydroxide to obtain a multichain polyhydrophilic compound. A formulation containing this material is shown in **Formula 3**.

Formula 3. Oily gel composition[16]

Multichain polyhydrophilic compound	2.00% w/w
Glycerin	20.00
Decylglucoside	0.40
Jojoba oil	6.70
Hydrogenated lysolecithin	2.70
Squalane	40.30
Tetraoctanoylpentaerythritol	20.10
Water (*aqua*)	qs to 100.00

Formula 4. Transparent lotion emulsion[18]

Vitamin A	0.005% w/w
Phenoxyethanol	0.005
Ethoxylated hydrogenated castor oil	0.100
Citric acid	0.020
Sodium citrate	0.100
Glycerin	5.000
Water (*aqua*)	qs to 100.000

Transparent cosmetics: Noevir Co., Ltd. has disclosed transparent aqueous cosmetics containing oil-soluble components.[18] This invention also relates to a method for manufacturing storage-stable transparent cosmetics that contain oil soluble components. The oil soluble components, such as perfumes and essential oils, are dissolved in phenoxyethanol and surfactants and water are added to obtain a stable solution. An example is shown in **Formula 4**.

Published April 2009 *Cosmetics and Toiletries* magazine

References

1. S Kezic et al., Loss-of-function mutations in the fillaggrin gene lead to reduced level of natural moisturizing factor in the stratum corneum, *Journal of Investigative Dermatology* 128(8) 2117–2119 (2008) (in English)

2. JP 2008 239,714, Antioxidants containing carotenes, tocopherols or tocotrienol, and coenzyme Q10, and antioxidant compositions, Lion Corp., Japan, Oct 9, 2008

3. JP 2008 195,629, Skin photoaging inhibitors containing proteoglycan-related substances, and cosmetics containing them, Narisu Cosmetic Co., Ltd., Japan, Aug 28, 2008

4. JP 2008 201,753, Skin compositions containing gamma-oryzanol and N-acyl glutamic acid diesters, Kosei Co., Ltd., Japan, Sep 4, 2008

5. JP 2008 247,894, Sweet orange oils as stress response improvers and cosmetics, Shiseido Co., Ltd., Japan, Oct 16, 2008

6. C Lenaers et al., Triple target for a high anticellulite action: fat storage, inflammation and adipose tissue degradation, *Frag Jrnl* 36(9) 53–58 (2008) (in Japanese)

7. US 2008 248,130, Composition and method for the promotion of hair growth on a mammal, Matthias Rath, Aleksandm Niedzwiecki and Waheed Roomi, Netherlands, Oct 9, 2008

8. T Shinpou et al., Control of life cycle of human melanocytes by paracrine factors, *Frag Jrnl* 36(9) 42–47 (2008) (in Japanese)

9. K Jimbow, Aging and skin pigmentation: molecular targets for management, *Frag Jrnl* 36(9) 17–25 (2008) (in Japanese)

10. WO 2008 102,875, Sunscreens comprising dibenzoylmethane derivatives in combination with alkyl diphenylacrylate and benzalmalonate derivative, Shiseido Company Ltd., Japan, Aug 28, 2008

11. B Herzog, et al., Development of new broad-spectrum UV filter for cosmetic application, *Frag Jrnl* 36(8) 72–76 (2008) (in Japanese)

12. JP 2008 195,614, Stick-type makeup removers containing solid fats, dialkyl carbonates, and powder, Kosei Co., Ltd., Japan, Aug 28, 2008

13. JP 2008 195,659, Two-phase aqueous cosmetics comprising surface-treated powders and fluoro oils, Kao Corp., Japan, Aug 28, 2008

14. JP 2008 247,854, Plant exts. as antioxidants, DNA damage inhibitors, and topical drugs and cosmetics, Shiseido Co., Ltd., Japan, Oct 16, 2008

15. S Yamanouchi et al., The properties of the marine wax ester and its effects on human skin, *Frag Jrnl* 36(8) 83–87 (2008) (in Japanese)

16. JP 2008 195,624, Oily bases containing esters of amino acids with dimer diols and optional fatty acids, and cosmetics or topical preparations containing them, Nippon Emulsion Co., Ltd.; Ajinomoto Co., Inc., Japan, Aug 28, 2008

17. JP 2008 195,665, Oily gel compositions containing multichain polyhydrophilic compounds, polyhydroxyl compounds, and surfactants, Asahi Kasei Chemicals Corp., Japan, Aug 28, 2008

18. JP 2008 195,676, Transparent aqueous cosmetics containing oil-soluble components, Noevir Co., Ltd., Japan, Aug 28, 2008

CHAPTER 28

An ECM-derived Tetrapeptide to Counterbalance ECM Degeneration

Mike Farwick, Ursula Maczkiewitz and Peter Lersch
Evonik Goldschmidt GmbH, Essen, Germany

Tim Falla
Helix Biomedix Inc., Bothell, Wash. USA

Susanne Grether-Beck and Jean Krutmann
Institut für Umweltmedizinische Forschung, Heinrich-Heine-University
Düsseldorf, Germany

KEY WORDS: *peptides, antiaging, collagen, hyaluronic acid, fibronectin*

ABSTRACT: *Degradation of dermal and epidermal proteins and the reduced proliferation of collagen and hyaluronic acid in the dermis occur during aging. Thus, antiaging technologies must to correct these deficiencies to induce skin regeneration and combat the signs of aging. Data presented here demonstrates that ECM-derived tetrapeptides have the potential to counterbalance ECM degeneration.*

The extracellular matrix (ECM) is the structural backbone of many tissues, especially the skin, and represents a main target for cosmetic applications. ECM proteins are believed to play a pivotal role in cellular migration, proliferation and gene regulation during wound healing. Fragments from ECM constituents have been found capable of stimulating ECM biosynthesis to compensate for tissue destruction.[1] Their mechanisms have been implicated in wound healing, skin aging and skin's response to UV irradiation;[2, 3] from this knowledge, new actives have evolved, as the authors describe here.

Building from the concept that ECM constituents stimulate ECM biosynthesis, bioinformatic methods were employed to identify highly repetitive amino acid motifs with inherent antiaging activities. Several dozens of tetrapeptides were found scattered across sequences of the major ECM macro-molecules.[4] Ten peptides showed the desired effect of significantly increasing collagen protein in supernatant, thus verifying the underlying assumption that breakdown products of ECM proteins stimulate the ECM neosynthesis.

Of the ten peptides, the five most promising were subjected to further analysis including concomitant collagen determination in the supernatant, as well as gene expression analysis of the ECM marker genes: collagen (COL1A1), fibronectin (FN1) and hyaluronic acid synthetase (HAS1).

Collagen, being a dermal protein responsible for skin strength and elasticity, was examined since its degradation leads to wrinkles that accompany aging.[5] Hyaluronic acid, one of the main components of the ECM, is a nonsulfated glycosaminoglycan that binds water, also ensuring the elasticity of the skin.[6] Fibronectin, a glycoprotein that helps to create a cross-linked network within the ECM, was also of interest since it provides binding sites for other ECM components such as hyaluronic acid and collagen.[7]

In the end, one tetrapeptide, glycine-glutamic acid-lysine-glycine (GEKG, or INCI: tetrapeptide-21)[a], was evaluated in vivo for effects on these genes.

Material and Methods

Human dermal fibroblasts (HDFs) prepared from neonatal foreskin were cultured for four days in a humidified 5% carbon dioxide atmosphere in Eagle's minimal essential medium[b] supplemented with: 5% fetal calf serum[c], 0.1% l-glutamine, 2.5% sodium bicarbonate, and 1% streptomycin/amphotericin B, until they reached confluence. For the studies described here, only early passage fibroblasts (< 12) were used so as to avoid any changes in their original phenotype during subculture. Cells were kept in 6-well plates for culture.

---

[a] Tego Pep 4-17 (INCI: Tetrapeptide-21 (and) Glycerin (and) Butylene Glycol (and) Water (aqua)), is a product of Evonik Goldschmidt GmbH.
[b] EMEM is a product of Life Technologies GmbH, Eggenstein, Germany.
[c] Fetal Calf Serum is a product of Greiner, Frickenhausen, Germany.

For isolation of total RNA, kits[d] were used according to manufacturer instructions. The RNA concentration was determined via photometric measurement[e] at 260/280. To avoid repeated free-thaw cycles for the prepared RNA for multiple experiments, aliquots of total RNA (100 ng) were applied for cDNA synthesis using a synthesis system[f] for the reverse transcription step with random healers. For each gene, a specific primer pair was designed[g] based on the cDNA sequence published as indicated. For each gene expression determination, three independent experiments were performed and the mean value of these was calculated.

PCR reactions were carried out using a continuous fluorescence detection device[h] and software[j]. Each sample was analyzed twice, employing the universal protocol over 46 cycles. Detailed reaction conditions included: 10 min 94°C of hot-start taq polymerase activation, 20 sec 95°C denaturation, 20 sec 55°C annealing, and 30 sec 72°C extension. For comparison of relative expression in real time PCR control cells and treated cells, the 2 (-$\Delta\Delta C(T)$) method was used.

The tested peptides were applied at concentrations of 1 µg/mL for 24 hr to human dermal fibroblast cell cultures, and RNA was extracted to perform gene expression profiling. Induction of hyaluronic acid-synthase-1 and collagen was analyzed by real time PCR with the primer pairs shown in **Table 1**. Since collagen production depends not only on stimulated gene

Table 1. Primer pairs	
18S rRNA	5´-GCCGCTAGAGGTGAAATTCTTG-3´
	5´-CATTCTTGGCAAATGCTTTCG´-3´
Collagen 1A1	5´-CCTGCGTGTACCCCACTCA-3´
	5´-ACCAGACATGCCTCTTGTCCTT-3´
HAS-1	5´-GCGGGCTTGTCAGAGCTACT-3´
	5´-AACTGCTGCAAGAGGTTATTCCTATAT-3´
Fibronectin	5´-GAAAGTACACCTGTTGTCATTCAACA-3´
	5´-ACCTTCACGTCTGTCACTTCCA-3´

---

[d] The RNeasy Total RNA Mini Kit is a product of Qiagen.
[e] BioPhotometer is a product of Eppendorf.
[f] SuperScript III First-Strand Synthesis System is a product of InVitrogen.
[g] Primer Express 2.0 Software is a product of Applied Bio Systems.
[h] The Opticon 1 machine is a device from MJ Research, Waltham, MA, USA.
[j] The SYBR Green PCR Master Mix software is a product of Applied Biosystems.
[k] The Sircol Collagen Assay is a product of Biocolor.

expression, but also on a complex process of post-translational modification, researchers further quantified the collagen concentration in the fibroblast cell culture supernatants using a collagen assay[k].[8] All samples were incubated in the presence of β-aminopropionitrile (50 µg/mL) to increase the stability of the collagen.

In addition, an in vivo study was conducted with a panel of 60 volunteers divided into four groups. Four variations of a test cream were developed (see **Formula 1**), including a placebo cream without the active, a positive control cream incorporating 10 ppm palmitoyl pentapeptide-4,[2,3] a cream with 10 ppm GEKG, and a cream with 100 ppm GEKG. The samples were applied to the inner forearms of subjects twice daily for eight weeks. Before and after eight weeks of application, skin volume and roughness were analyzed using a skin surface characterization device[m].

Formula 1. Sample cream used for in vivo tests	
Polyglyceryl-3 methylglucose distearate	3.0%
Glyceryl stearate	2.0%
Stearyl alcohol	1.0%
C12-15 alkyl benzoate	9.5%
PPG-3 myristyl ether	9.5%
Glycerin	2.5%
1,2-Butanediol	0.25%
Polysorbate 20	0.025%
Peptide	varied
Preservative	0.8%
Fragrance (*parfum*)	0.1%
Water (*aqua*)	qs to 100.0%

Results

Of all those tested, the most active peptide found had the sequence GEKG (see **Figure 1**). At a concentration of 1 µg/mL, the peptide increased the amount of secreted collagen protein in the supernatant approximately 2.5-fold. On the mRNA level, all three tested ECM marker genes were induced, resulting in a 2.5-fold increase of COL1A1 expression. In addition, HAS1 encoding for the hyaluronic acid was 5.7-fold, and the gene encoding for fibronectin was induced by 10.5-fold. The well-balanced induction of these important ECM constituents by the GEKG peptide suggests strong antiaging effects.

Although the palmitoyl pentapeptide-4 positive control showed a stronger induction in COL1A1 gene expression, the effect was not completely translated into collagen protein. This could be due to different gene induction kinetics. For instance, GEKG may cause a faster response on expression levels that is immediately translated into protein production, and that afterward diminishes to minor levels; whereas the positive control peptide could take longer to react to the stimulus, thus delaying the response.

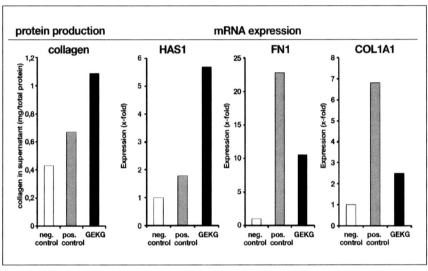

Figure 1. In vitro effects of GEKG on secreted collagen levels and ECM marker gene expression in human dermal fibroblasts

The in vivo relevance of GEKG activity was additionally tested by a vehicle-controlled biopsy and elasticity study. After eight weeks' application of a cream formulation containing 50 ppm GEKG, both collagen gene expression and skin elasticity significantly increased, compared with the vehicle and untreated skin (data not shown but available).

Thus, to demonstrate the proposed antiaging effect of GEKG in vivo, a parameter "volume" measurement was taken of the previously mentioned 60 volunteers. This software-based method compares the distribution of gray scales in photographs taken of the volunteers' skin before and after the eight-week application period. It calculates the theoretical amount of liquid that would be necessary to fill the wrinkles and generate a plain surface. A reduction of the parameter volume is interpreted as an overall improvement in skin structure resulting from the reduction of skin wrinkles in number and depth.

With an increasing concentration of GEKG, an increased reduction of the volume was observed. Compared with the positive control, a significant increase was obtained with 100 ppm GEKG (see **Figure 2a**).

Besides parameter volume measurements, parameter roughness was assessed via the same skin texture analysis device[m].[9,10] These roughness parameters originate from the DIN-parameters Ra–Rz, and describe the depth of fine and coarse wrinkles. R1–R5, for instance, describe the maximum and average amplitude of a surface structure, as well as the mean height level. In the case of GEKG in skin, **Figure 2b** again demonstrates a dose-dependent effect; increasing concentrations of GEKG increased the reduction of skin roughness. Compared with the positive control, 10 ppm GEKG showed comparable efficacy whereas 100 ppm GEKG doubled the effect.

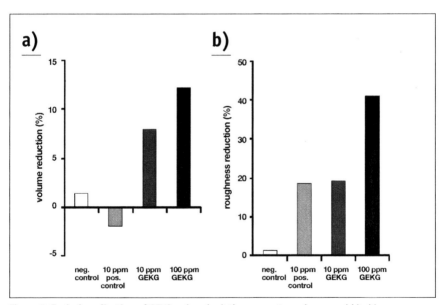

Figure 2. Topical application of GEKG reduced: a) the parameter volume, and b) skin roughness in vivo

Only 10 ppm of palmitoyl pentapeptide was tested, which is closer to its maximum suggested use level. GEKG at 10 ppm and 100 ppm translates to approximately 0.5–5.0% of the tetrapeptide-21 use concentration, which contains 2,000 ppm peptide.

Figure 3 shows the skin structure of one volunteer who applied the formulation containing 100 ppm GEKG for eight weeks. The pictures demonstrate an overall improvement of the skin structure; the wrinkles are less deep and less pronounced and the skin roughness is decreased.

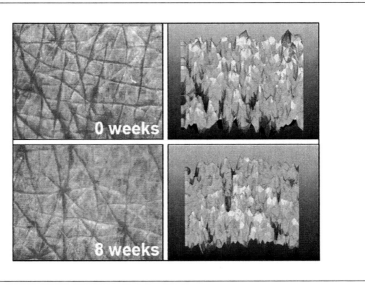

Figure 3. Photographs of one volunteer's skin taken before and after eight weeks of topical application of 100 ppm GEKG; for software-supported analysis, each photograph was digitalized and the differences were calculated

Conclusion

Aging is associated with changes in the skin at all levels. For instance, degradation of key dermal-epidermal and dermal proteins occur, together with reduced epidermal proliferation and collagen and hyaluronic acid synthesis in the papillary dermis. Antiaging technologies must correct these deficiencies in order to induce skin regeneration to combat the resulting signs of aging.

The data presented in this study demonstrates that ECM-derived tetrapeptides have the potential to counterbalance the ECM degeneration observed during skin aging. In silico analysis identified approximately 30 abundant tetrapeptide motifs in ECM proteins, and in vitro analysis showed that 10 of these motifs can stimulate collagen synthesis.

GEKG was identified as a highly active tetrapeptide that is able to stimulate dermal repair and renewal mechanisms. An increased expression of ECM-synthesizing enzymes like hyaluronic acid synthethase, as well as expression and production of ECM proteins like collagen and fibronectin, was observed. Finally, in vivo data confirmed the efficacy of GEKG, leading to an improved skin structure and reduced wrinkles.

Published June 2009 *Cosmetics and Toiletries* magazine

References

1. LR Robinson, NC Fitzgerald, DG Doughty, NC Dawes, CA Berge and DL Bissett, Topical palmitoyl pentapeptide provides improvement in photoaged human facial skin, *Int J Cosm Sci* 27(3) 155–160 (2005)
2. KT Tran, P Lamb and JS Deng, Matrikines and matricryptins: Implications for cutaneous cancers and skin repair, *J Dermatol Sci Oct* 40(1) 11–20 (2005)
3. KT Tran, L Griffith and A Wells, Extracellular matrix signaling through growth factor receptors during wound healing, *Wound Repair Regen* 12(3) 262–8 (May-Jun 2004)
4. US 20070299105, Peptide fragments for inducing synthesis of extracellular matrix proteins
5. M Yaar and BA Gilchrest, Photoaging: Mechanism, prevention and therapy, *Br J Dermatol*, 157(5) 874–87 (Nov 2007)
6. L Baumann, Skin aging and its treatment, *J Pathol* 211(2) 241–51 (Jan 2007)
7. M Larsen, VV Artym, JA Green andKM Yamada, The matrix reorganized: Extracellular matrix remodeling and integrin signalling, *Curr Opin Cell Biol* 18(5) 463–71 (Oct 2006)
8. VV Yurovsky, Tumor necrosis factor-related apoptosis-inducing ligand enhances collagen production by human lung fibroblasts, *Am J Respir Cell Mol Biol* 28(2) 225–31 (2003)
9. K De Paepe, JM Lagarde, Y Gall, D Roseeuw and V Rogiers, Microrelief of the skin using a light transmission method, *Arch Dermatol Res* 292(10) 500–10 (2000)
10. A Pagoni, Photo-aging and photodocumentation, *Cosmet Toil* 117(1) 39–46 (2002)

CHAPTER 29

Mitochondrial Nourishment and Protection for Antiaging Effects

KG Sabarinathan, PhD
CoValence Inc., Chandler, Ariz. USA

KEY WORDS: *mitochondria, antioxidant, nutrition, antiaging, DNA*

ABSTRACT: *Multiple factors affect the integrity of cell mitochondria, leading to loss of cell function, aging and apoptosis. In skin, this is expressed in the form of wrinkles, loss of tone, etc. To combat these effects, the author describes a technology that contains mitochondria-nourishing compounds to deliver antiaging benefits.*

Virtually everything that human cells need to maintain health requires energy. Each cell contains hundreds to thousands of mitochondria, and each mitochondrion contains multiple copies of mitochondrial DNA (mtDNA). Mitochondrial proteins take food molecules and combine them with oxygen to create chemical energy. This chemical energy produced by the mitochondria through the cellular respiration process is called adenosine triphosphate (ATP) (see **Figure 1**).

Generally the duration of life varies inversely with the rate of energy expenditure during life. Bio-gerontologist Denham Harman, PhD, the "father of the free radical theory of aging," once suggested that mitochondria are the crucial component of cells whose rate of decline dictates the overall rate of aging.[1] In addition to supplying cellular energy, mitochondria are involved in a range of other processes such as signaling, cellular differentiation and cell death, as well as controlling the cell's cycle and growth.[2]

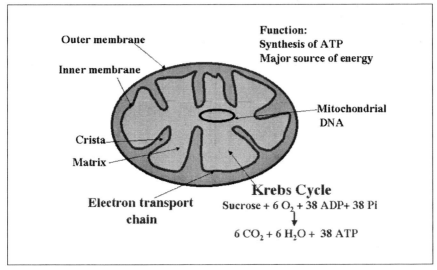

Figure 1. The chemical energy produced by the mitochondria through the cellular respiration process is called adenosine triphosphate (ATP).

In human cells and eukaryotic cells in general, DNA is found in two cellular locations: inside the nucleus and inside the mitochondria. The generation of reactive oxygen species (ROS) such as superoxide anion, hydrogen peroxide and hydroxyl radicals as by-products of mitochondrial oxidative phosphorylation (see **Figure 2**) damages mitochondrial macromolecules including the mtDNA, leading to deleterious mutations.

MtDNA damage is more extensive and persists longer than nuclear DNA damage

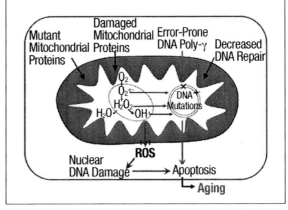

Figure 2. By-products of mitochondrial oxidative phosphorylation damage the mitochondrial macromolecules, including the mtDNA, and lead to deleterious mutations.

in human cells,[3] so when ROS have damaged the mitochondrial energy-generating apparatus beyond a functional threshold, rather than restoring it to a healthy condition, the mitochondria releases proteins that activate the caspase pathway, leading to aging and apoptosis.[4] In skin, this aging is expressed in the form of wrinkles, loss of tone, thinning and abnormal collagen accumulation.

The human mitochondrial genome was sequenced in 1981, facilitating the isolation of mutant mtDNA and eventually its quantification. These experiments confirmed that mtDNA damage increases aging in humans and other mammals.[5] Recent work by Trifunovic et al.[6] also supports the mitochondrial theory of aging, showing that in prematurely aged mice, defective mitochondrial DNA polymerase is expressed. This work provides a causative link between mtDNA damage and aging phenotypes in mammals.[6]

Delivering Mitochondria Nutrition

An approach to the mitochondrial theory of aging, as will be described, is a technology focused on mitochondria-nourishing compounds. However, since the efficacy of functional ingredients fundamentally is determined by their delivery and influenced by the vehicle and molecules themselves,[7] it is important first to consider the delivery aspect; in this case, the technology was encapsulated for controlled delivery.

A free-flowing powder of solid, hydrophobic nanospheres containing the mitochondria-nourishing compounds was further encapsulated in moisture-sensitive microspheres averaging 100–300 nm in diameter to deliver them to the epidermal level. These spheres adhere to skin as a result of lipophilic properties and electrostatic forces. While they are unable to penetrate the stratum corneum (SC), once they are deposited on skin, they form a reservoir, and moisture in the skin triggers the release of the nanospheres, which penetrate the lower layers of the SC. The incorporation of this controlled release system into anhydrous cosmetic formulations was found to provide moisture-triggered and prolonged release of the active ingredients (data not shown).

Mitochondria-nourishing Components

The nano-encapsulated, chirally active ingredients[a] at the core of the described technology (see **Chirality in Chemistry**) were used to nourish mitochondria and stimulate the mitochondria support enzymes,[8–10] to protect against endogenous and exogenous ROS, in turn slowing the aging of skin cells and other cellular material.

Spin-trap phenyl-butyl-nitrone (PBN): Research has shown that spin-trap PBN provides neuroprotective, cytoprotective, anti-inflammatory, oxidative stress recovery and free radical scavenging properties.[11] Spin-traps originally were used to measure free radical activity both in vivo and in vitro by their ability to form stable complexes. Reactive free radicals are attracted and bound to the beta carbon atom in the spin trap, forming a spin adduct and effectively "trapping" the free radical, allowing the structure of the trapped radical to be deduced, and returning it to a normal orbit before it causes damage to the mitochondria.[12] The material acts to prevent free radical damage caused endogenously through normal metabolic processes or exogenously by sources such as UV radiation, NO and other air pollutants by absorbing electrons as they spin out of control.

Coenzyme Q10 (CoQ10): CoQ10 or ubiquinone is a naturally occurring compound found in all cells in the human body that plays a key role in

Chirality in Chemistry

Chirality or *handedness* refers to a molecule that is not superimposable on its mirror image. This positioning is described in chemistry using *L* to define the left side of a molecular twin—i.e., the *L-isomer*, and *D* to define the right side, or *D-isomer*. One version of the molecule may interact with a cell receptor to produce the desired outcome, while the other may have no useful application, or even unwanted effects.

In the present invention, the company used chirally active ingredients by selecting the effective isomer from the racemic mixture of the ingredient. The efficiency of the percutaneous absorption of cosmetic products is also influenced by the chirality of the ingredients; this is well-documented by Heard and Brain (1995) and Heard et al. (1993).

---

[a] Mitoprotect (INCI: Phenyl-butyl-nitrone (PBN) (and) Ubiquinone (and) 1,2-Dithiolane-3-Pentanoic Acid (and) Adenine (and) Acetyl Carnitine (and) antioxidants) is a product and registered trademark of CoValence.

the mitochondria by converting food into energy. Ninety-five percent of all human body energy requirements are converted to ATP with the aid of CoQ10, and the depletion of CoQ10 levels in skin cells leads to the premature aging as well as a decrease in the formation of new cells.[13, 14] Studies have shown that low doses of CoQ10 applied topically reduce oxidation and DNA double-strand breaks. In addition, CoQ10 supplements have been shown to extend the lifespan of human cells. In the described technology, CoQ10 stabilizes the CoQ10 content in the skin cells to increase their longevity.[15]

R-lipoic acid: Normally only the R-enantiomer of lipoic acid occurs naturally and in miniscule amounts in animal and plant tissues. Due to the difficulty and high cost of isolating natural R-alpha lipoic acid (ALA), studies and products were initially conducted and produced using synthetic lipoic acid. Unlike natural R-ALA, however, synthetic lipoic acid contains a 50/50 mixture of both R-ALA and S-ALA. Thus, most cosmetic products on the market containing ALA in fact contain both forms of lipoic acid—the synthetic S form and the natural R form.

However, Loffelhardt and co-workers have shown[16] the S-enantiomer to have an inhibiting effect on the R-enantiomer since they are isomers, and with their atomic arrangements reversed, the biological activity of the R-enantiomer is substantially reduced, creating oxidative stress in human cells.

R-lipoic acid is water- and fat-soluble[8] and therefore can neutralize free radicals both in membranes and within cells; it can also mimic other antioxidants and improve their performance by replenishing them.[17] When an antioxidant neutralizes a free radical, it turns the radical into a stable form. In the chemical reaction that follows, the free radical is eventually passed off to lipoic acid or a glutathione molecule, which allows the original antioxidant to regenerate and continue to neutralize more free radicals while ALA washes out the offending free radical.[18] This provides protection to the mitochondria.

In addition to its antioxidant function, R-lipoic acid has been shown to remodel collagen synthesis; to inhibit the abnormal attachment of sugar to protein and collagen, which makes skin inflexible and stiff (glycosylation); and to provide an anti-inflammatory function.[19, 20] Research also has shown that R-lipoic acid increases the mitochondrial membrane potential of aged rats by up to 50%, compared with unsupplemented, aged rats.[8]

Adenine: Adenine is one of the two purine nucleobases used in forming nucleotides of the nucleic acids. In DNA, adenine binds to thymine via two hydrogen bonds to assist in stabilizing the nucleic acid structures. Some scientists have proposed that during the origin of life on Earth, the first molecule formed was adenine by polymerization reaction.[21] Adenine performs a variety of roles in cellular biochemistry including cellular respiration in the form of energy-rich ATP and other cofactors such as nicotinamide adenine dinucleotide and flavin adenine dinucleotide, thus increasing the longevity and proper functioning of the mitochondria.[22]

Acetyl-L-carnitine (ALC): ALC regulates the mitochondrial cytochrome-C oxidase level in the human body, including skin cells; cytochrome-C oxidase is a vital component of cellular energy processes and is responsible for virtually all oxygen consumption in mammals.[23] ALC transports long-chain acyl groups from fatty acids into the mitochondrial matrix so they can be broken down to acetate via β-oxidation to obtain usable energy through the citric acid cycle. Throughout human aging, carnitine concentration in cells diminishes, affecting energy production by the mitochondria. Recently reported data clarifies the role of ALC and the carnitine transport system in the interplay between peroxisomes and mitochondrial fatty acid oxidation.[24]

Thus, the combination of R-lipoic acid with ALC can significantly improve metabolic function; at the same time, this combination lowers oxidative stress and free radical production.[25]

Antioxidant Activity

The antioxidant potential and activity of the enzymes in the complex[a] were evaluated through the Oxygen Radical Absorbance Capacity (ORAC) assay[b] developed at the National Institute on Aging in the National Institutes of Health (NIH). This assay is based on a hydrogen atom transfer (HAT) reaction mechanism, which is relevant to human biology (see **HAT Assays**). The stimulation by antioxidant

---

[b] The ORAC assay is a patented technology from Brunswick Laboratories.

enzymes thus served as an indicator of the nutritional effects of the complex on the mitochondria.

The ORAC assay based on Glazer's study measures the oxidative degradation of a fluorescent molecule (either β-phycoerythrin or fluorescein) after being mixed with free radical generators such as azo-initiator compounds. Azo-initiators are considered to produce peroxyl free radicals by heating, which damages the fluorescent molecule, resulting in the loss of fluorescence. Antioxidants protect the fluorescent molecule from oxidative degeneration, and this degree of protection is quantified using a fluorometer.

HAT Assays

HAT-based assays measure the capability of an antioxidant to quench free radicals (generally peroxyl radicals) by H-atom donation. The HAT mechanisms of antioxidant action in which the hydrogen atom (H) of a phenol (Ar-OH) is transferred to an ROO radical can be summarized by the reaction:

$$ROO + AH/ArOH \rightarrow ROOH + A/ArO$$

The water-soluble vitamin E analog Trolox[c] was used as a calibration standard and the ORAC result is expressed as micromole Trolox equivalent (TE)/g (see **Figure 3**).[1] Caffeic acid also served as a calibration standard and the hydroxyl radical antioxidant capacity (HORAC) result is expressed as µmole caffeic acid equivalent (CAE)/g.[2] The acceptable precision of the ORAC assay is 15% relative standard deviation.

---

[c] 6-Hydroxy-2,5,7,8-tetramethylchroman-2-carboxylic acid (Trolox, Hoffman-LaRoche) is a water-soluble derivative of vitamin E.

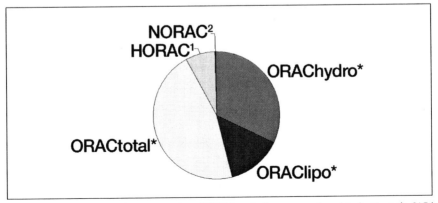

Figure 3. The radical absorbance capacity of HORAC and nitrogen was found to be 7 µmole CAE/g and 0.3 µmole TE/g, respectively.

Results of the ORAC assay indicated that the water-soluble or hydrophilic antioxidant capacity and the lipid-soluble or lipophilic antioxidant capacity of the text complex were 30 and 13 μmole TE/g, respectively. In addition, the HORAC and nitrogen radical absorbance capacity was found to be 7 μmole CAE/g and 0.3 μmole TE/g, respectively (see **Figure 3**).

The Singlet Oxygen Absorbance Capacity (SOAC) using α-tocopherol as a calibration standard showed that the tested complex possessed the antioxidant power of 198 μmole VtE/g— higher antioxidant power than anti-oxidants currently used in the cosmetics industry. As a comparison, apples, evaluated for their ORAC activity by the USDA, generally have measured 22.10 to 42.75 micromoles TE/g.

Stimulating SC Antioxidant Enzymes

The skin is constantly exposed to environmental sources, producing reactive oxygen species (ROS). To protect against oxidative damage, the skin is equipped with a large network of enzymatic antioxidant defense systems such as catalase, superoxide dismutase (SOD), and tissue GSH.[26] In human SC, SOD and catalase are considered major antioxidant enzymes.[27] In various skin disorders, the decreased antioxidant enzyme activity could be considered a marker for the increased susceptibility of the skin to external stimuli.[28]

The ability of the test complex to induce SC antioxidant enzymes was evaluated by the protocol standardized by Hellemans et al.[27] In this study, 40 albino guinea pigs of the same age weighing 350–430 g were selected. The dorsal skin of the guinea pigs was washed and a 35 cm^2 area was shaved before exposing it to a single dose of UVB (290–320 nm) irradiation. The total energy exposure of the guinea pig was 0.9 J/cm^2. The irradiation time was approximately 30 sec.

The test complex was applied in the irradiated area and the anti-oxidant enzyme expression was studied by taking noninvasive tape strippings to determine SOD and catalase activity in guinea pig SC in vivo. In each study, 5 successive tape strippings were collected on the abdomen region, and stored at -80°C until analysis.

Detection of the catalase and SOD activity on the tape strippings from the SC was estimated as described by Giacomoni et al.[29] and

Hellemans et al.,[27] respectively. The total protein amount on the tape stripping was quantified as the total amount of amino acids after acid hydrolysis at elevated temperature.

The GSH activity was estimated through Beutler et al.[30] and showed an increase in SOD (see **Figure 4a**), catalase (see **Figure 4b**), and tissue GSH level (see **Figure 4c**) in skin cells, up to 3.33-, 4.3- and 2.7-fold higher than the control treatment.

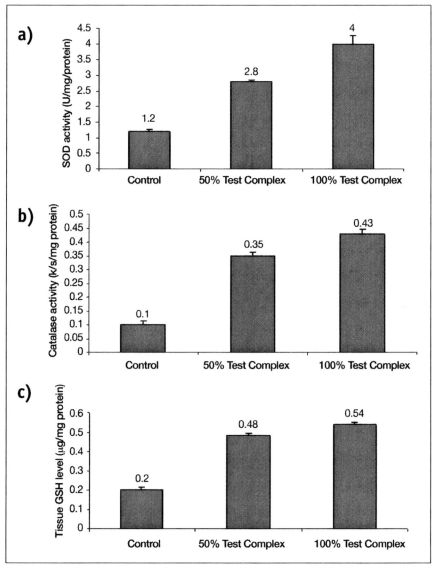

Figure 4. The GSH activity showed an increase in a) SOD, b) catalase, and c) tissue GSH levels in skin cells.

Conclusion

Mitochondria are a key organelle to the health of skin, producing important proteins necessary to control the cell energy release process. Oxidative damage has been implicated as a major factor in the decline of physiological functions of the mitochondria, which leads to the aging process.

The free radical scavenging and antioxidant abilities shown in the data for the test complex[a] suggest its ability to scavenge a range of deleterious free radicals and stimulate antioxidant enzymes to delay the aging symptoms. In addition to its antioxidant mechanisms, the complex prompts DNA repair abilities and mitochondrial nutrition through mobilization of acyl groups from fatty acids, and enhanced ATP production. In short, these effects and formulation benefits suggest a new, mitochondrial approach for targeting young and mature skin alike.

Published June 2009 *Cosmetics and Toiletries* magazine

References

Send e-mail to sabari@covalence.com.

1. D Harman, A biologic clock: The mitochondria? *J of the Amer Geriatrics Soc* 20 (4) 145–147 (1972)
2. HM McBride, M Neuspiel and S Wasiak, Mitochondria: More than just a powerhouse, *Curr Biol* 16(14) 551–560 (2006)
3. FM Yakes and B Van Houten, Mitochondrial DNA damage is more extensive and persists longer than nuclear DNA damage in human cells following oxidative stress, *Proc Natl Acad Sci USA* 94(2) 514–9 (Jan 21, 1997)
4. LA Loeb, DC Wallace and GM Martin, The mitochondrial theory of aging and its relationship to reactive oxygen species damage and somatic mtDNA mutations, *PNAS* 102(52) 18769–18770 (2005)
5. A Trifunovic, Mitochondrial DNA and aging, *Biochim Biophys Acta* 1757(5-6) 611–617 (2006)
6. A Trifunovic et al, Premature aging in mice expressing defective mitochondrial DNA polymerase, *Nature* 429 357–359 (2004)
7. S Richert, A Schrader and K Schrader, Transdermal delivery of two antioxidants om different cosmetic formulations, *Intl J Cos Sci* 25 (1–2) 5–13 (2003)
8. TM Hagen et al, (R)-α-*Lipoic* acid-supplemented old rats have improved mitochondrial function, decreased oxidative damage, and increased metabolic rate, *The FASEB J* 13 411–418 (1999)
9. B Cohen and D Gold, Mitochondrial cytopathy in adults: What we know so far, *Cleveland Clinic J Medicine*, 68 7 625–642 (2001)
10. M Sugrue and W Tatton, Mitochondrial membrane potential in aging cells, *Biol Signals Recept* 10 3–4, 176–188 (2001)
11. CE Thomas et al, Characterization of the radical trapping activity of a novel series of cyclic nitrone spin traps, *J Biol Chem* 271 3097–3104 (1996)
12. N Perricone, Spin traps: Stopping free-radical damage before it begins, in *The Wrinkle Cure,* NY: Warner Books, (2001) 181-183

13. L Ernster and G Dallner, Biochemical, physiological and medical aspects of ubiquinone function, *Biochim Biophys Acta* 1271:195-204 (1995)

14. PL Dutton et al, Coenzyme Q oxidation reduction reactions in mitochondrial electron transport, in *Coenzyme Q: Molecular mechanisms in health and disease* VE Kagan and PJ Quinn (eds), Boca Raton: CRC Press (2000) 65–82

15. J Herschthal and J Kaufman, Cutaneous aging: A review of the process and topical therapies, *Expert Review of Derm* 2(6) 753–761(2007)

16. S Loffelhardt, C Bonaventura, M Locher, HO Borbe and H Bisswanger, Interaction of alpha-lipoic acid enantiomers and homologues with the enzyme components of the mammalian pyruvate dehydrogenase complex, *Biochem Pharmacol* 50(5) 637–46 (1995)

17. JH Suh et al, Oxidative stress in the aging rat heart is reversed by dietary supplementation with (R)-(alpha)-lipoic acid, *FASEB J* 15(3) 700–706 (2001)

18. S Jacob, K Rett, EJ Henriksen and HU Haring, Thioctic acid—effects on insulin sensitivity and glucose-metabolism, *Biofactors* 10(2–3) 169–174 (1999)

19. H Beitner, Randomized, placebo-controlled, double blind study on the clinical efficacy of a cream containing 5% alpha-lipoic acid related to photo-aging of facial skin, *Br J Dermatol* 149(4) 841–9 (Oct 2003)

20. RM Moore et al, Alpha-lipoic acid inhibits tumor necrosis factor-induced remodeling and weakening of human fetal membranes, *Biol of Reproduction*, 80 781–787 (2009)

21. Shapiro and Robert, The prebiotic role of adenine: A critical analysis, *Origins of Life and Evolution of Biospheres* 25 83–98 (1995)

22. Adenine, Genetics Home Reference, available at: *http://ghr.nlm.nih.gov/ghr/glossary/adenine* (accessed Apr 29, 2009)

23. TM Hagen, J Liu, J Lykkesfeldt and BN Ames, Feeding acetyl-L-carnitine and lipoic acid to old rats significantly improves metabolic function while decreasing oxidative stress, *Proc Natl Acad Sci* USA, 19; 99(4)1870–1875 (2002)

24. A Steiber, J Kerner and CL Hoppel, Carnitine: A nutritional, biosynthetic and functional perspective, *Molecular Aspects of Medicine* 25 (5–6) 455–473 (2004)

25. J Liu, DW Killilea and BN Ames, Age-associated mitochondrial oxidative decay: Improvement of carnitine acetyltransferase substrate-binding affinity and activity in brain by feeding old rats acetyl-L- carnitine and/or R-alpha -lipoic acid, *Proc Natl Acad Sci* USA 19 99(4) 1876–1881 (2002)

26. HO Yang, G Stamatas, C Saliou and N Kollias, A chemiluminescence study of UVA-induced oxidative stress in human skin in vivo, *J of Investigative Derm* 122 1020–1029 (2004)

27. L Hellemans, H Corstjens, A Neven, L Declercq and D Maes, Antioxidant enzyme activity in human stratum corneum shows seasonal variation with an age-dependent recovery, *J of Investigative Derm* 120 434–439 (2003)

28. S Briganti, A Cristaudo and V D'Argento, Oxidative stress in physical urticarias, *Clin Exp Dermatol* 26 284–288 (2001)

29. PU Giacomoni, L Declercq, L Hellemans and D Maes, Aging of human skin: Review of a mechanistic model and first experimental data, *IUBMB Life* 49 259–263 (2000)

30. E Beutler, O Duron and BM Kelley, Improved method for the determination of blood glutathione, *J Lab Clin Med* 61 882 (1963)

CHAPTER 30

Nature's Answer to Insect Repellent

Katie Schaefer

Cosmetics and Toiletries Magazine, Carol Stream, IL, USA

KEY WORDS: *fragrance, natural, DEET, active, skin*

ABSTRACT: *Researchers have sourced fragrance ingredients that could provide a natural alternative to N,N-diethyl-m-toluamide (DEET), one of the most frequently used actives in insect repellents. Although DEET effectively repels mosquitoes and ticks, some agencies have questioned its effects on the environment and its skin irritation potential.*

Researchers have sourced fragrance ingredients that could provide a natural alternative to N,N-diethyl-m-toluamide (DEET), one of the most frequently used actives in insect repellents. Although DEET effectively repels mosquitoes and ticks, some agencies have questioned its effects on the environment and its skin irritation potential.

In May 2008, the US Centers for Disease Control recommended the use of DEET, picardin, lemon eucalyptus and IR3535 to repel mosquitoes from human skin.[1] However, both the US Environmental Protection Agency (EPA)[2] and the Pesticide Information Project of Cooperative Extension offices at Cornell University[3] have found DEET to produce dermal and neurological reactions in humans. With ongoing debate regarding the safety of DEET, an equally effective but safer alternative would prove beneficial (and lucrative).

While searching for a compound to repel insects from coffee beans, Aijun Zhang, PhD, and his team at the US Department of Agriculture (USDA) stumbled upon what they believe to be a safe, cost-effective active for insect repellents. "We discovered a fungus that repelled insects from the coffee bean," explained Zhang, who added that a volatile or some other chemical from the fungus was providing this effect. After comparisons with a control, the team isolated the compound: isolongifolenone.

Zhang then explored sources from which the compound could economically be obtained. "I did some research to see if it existed naturally," said Zhang, who found the compound present in the leaves of *Humiria balsamifera* (tauroniro), a tree from South America. However, according to Zhang, isolating the compound from the tauroniro tree can be expensive, so he sought other sources.

An Ever*green* Answer

"When I [searched the] literature, I found that isolongifolenone is not used in the pharmaceutical or cosmetic industry," said Zhang "but its derivative, isolongifolene, was discovered by the USDA 50 or 60 years ago, and has been used by the perfumery industry for a long time." In perfumery, isolongifolene is incorporated into products for its woody scent. Zhang adds, "We [also] discovered that ... isolongifolene can be synthesized from pine oil."

Zhang currently is seeking a pine oil with a high enough isolongifolene content to synthesize isolongifolenone for commercial use. "If it contained 50% isolongifolene, I could easily make the compound," said Zhang. In the meantime, he is testing pine oil from the *Humiria balsamifera* (tauroniro) tree to determine the material's efficacy.

Efficacy Testing

If evidence of the efficacy of isolongifolenone as an insect repellent could be shown, Zhang reasoned he could synthesize isolongifolenone from isolongifolene. Tests were thus conducted against two species each of ticks and mosquitoes. First, a mosquito bioassay involved maintaining mosquitoes on skin with sucrose and water before applying the test compound to the skin. After application, if the mosquitoes fed, the repellent was deemed ineffective.

The researchers also conducted the Klun and Debboun assay.

"This method included a module of six small wells containing warmed red blood cells covered with a collagen membrane," explained Zhang. Researchers placed a cloth on top of the membrane treated partially with the compound and partially with a control. The experiment was repeated with DEET. In both tests, the researchers found the isolongifolenone compound effectively deterred the mosquitoes from biting, almost 10% more than DEET.

"The average feeding deterrent of DEET is about 80% for *Aedes aegypti* [the yellow fever mosquito], whereas the test compound averaged about 90% for that mosquito. For *Anopheles stephensi* [the malaria mosquito], nearly 65% were deterred by DEET, compared with 75% by isolongifolenone."

In addition to mosquito assays, the team conducted a tick bioassay with *Ixodes scapularis*, the deer tick. In this assay, a human finger is treated with either a repellent or a control and ticks either bite or drop off. The results showed that isolongifolenone effectively deterred ticks from biting.

The researchers investigated other repellent functions for the compound as well, noting it effectively deterred stable flies and could therefore be formulated into products to protect horses. His team currently is collaborating with Rutgers University to determine whether the compound could repel bedbugs, which Zhang says are "very difficult to control."

The benefits of the compound are many, according to Zhang. In addition to its natural origin, the compound does not dissolve materials like plastic, which DEET can. Zhang also notes the compound is safe on skin and does not pose a hazard to the environment.

Published June 2009 *Cosmetics and Toiletries* magazine

References

1. Updated information regarding insect repellents, Centers for Disease Control and Prevention, May 8, 2008, available at: *www.cdc.gov/ncidod/dvbid/westnile/repellentupdates.htm* (Accessed Apr 17, 2009)
2. Reregistration eligibility decision: DEET, US Environmental Protection Agency, Office of Prevention, Pesticides and Toxic Substances, Sep 1998, 39–40, available at: *www.epa.gov/oppsrrd1/REDs/0002red.pdf* (Accessed Apr 17, 2009)
3. DEET, available at: *http://pmep.cce.cornell.edu/profiles/extoxnet/carbaryl-dicrotophos/deet-ext.html* (Accessed Apr 17, 2009)

CHAPTER 31

Leucojum aestivum Bulb Extract for Antiaging Benefits

Liki von Oppen-Bezalel, PhD

IBR Ltd., Ramat Gan, Israel

KEY WORDS: Leucojum aestivum, *antiwrinkle, muscle contraction, antiaging, SOD*

ABSTRACT: *Dormant* Leucojum aestivum *bulb extract is shown by the author to provide antiaging benefits including: slowing the proliferation of melanocytes and keratinocytes potentially to reduce age spots and slow cellular aging; reducing wrinkle formation by inhibiting muscle cell contractions; and increasing SOD expression in the skin to boost its natural defenses.*

The skin is the outermost covering of living tissue. It is the largest organ of the body and it is made up of multiple layers of epithelial tissues to guard the underlying muscles, bones, ligaments and internal organs. The skin contains various functional systems and cell types to provide comprehensive protection against external elements and as such, it is excessively exposed to harsh and damaging environmental aggressions including sunlight (UV exposure), free radicals and other hazardous molecules that lead to the expression of wrinkles and pigmentation (age spots), loss of elasticity and flexibility, and higher susceptibility to the buildup of damage.

Skin is composed primarily of the epidermis and the dermis. The outermost epidermis is made up of stratified squamous epithelium with an underlying basement membrane. It contains no blood vessels and is nourished by diffusion from the dermis. The epidermis is composed mainly of keratinocytes with melanocytes as well as langerhans cells. This layer of skin functions as a barrier between the body and the external environment, maintaining water inside the body and keeping out harmful chemicals and pathogens.[1]

The dermis lies below the epidermis and contains a number of structures including blood vessels, nerves, hair follicles, smooth muscle, glands and lymphatic tissue. The dermis is typically 3–5 mm thick and is the major component of human skin. It is composed of a network of connective tissue, predominantly collagen fibrils that provide support, and elastic tissue that provides flexibility. The main cell types in the dermis are fibroblasts, adipocytes (fat storage) and macrophages. The purpose of the hypodermis, which lies below the dermis, is to attach the skin to underlying bone and muscle as well as supply it with blood vessels and nerves.[1]

Considering the various layers and structures within skin, facial aging occurs as a result of several factors including inherent changes and intrinsic aging factors such as: effects of gravity, facial muscles acting on the skin (dynamic lines), soft tissue loss or shift and bone loss, and loss of tissue elasticity; as well as extrinsic aging factors such as exposure to harsh environmental conditions, particularly UV radiation and pollutants. The skin ages as the epidermis begins to thin, causing its junction with the dermis to flatten.[2-4] Collagen decreases as individuals age and bundles of collagen, which give the skin turgor, become looser and lose strength. When the skin loses elasticity, it is less able to resist stretching. Coupled with gravity, muscle contractions and tissue changes, the skin begins to wrinkle. Water loss and the breaking of bonds between cells also reduce the barrier function of skin.[2-4]

These intrinsic factors are natural and a "programmed" type of aging, based on Hayflick's theory that cells have an internal clock that predetermines their number of replications.[5,6] Thus, slowing cell proliferation could provide one approach to delaying the aging process.[7-13]

Another intrinsic mechanism behind the appearance of wrinkles is sub-cutaneous muscle contraction. When damage to the skin reduces collagen levels and the cell matrix and decreases skin's elasticity, subcutaneous muscle contractions generate folding in the skin that is not easily or automatically smoothed back to its original state. These folds are, in effect, wrinkles. Therefore, inhibiting the contraction of subcutaneous muscle cells may also stave off wrinkles by preventing the folds from forming, thus allowing the skin more time to regenerate collagen, increase moisture levels and rebuild skin layers. Botulinum Toxin Type A[a] is based on this approach and works by relaxing the muscles to flatten wrinkles.

In addition to intrinsic factors, extrinsic factors including reactive oxygen species (ROS), UV radiation and free radicals contribute to accumulated collagen damage and cell matrix degradation. Further, according to Harman, cells accumulate free radical damage over time.[14–17] Thus, antioxidants are used to fight the signs of aging in skin. To address these three approaches to antiaging—inhibiting cell proliferation, reducing subcutaneous muscle contractions and acting as an antioxidant—the author describes a dormant *Leucojum aestivum* bulb extract[b], offering product formulators novel strategies for advanced skin care.

Slowing Cell Proliferation

Previous work[18] has shown that, in order for plants to protect and rejuvenate themselves from unfavorable conditions, they enter a state of dormancy. During this time, growth functions are slowed and cell proliferation is inhibited. The inhibition of cell proliferation during dormancy is achieved by dormins, which occur in natural extracts taken from plants and plant organs during their dormant stage.

An extract from dormant *Leucojum aestivum* bulb was shown[18] to slow cell proliferation of active plant root meristems and human skin cells by employing the Hayflick limit theory (see **Figure 1**). Internal studies also suggest that dormins from *Leucojum aestivum* bulb extract slow cell proliferation in a nonspecific manner, transferring dormancy from the flower bulb to skin cells such as melanocytes, which could reduce pigmentation and the appearance of age spots (data not shown); additional studies in this area are under way.

---

[a] Botox is a registered trademark of Allergan Inc.
[b] IBR-Snowflake (INCI: *Leucojum aestivum* Bulb Extract) is a product and registered trademark of IBR Ltd.

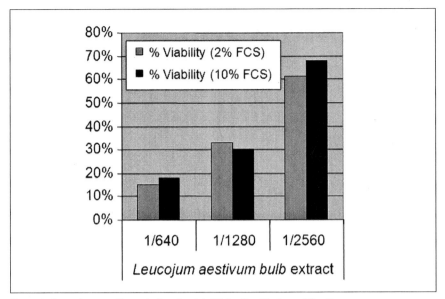

Figure 1. **Leucojum aestivum** bulb extract inhibits fibroblasts proliferation.

In vitro Muscle Contraction

Building on the described work, researchers also evaluated dormant *Leucojum aestivum* bulb extract for its effect on muscular contractions. Human muscular cells were co-cultivated with motor neurons in 24-well plates for 21 days until maturity so that the fibers were functional and exhibited contractions. This system was used to determine the material's myo-relaxing or antiwrinkle potential. The muscular contractions can be observed with an inverted microscope and counted.

By counting the muscular contractions during a given time before and after applying the test extract, the number obtained in the presence of the extract is expressed as a percentage of the initial number of contractions. The extract was considered to provide an inhibitory effect on muscle contraction when it significantly reduced or blocked the muscular contraction frequency in at least two of three well cultures.

The *Leucojum aestivum* bulb extract was applied at 1.5% and compared with both the culture medium alone as the negative control, and carisoprodol—a drug that reversibly blocks muscular contraction frequencies—as the positive control.

Results

Figure 2 shows the number of contractions with the negative (culture media) control, positive control (carisoprodol 5 x 10⁻³M) and *Leucojum aestivum* bulb extract. In the case of *Leucojum aestivum* bulb extract at 1.5%, the material blocked the muscular contraction frequency at 2 hr, 6 hr and 24 hr after application. Although some contraction frequency variations were observed with the negative control at 6 hr and 24 hr, the procedure was validated since the test product blocked the contractions (**Figure 2**) rather than partially decreasing them. The effect continued 1 hr after removal, indicating a lasting effect. Thus, the tested extract showed the ability to reduce contractions of muscular contractions in vitro.

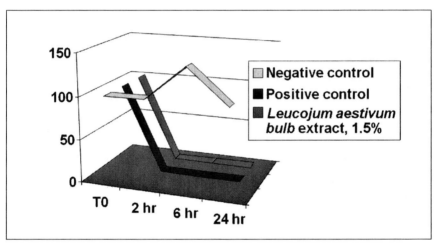

Figure 2. The number of muscle contractions measured with the application of *Leucojum aestivum* bulb extract, culture media as a negative control, and carisoprodol 5 x 10⁻³M as a positive control.

In vivo Wrinkle Reduction

A clinical efficacy study was then performed with 21 healthy female volunteers aged 42–64 (median age of 60) to test *Leucojum aestivum* bulb extract as an antiwrinkle active. The randomized double-blind study was placebo-controlled and randomized. Test subjects received a 2% hemi-face application of the *Leucojum aestivum* bulb extract (the maximum recommended use level) in a simple cream base to use twice daily for 28 days (see **Formula 1**). Half-face comparisons were made using a placebo treatment of the same cream without the

Leucojum aestivum bulb extract. Wrinkles were measured using
a skin image analyzer[c] at time 0 and after 28 days of twice daily
application (see **Figure 3**).

[c] The Skin Image Analyser (SIA) with a QuntiRides software (Monaderm, Monaco) and 3D
PRIMOS Compact were used for this study.

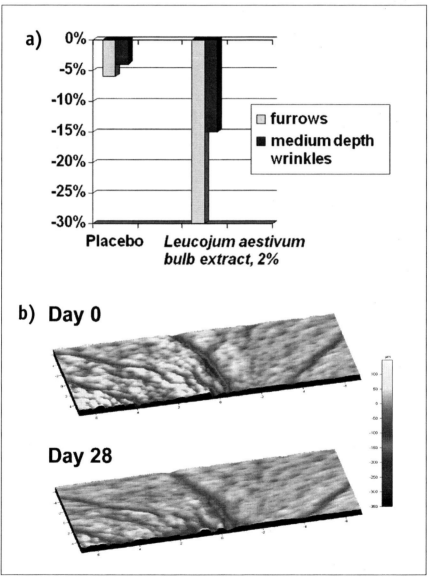

Figure 3. a) After 28 days, the number of micro relief furrows decreased by 30% (p < 0.05)
in 86% of panelists, and medium depth wrinkles decreased by 15% (p < 0.07) in 62% of
panelists; b) improvement of wrinkles visible via 3D imaging.

Formula 1. Antiwrinkle day cream with *Leucojum aestivum* bulb extract

Note: This formula is a suggestion and while it is similar to the formula used in the described study, it is not the same.

A.	Water (*aqua*)	qs to 100.00%
B.	Xanthan gum	0.20
	Glycerin	2.00
	Magnesium aluminum silicate	2.00
C.	Potassium palmitoyl hydrolyzed wheat protein (and) glyceryl stearate (and) cetearyl alcohol	10.00
	Isohexadecane	8.00
	Caprylic/capric triglyceride	8.00
	Cetearyl alcohol	0.50
	PPG-15 stearyl ether	2.00
D.	Glycerin (and) water (*aqua*) (and) *Leucojum aestivum* bulb extract (IBR-Snowflake, IBR Ltd.)	2.00
	Benzyl alcohol (and) dehydroacetic acid (and) benzoic acid (and) sorbic acid	1.00

Procedure: Heat A 40–45°C and add B to A. Stir for 20–30 min. Heat C and AB to 75°C, then add C to AB while stirring moderately. Homogenize ABC for 90 sec (Silverson: 3,000 rpm). Allow to cool to 40–45°C while stirring slowly. Add D in order and adjust final pH to 5.5–6.0.

Results

The number of micro-relief furrows measured in panelists with the test cream containing *Leucojum aestivum* bulb extract was decreased by 30% over the placebo and these results were seen in 86% of panelists; results of the tested extract vs. placebo were highly significant ($p < 0.05$). In addition, the number of medium depth wrinkles was decreased by 15% with the test cream containing *Leucojum aestivum* bulb extract over the placebo, and these results were seen in 62% of panelists; results of the tested extract vs. placebo again were significant ($p < 0.07$).

In vitro Antioxidant Activity

Leocojum aestivum bulb extract also was evaluated for its effect on the skin's natural antioxidant defenses. The expression of the antioxidant enzyme MnSOD was evaluated by flow cytometry (fluorescence-activated cell sorting, or FACS) on normal human epidermal keratinocyte (NHEK) cells in culture. The study was carried out based on published methods.[14, 15] The extract was added to the cell-based test system in several concentrations and compared with culture media as a control, which was used as the baseline for the expression of SOD.

Leucojum aestivum bulb extract was found to increase the expression of the antioxidant enzyme MnSOD in keratinocytes using the FACS-based testing system with fluorescently marked MnSOD antibodies. The effect of the extract was significant ($p < 0.05$); at a low concentration (0.15%), the extract increased SOD expression by 20% (see **Table 1**).

The fact that the extract is water-based increases the probability of its delivery to the skin to provide activity. These results indicate that *Leucojum aestivum* bulb extract could increase the protection of the skin when applied topically to reduce oxidative damage caused by super oxide unions.

Table 1. The effect of *Leucojum aestivum* bulb extract on MnSOD expression in keratinocytes

Treatment	Concentration	% of Control
Control	---	100
Leucojum aestivum bulb extract	0.075%	109
	0.15%	121

Conclusions

In the described work, *Leucojum aestivum* bulb extract was shown to smooth skin and reduce wrinkles. These results suggest the material acts via the combination of inhibiting subcutaneous muscle contraction and cell proliferation, as well as by enhancing skin's natural defenses by inducing expression of SOD in the skin. *Leucojum aestivum* bulb extract could thus provide formulators with a new dimension and approach to antiaging actives.

Published July 2009 *Cosmetics and Toiletries* magazine

References

1. Wikipedia Web site, available at *en.wikipedia.org/wiki/skin* (Accessed May 15, 2009)
2. Causes of aging skin, AAD Web site, available at *www.skincarephysicians.com/agingskinnet/basicfacts.html* (Accessed May 15, 2009)
3. BA Gilchrest et al, Premature aging affecting the skin, in: *Skin and aging process*, CRC Press Inc.: Boca Raton, FL (1984) pp 57–66
4. Skin care and aging, National Institute on Aging Web site, available at *www.niapublications.org/agepages/skin.asp* (Accessed May 15, 2009)
5. AG Bondar et al, Extension of life span by introduction of telomerase into human cells, *Science* 279 349–352 (1998)
6. KH Buchkovich, Telomeres, telomerase and cell cycle, *Prog Cell Cycle Res* 2 187–195 (1996)
7. L Hayflick and PS Moorhead, The serial cultivation of human diploid cell strains, *Exp Cell Res* 25 585–621 (1961)
8. L Hayflick, Current theories of biological aging, *Fed Proc* 34 9–13 (1975)
9. L Hayflick, The cell biology of aging, *Clin Geriatr Med* 1(1) 15–27 (1985)
10. L Hayflick, *How and Why We Age*, Ballantine Books: New York (1994)
11. L Hayflick, The future of ageing, *Nature* 408 6809 267–269 (2000)
12. L Hayflick, Antiaging is an oxymoron, *J Gerontol A Biol Sci Med Sci* 59(6) B573–578 (2004)
13. J Campisi, Replicative senescence and old lives' tale?, *Cell* 84 497–500 (1996)
14. D Harman, Aging: A theory based on free radical and radiation chemistry, *J Gerontol* 11(3) 298–300 (1956)
15. D Harman, Free radical theory of aging: Effect of free radical reaction inhibitors on the mortality rate of male LAF mice, *J Gerontol* 23(4) 476–482 (1968)
16. D Harman, The biologic clock: The mitochondria?, *J Am Geriatr Soc* 20(4) 145–147 (1972)
17. D Harman, The aging process, *Proc Natl Acad Sci USA* 78(11) 7124–7128 (1981)
18. L von Oppen-Bezalel, Slowing intrinsic and extrinsic aging: A dual approach, *Cosm & Toil* 124(5) 80–84 (May 2009)

CHAPTER 32

Liquid Crystal O/W Emulsions to Mimic Lipids and Strengthen Skin Barrier Function

In-Young Kim, PhD; Sayaka Nakagawa; Kinka Ri, PhD; Satoru Hashimoto, PhD; and Hitoshi Masaki, PhD

Nikkol Group, Tokyo, Japan

KEY WORDS: *liquid crystal, multilayer, bound water, barrier function, emulsifier, moisturizing effect*

ABSTRACT: *In the present study, the authors produced liquid crystalline (LC) o/w emulsions whose structure mimics the skin's intercellular lipids. These emulsions are shown in cosmetic formulations to strengthen skin barrier functions while maintaining stability at higher temperatures than that of the skin.*

Intercellular lipids of the stratum corneum (SC) form a lamellar structure (LS) that consists mainly of ceramides, cholesterols and fatty acids as amphiphilic substances, and that demonstrates significant skin barrier function.[1,2] This natural liquid crystalline (LC) structure has a bi-continuous composition of water and amphiphilic lipids, and simultaneously possesses high moisturizing and water loss prevention effects.[3]

In the past, much work has been devoted to preparing emulsions using the self-organization of structures formed in mixed systems of surfactants and amphiphilic lipids—such as fatty alcohols, fatty acids, lecithin, polyglycerol alkyl ethers and mono alkyl phosphates, among others—to develop bio-mimetic LC emulsions.[4-7] In relation, Suzuki et al. disclosed work in this field describing a bio-mimetic lamellar LC system based instead on synthetic ceramides.[8] **Figure 1** exemplifies a schematic illustration of oil droplets surrounded by liquid crystals, forming LC o/w emulsions.

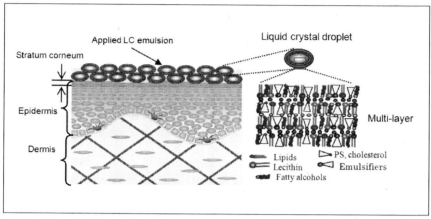

Figure 1. Schematic illustration of oil-in-liquid, crystalline-in-water emulsion systems (LC o/w emulsions).

It has been reported that the advantages to using this type of system include higher moisturizing effects, as well as enhanced barrier function of the SC.[2,4,5] However, few successful systems exist due to the poor stability of the LC structure during application to the human skin; i.e., the liquid crystals surrounding the oil droplets break and disappear quickly at skin temperature. Thus, the aim of the present study was to produce an optimized system for the preparation of LC o/w emulsions that are stable at temperatures higher than that of the skin, and to confirm their efficacy and function as bio-mimetics of intercellular skin lipids.

Materials and Methods

Materials: To prepare the LC base (LCB), the following materials were obtained[a]: phytosterol (PS), PEG_{10-30} soy sterol (PEG10-30-SS), hydrogenated lecithin (HL), oils including squalane and caprylic/capric triglyceride, and waxes such as fatty alcohol. (See **Figure 2.**) All materials were technical grade and used without further purification.

---

[a] All materials used to prepare the LC base were obtained from Nikko Chemicals, Japan.

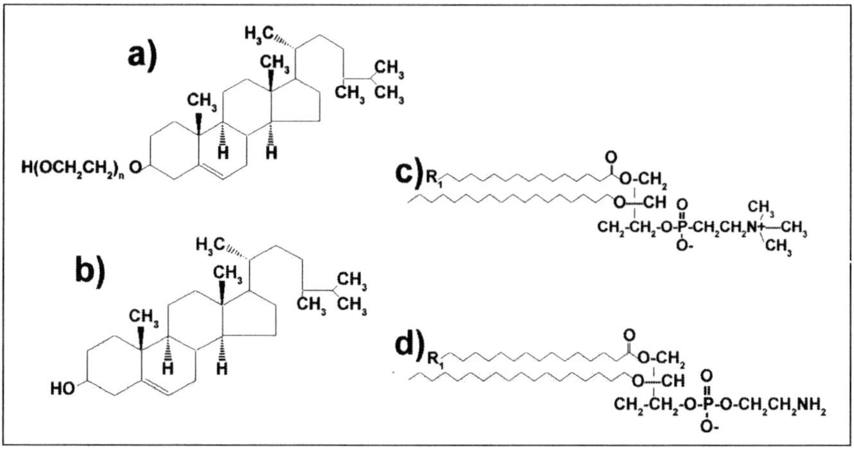

Figure 2. Molecular structures of materials for preparation of the LCB: a) poly-oxyethylene 10-30 phytosterol (POE(10-30)-PS); and b) phytosterol (PS; β-sitosterol, stigmasterol and campesterol at 2:1:1); the hydrogenated lecithin (HL) mainly consisted of: c) phosphatidyl choline and d) phosphatidyl ethanolamine (c:d = approximately 7:3)

Preparing the LCB: The LCB was prepared in a wax form by mixing the HL, PEG10-30-SS, PS and fatty alcohols (C_{16}-C_{22}) at 80°C, a temperature above their melting points, then cooling the batch to room temperature. After several trial variations, the optimized weight ratio of each component was determined to be 1:2:1:6.

Phase diagram study: Various amounts of the LCB, oil (squalane) and water were sealed in ampoules. The phase states and presence of liquid crystals at 25°C were determined by direct visual inspection and polarization microscopy, respectively.

Repeat distance of the LC system: The interlayer spaces of the lamellar structure were examined using small angle x-ray scattering (SAXS)[b] with a Cu-Kα wavelength of λ = 0.1542 nm at 25°C. Two test samples were measured—an LCB aqueous system, 20% w/w, and the same concentration LCB in water with 20.0% w/w squalane system. Their LC phases were distinguished by SAXS peaks. Specifically, the ratios of interlayer spaces (d; repeat distance) from the first to the second and third peaks were 1:1/2:1/3 for the lamellar type.

Preparing LC o/w and control emulsions: LC o/w emulsions were prepared with the LCB, oils, polyols and water by high speed

---

[b]The TKS1706 SAXS device used was from Anton Paar in Germany.

homogenizing emulsification at 70 ± 5°C using a homomixer[c]. The LCB was first added to the oil phase and agitated to dissolve. This mixture of LCB with oils was then added into a water phase to obtain LC o/w emulsions. Meanwhile, non-LC o/w emulsions were prepared as controls, using polysorbate-60 as an emulsifier and following the same mixing procedure.

Confirming the structure of LC o/w emulsions: The structure of LC o/w emulsions was confirmed by two types of observation: polarized light microscopy attached to a digital camera[d] and transmittance electron microscopic (TEM) analysis[e]. The structural stability also was confirmed at 30°C, 35°C, 37°C and 40°C.

Verifying liquid crystal stability on skin: The structural stability of LC o/w emulsions on the skin was confirmed by applying 20 μg/cm^2 of LC o/w emulsions on the inside forearms of volunteers as described below; samples were left on the skin for 6 hr, after which the emulsions were recovered by tape stripping. The recovered test emulsion on the tape was transferred to a slide glass and observed by polarized light microscopy to determine whether the LC structures remained present.

Measurement of water content: Bound water content within LC o/w emulsions or non-LC o/w emulsions was measured by differential scanning calorimetry (DSC) analysis[f].[9]

Clinical evaluation of moisturizing effect: 2.5 mg/cm^2 of LC o/w emulsions or non-LC o/w emulsions were applied on the inside forearms of 6 volunteers, 25-45 years. The volunteers were first initialized for 15 min in an incubation room at 22°C and 45% relative humidity (RH). The conductance (μS) of the applied and non-applied areas was measured at 22°C and 45% RH[g]. Measurements were taken initially and at 15 min, 30 min, 45 min and 60 min after application. The moisturizing effect was evaluated by comparing the changes of conductance between the initial measurement and each time interval.[10, 11]

---

[c] The T.K. Homomixer used for this study is a device from Tokushu Kika Kogyo Co. Ltd., Japan.
[d] The BX50 polarized light microscope and FX380 CCD digital camera used for this study are devices from Olympus, Japan.
[e] The JEM1200EX transmittance electron microscopic used in this study is a device from JEOL Co. Ltd., Japan.
[f] The 220C DSC analysis meter used for this study is a device from Seiko Instruments Inc., Japan.
[g] The SKICON 200 hydrometer used for this study is a device from I.B.S. Co., Ltd.

TEWL-reducing effect: LC o/w emulsions and non-LC o/w emulsions were applied twice daily on the inner thighs of 12 male volunteers, 28–55 years, for 21 days and the TEWL of the area was then calculated. Measurements were taken initially and at 1 week, 2 weeks and 3 weeks after application. The TEWL was evaluated using a water loss meter[h] in the incubation room maintained at 21°C and at 50% RH.[12] The skin condition of the inner thighs before and after application was evaluated by tape-stripping a few layers of the SC using cellophane tape. The skin condition was observed by BG dye method.[13]

Results and Discussion

Phase diagram study: The schematic phase diagram of the LCB/squalane/water system in the whole concentration range at 25°C is shown in **Figure 3**. Confirmation of phase states depending on the compositions was determined by a polarization microscope. As shown in the water/LCB line, a lamellar liquid crystal phase is formed at 3–30% LCB, and this lamellar phase was confirmed to change to a hexagonal phase with increasing concentrations of LCB.

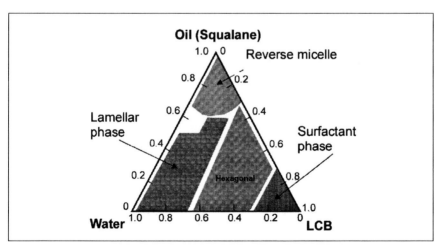

Figure 3. Schematic phase diagram of the LCB/squalane/water phase system

This hexagonal phase was present at up to 70% LCB but above 70%, a reverse micellar phase having a gel formation appeared.

---

h The AS-TW2 water loss meter used for this study is a device from Asahi Biomed, I.B.S. Co., Ltd.
j The TVB-10 viscometer used for this test is a device from Toki Sangyo Co. Ltd.

The lamellar liquid crystal phase that was formed in the range of 11–30% LCB was too viscous[j] and, according to evaluation by 5 panelists, felt too greasy for cosmetic formulations. Therefore, the most suitable condition for lamellar phase formation was determined to be in the range of 4% to 10% of LCB.

Repeat distance of the LC system: The SAXS measurement of the 20% LCB aqueous system showed three sharp peaks with interlayer spaces (d) of: 5.712 nm, 2.870 nm and 1.917 nm, whose ratios from the first to the second and third peaks were 1:1/2:1/3. The same concentration of LCB in water with 20.0% squalane system showed similar interlayer spaces (d) of: 5.770 nm, 2.885 nm and 1.923 nm, having the ratios of 1:1/2:1/3. Therefore, the liquid crystal system prepared with the LCB was characterized as a lamellar structure.

Table 1. Compositions (% w/w) of the tested emulsions

Ingredients	Non-LC O/W Emulsions		LC O/W Emulsions	
	a)	b)	c)	d)
Water (*aqua*)	62.6	52.6	62.6	52.6
Glycerin	5.0	-	5.0	-
1,3-Butylene glycol	5.0	-	5.0	-
Carbomer	0.1	0.1	0.1	0.1
Methylparaben	0.1	0.1	0.1	0.1
Arginine	0.1	0.1	0.1	0.1
LCB	-	-	5.0	5.0
Polysorbate 60	5.0	5.0	-	-
Squalane	10.0	30.0	10.0	30.0
Caprylic/capric triglyceride	10.0	10.0	10.0	10.0
Cetearyl alcohol	2.0	2.0	2.0	2.0
Propylparaben	0.1	0.1	0.1	0.1

Confirming the structure of LC o/w emulsions: Test samples of LC o/w emulsions or non-LC o/w emulsions (see **Table 1**) were observed first by polarized light microscopy to confirm the existence of liquid crystalline structures. As seen in **Figure 4,** LC o/w emulsions showed the Maltese cross image of emulsion droplets (**4c-d**); however, non-LC o/w emulsions did not (**4a-b**). Therefore, LC o/w emulsions based on the LCB were confirmed as having liquid crystalline structures that could be identified as a lamellar form. On the other hand, non-LC o/w emulsions prepared with polysorbate-60 did not form a liquid crystalline structure.

The structure of liquid crystals surrounding the oil droplet of LC o/w emulsions (**Table 1c**) was then observed by TEM. As shown in **Figure 5**, the existence of multi-lamellar structures around oil droplets was confirmed (**5a**) and this multi-lamellar structure is similar to intercellular lipid layers in the SC (**5b**).[14, 15] This result can be explained by the equation below, known as the critical packing parameter (CPP):

$$CPP = v/(a_o l_c) \; \textbf{Eq. 1}$$

where ao is the optimal surface area; v is the hydrocarbon chain volume; and lc is the critical length of the lipids.

The CPP determines whether lipids will form spherical micelles (CPP<1/3), nonspherical micelles (1/3<CPP<1/2), bilayers (vesicles) (1/2<CPP<1) or lamellar (CPP~1) structures. Here, HL itself is in the range of 1/2<CPP<1, which is not favored to form lamellar structures. In the case of PS, it has a CPP>1. By mixing HL with PS, the CPP of the mixture will be close to 1, which is favorable for

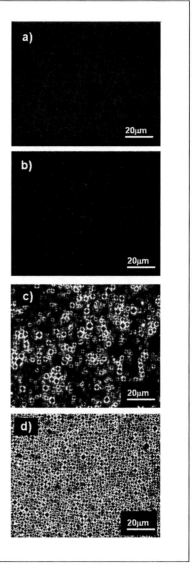

Figure 4. Optical micrographs of LC o/w emulsions and non-LC o/w emulsions, observed by polarized light microscopy; a) and b) = non-LC o/w emulsions; c) and d) = LC o/w emulsions

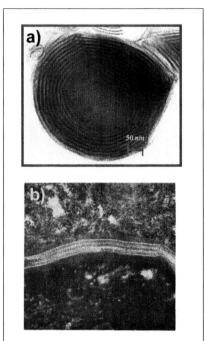

Figure 5. TEM micrograph of:
a) LC o/w emulsions (Table 1c),
and b) TEM micrograph of the SC[15]

lamellar formation. Therefore, it is suggested that LC o/w emulsions based on the LCB could form sufficiently stable lamellar structures even at low LCB concentrations.

Finally, the similarities between the LCB system and SC lipids were compared. Previous studies indicate that SC lipids have an LC structure that consists mainly of ceramides, cholesterols and fatty acids.[1,2] Moreover, the schematic diagram of the proposed model of lamellar phase formation of the epidermal barrier has been reported as well.[16] Therefore, although the individual components of the LCB do not have exactly the same structure as SC lipids, the LC system with the LCB having a lamellar form can be regarded as showing great similarities to SC lipids.

Stability of the LC Structure

Temperature stability: The stability of LC o/w emulsions (see **Table 1c**) at different temperatures is shown in **Figure 6.** Each image shows a change in the LC form as the temperature increases from 30°C to 35°C, 37°C and 40°C, confirming that the LC form is maintained even up to 40°C—higher than the normal skin temperature of ~33°C. Therefore, the LC o/w emulsions could be expected to maintain their LC form in practical applications on the skin surface.

Presence of LC on skin: As shown in **Figure 7**, the recovered LC o/w emulsions (see **Table 1c**; applied amount = 20 µg/cm^2) from the inside forearms of volunteers demonstrated Maltese cross images after 6 hr, suggesting the LC form is stable against skin temperature. Therefore, LC o/w emulsions were concluded to act as an artificial SC lipids.

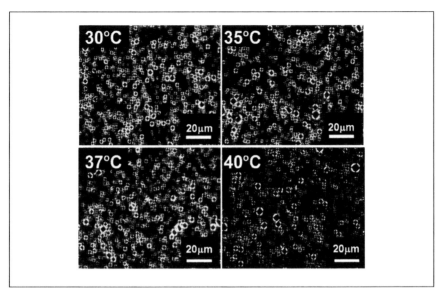

Figure 6. Micrographs of LC o/w emulsions (Table 1c) at increasing temperatures

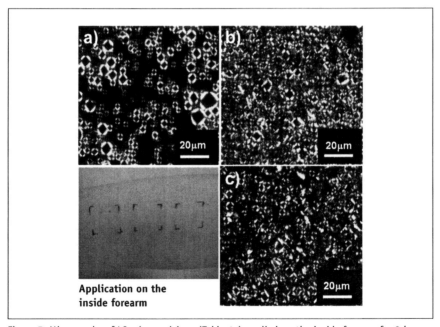

Figure 7. Micrographs of LC o/w emulsions (Table 1c) applied on the inside forearm for 3 hr and 6 hr

Bound water content: Generally, water within intercellular lipids, or bound water, exists in a different form than free water, which easily evaporates from the skin surface. Bound water in intercellular lipids is retained tightly in the lipid structure and protects the skin against over-drying. The bound water content in LC o/w emulsions (**see Table 2**) was quantified and compared with the water content in non-LC o/w emulsions by enthalpy measurements of melted test samples containing various amount of water—20%, 30%, 40%, 50% and 60%. Here, total content of water (bound water + free water) in the test samples was quantified by the Karl Fisher method. The results are shown in **Figure 8**.

Table 2. Composition of the tested emulsions containing various amounts of water

Ingredients	LC O/W Emulsions (%)					Non-LC O/W Emulsions (%)				
Water (*aqua*)	20	30	40	50	60	20	30	40	50	60
LCB	5	5	5	5	5	-	-	-	-	-
Polysorbate-60	-	-	-	-	-	5	5	5	5	5
Caprylic/capric triglyceride	20	20	20	20	20	20	20	20	20	20
Squalane	53	43	33	23	13	53	43	33	23	13
Cetearyl alcohol	2	2	2	2	2	2	2	2	2	2

Figure 8a depicts the relationship between the enthalpy changes and the total water content. The y axis gives an estimate of the bound water content; the LC o/w emulsions showed that the y axis was 12.7%, and the correlation coefficient (R^2) was 0.9968. In non-LC o/w emulsions, the y axis was 8.3%, and the correlation coefficient (R^2) was 0.9967. According to the results, LC o/w emulsions were estimated to have almost 53% more bound water than non-LC o/w emulsions. Consequently, LC o/w emulsions were expected to provide better moisturization than non-LC o/w emulsions.

Clinical Evaluation

Moisturizing effect: The moisturizing activity of LC o/w emulsions (see **Table 1c**) was evaluated and compared with non-LC o/w emulsions (see **Table 1a**) by measuring the skin conductance of the volunteers. **Figure 9** shows the changes in skin conductance as a

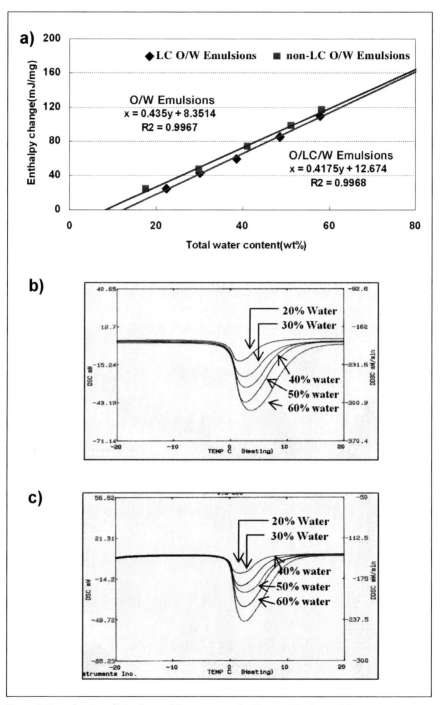

Figure 8. Bound water of LC o/w emulsions compared with non-LC o/w emulsions;
a) relationship between total water content and enthalpy change; b) DSC curve of non-LC
o/w emulsions; c) DSC curve of LC o/w emulsions

function of time. After 1 hr, the conductance of LC o/w emulsions was 100.0 μS ± 9.6; for non-LC o/w emulsions, it was 61.2 μS ± 8.2. According to *t*-test, the conductance of LC o/w emulsions was confirmed as being significantly higher than non-LC o/w emulsions (p < 0.05). Hence, LC o/w emulsions were concluded to provide more moisturization than conventional, non-LC o/w emulsions.

Reducing TEWL: LC o/w emulsions (**see Table 1d**) and non-LC o/w emulsions (**see Table 1b**) were separately applied to skin (**see Figure 10**) and the TEWL of each was measured. After 2 weeks and 3 weeks of application twice daily, the TEWL of LC o/w emulsions was shown to significantly decrease, compared with non-LC o/w emulsions.

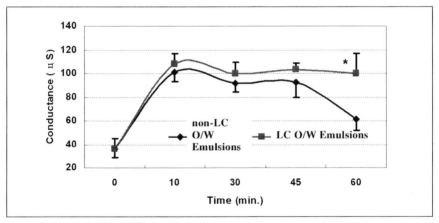

Figure 9. Changes in skin conductance as a function of time, male and female volunteers (n = 6), student's **t**-test (*p < 0.05)

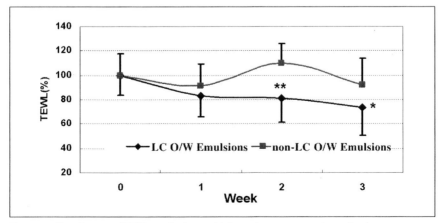

Figure 10. The changes of TEWL on the inner thighs; volunteers: n = 12, student's t-test (**p < 0.001, *p < 0.05)

Improvement of skin condition: The skin condition of volunteers after application of the test emulsions was observed by BG dye method. The results are depicted in **Figure 11**. As shown, before application, multiple desquamations of corneocytes were observed and after 4 weeks of application, LC o/w emulsions reduced this multiple desquamation. However, no improvement was shown in the number of corneocytes treated with non-LC o/w emulsions. These results suggest that LC o/w emulsions normalized the epidermal differentiation process due to their higher water-retaining ability, and that the normalization contributed to the improvement of skin barrier function.

Conclusion

The present study was conducted to find an optimized approach to enhance and strengthen the skin barrier function of cosmetic formulations. This study shows that skin barrier function of formulations can be

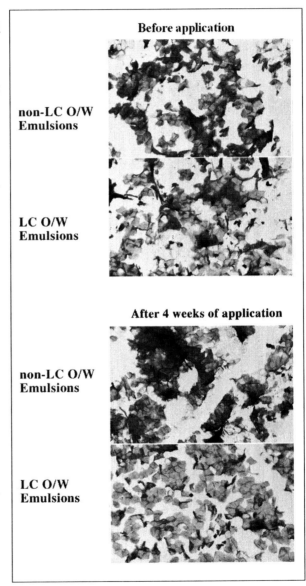

Figure 11. Images of the SC stripped off the skin, comparing LC o/w emulsions with non LC o/w emulsions

improved merely by focusing on the relationship between the structure and function of emulsion films, without the need for special active ingredients. Utilizing a hydrogenated lecithin, PEG10-30-SS, PS and fatty alcohols, an advanced LCB was achieved that can be incorporated into LC o/w emulsions. The structure of the LCB was confirmed as a multilayer LC form, surrounding oil droplets. In addition, LC o/w emulsions were shown to maintain stability as a multilayer LC structures on the skin surface in actual applications.

LC o/w emulsions were confirmed to possess moisturizing and water loss-prevention effects, and in clinical tests, such emulsions were shown to improve the skin moisture condition of volunteers and TEWL simultaneously. Thus, this study could contribute to the development of new tools for formulating advanced skin care cosmetics.

Published July 2009 *Cosmetics and Toiletries* magazine

References

1. S Nishiyama, H Komatsu and M Tanaka, A study on skin hydration with cream, *J Soc Cosmet Chem Japan* 16(2) 136-143 (1983)
2. L Norlen, Skin barrier Formation: The membrane folding model, *J of Invest Dermatol* 117(4) 823-829 (2001)
3. T Okamot, Y Matsushita, E Matsuura and M Masuda, The preparation of visible emulsion and its applications to cosmetics, *J Soc Cosmet Chem Japan* 39(4) 290-297 (1983)
4. T Suzuki, J Fukasawa and H Iwai, Multi-lamellar emulsion of stratum corneum lipid, *J Soc Cosmet Chem Japan* 27(3) 193-205 (1993)
5. Y Aoki and Y Sumida, Enhancement of moisturizing abilities of skin care products by a novel water retaining system, 22nd IFSCC congress, *Edinburgh*, podium presentation 38 1-8 (2002)
6. T Ochiai, H Sagitani and K Itho, Characteristics of polyglycerin copolymer type nonionic surfactants as cosmetic emulsifiers, *J Soc Cosmet Chem Japan* 22(3) 171-177 (1988)
7. T Suzuki, H Takei and S Yamazaki, Formation of fine three-phase emulsions by the liquid crystal emulsification method with arginine β-branched monoalkyl phosphate, *J Colloid Interface Sci* 129(2) 491-500 (1989)
8. T Suzuki and H Iwai, Formulation of liquid emulsions and clear gels by liquid crystal emulsion, *IFSCC* 9(3) (2006)
9. T Inoue, K Tsujii, K Okamoto and K Toda, Differential scanning calorimetric studies on the melting behavior of water in stratum corneum, *J Invest Dermatol* 86 689-693 (1986)
10. RS Summers, B Summers, P Chandar, C Feinberg, R Gursky and AV Rawlings, The effect of lipids with and without humectant on skin xerosis, *J Soc Cosmet Chem* 47 27-39 (1996)
11. T Suzuki, A Tsutsumi and A Ishida, Secondary droplet emulsion: Contribution of liquid crystal formation to physicochemical properties and skin moisturing effect of cosmetic emulsion, *J Soc Cosmet Chem Japan* 17(1) 6-70 (1983)
12. IY Kim, CK Zhoh and HC Ryoo, Liquid crystalline technology of cosmetic industry and moisturizing effect of skin, *J Soc Cosmet Sci Korea* 30(2) 279-294 (2004)
13. J Levin and HI Maibach, Correlation transepidermal water loss and percutaneous absorption, *Cosm Toil* 120(7) 28-31 (2005)

14. R Shukla, V Bansal, M Chaudhary, A Basu, RR Bhonde and M Sastry, Biocompatibility of gold nanoparticles and their endocytotic fate inside the cellular compartment, *Langmuir* 21 10644-10654 (2005)

15. DC Swartzendruber, PW Wertz, DJ Kitko, KC Madison and DT Downing, Molecular models of the intercellular lipid lamellae in mammalian stratum corneum, *J Invest Dermatol* 92(2) 251-257 (1989)

16. M Lynch and P Spicer, Bicontinuous liquid crystals: Cubic phase and human skin: Theory and practice, New York: Taylor & Fancis Group CRC Press (2005) 41-57

CHAPTER 33

Pisum Sativum Extract for Safe- and Self-tanning

**Isabelle Imbert, PhD; Anne Francoise Clay; Joel Mantelin
and Nouha Domloge, PhD**
ISP/Vincience, Sophia Antipolis Cedex, France

KEY WORDS: *pheomelanin, eumelanin, Skin Types I-VI, DHA, Maillard
reaction,* Pisum sativum *extract*

ABSTRACT: *The cosmetic industry is challenged to develop active
ingredients to provide the skin with a natural, healthy glow
without sunlight exposure. Here, the author examines the
effects of* Pisum sativum *extract on melanocytes and shows
a time- and dose-dependent increase in skin tone, also
suggesting the material could protect skin from UV damage.*

The desire for healthy, golden-brown skin has been uninterrupted
for years. This social phenomenon started when Coco Chanel traveled
to the French Riviera in the late 1930s and, after spending leisure
time in a bikini, returned with a tan. In relation, tanning is popular
because it indicates a social status—tanned skin implies that individuals have the means to take time off and relax in the sun.

In order to achieve a golden-brown tan, consumers expose
their skin to sunlight since this induces pigmentation, i.e., melanin
formation. An alternative to sun exposure is the application of a
self-tanning agent that reacts with the skin by producing a brown-
orange tone without exposure to sunlight.[1] In the past few years,
self-tanning agents have gained popularity due to improved
formulations allowing for better homogenization on the skin surface.
However, increased tanning often provides individuals
with a false sense of security.

Studies show that most individuals with darker skin feel uncon-
cerned about the risk of photo-aging and skin cancer.[2] Therefore,
the cosmetic industry faces a difficult challenge: to develop active
ingredients to provide the skin with a natural, healthy glow without
sunlight exposure—i.e., safe tanning. In addition, ideally this challenge should take into account the increased market demand for
nature-based technologies and eco-friendly products.

Skin Tones Worldwide

Human skin color ranges worldwide from a very dark brown in
some countries (Africa, Australia and Melanesia), to a near yellowish
pink in some North European countries. Research on skin color
variation indicates that color is governed by an adaptive mechanism
that protects skin against UV radiation. In the year 2000, a high
correlation between skin tone lightness (W) and annual exposure
to UV light (AUV) was established:[3]

$$W = 70 - (AUV/10)$$

Surprisingly, females were found to have lighter skin than males
in every population—a significant biological message emphasizing
the reproductive need for women to synthesize extra vitamin D3
for a developing fetus. Thus, skin tone variation seems to be a
compromise solution to the conflicting physiological requirements
of photo-protection and the reproduction of human beings.

Defining Skin Tone

Skin color is determined by the amount and type of melanin in the
skin. Melanin exists in two types: pheomelanin (almost colorless)
and eumelanin (dark brown to nearly black). Individuals with fair
skin mostly produce pheomelanin while those with dark-colored
skin mostly produce eumelanin. In addition, individuals differ in the
number and size of melanin particles, which are more important in
determining skin color than the percentages of melanin types present.
In lighter skin, color also is affected by red blood cells flowing close
to the skin surface. To a lesser extent, color also is affected by the
presence of fat beneath the skin and carotene, a reddish-orange
pigment in the skin.

Normal human skin can be classified into six skin types, which are determined by pigmentation response.[4] Skin Type I cannot achieve a tan, even with moderate and repeated exposure. This type creates pheomelanin, a pigment that is ineffective in producing a tan or protecting the skin against UV damage.[5] Skin Types II and III can tan but will generate only a light brown color. These types create eumelanin, the pigment known to protect against damage from subsequent exposure to UV.

Skin Types IV and V tan easily and profusely with minimal exposure, and Skin Type VI is extremely pigmented, even in the absence of UV. Both the amount and types of melanin are determined by several genes and result in the great variety of different skin tones.

Genetics of Skin Pigmentation

As noted, pigmentation is controlled by multiple genes in a complex fashion. While many of these genes are yet unknown, several that are key to pigmentation have been invoked to explain variations in skin. These genes include the Agouti-signaling protein precursor (ASIP), the Membrane Associated Transporter Protein (MATP), the tyrosinase gene (TYR) and the Oculocutaneous albinism II (OCA2) gene. Polymorphisms in ASIP and OCA2 may play a role in shaping light and dark pigmentation across the globe; MATP and TYR have a predominant role in the evolution of light skin in Europeans but not in East Asians.[6]

Variations in human skin tone have been correlated with mutations in the gene coding for the Melanocortin receptor MC1R, and variations in the amino acid sequence of this receptor result in lighter or darker skin. The genetic mutations leading to light skin among East Asians are different from those in Europeans, so although both ethnic groups experienced similar selective pressures by settling in northern latitudes,[7] the two groups became distinct populations.

Recent studies have also shown that the SLC24A5 gene was involved in differences in some of the melanin units between Europeans and Africans.[8] This gene is presumed to account for a 25% to 38% variation in skin pigmentation between black Africans and white Europeans.

Artificial vs. Physiological Tanning

Artificial tanning: Artificial tanning of the skin can be achieved by application of so-called self-tanning agents. The chemical structure of these compounds features keto or aldehyde groups that belong predominantly to the class of reducing sugars. One self-tanning substance employed rather frequently is 1,3-dihydroxyacetone (DHA), which reacts with the proteins and amino acids of the stratum corneum (SC) and induces a Maillard reaction. This reaction results in the formation of polymers that provide the skin with a brown/orange tone after about 4–6 hr.

Tan skin achieved in this way cannot be washed away; it is removed via normal skin desquamation. Therefore, self-tanning in this manner is more of a dyeing effect of the superficial keratinized layers than a tanning effect and it does not provide photo-protection for skin cells. Moreover, the use of self-tanning molecules without effective sun filters is not recommended since the enhanced tan provides individuals with a false sense of security.[2]

Physiological tanning: The tanning response of skin to UV radiation is unique in that its protective effects are generated in both short- and long-term events. Short-term tanning, called immediate tanning or immediate pigment darkening, is a process that occurs in only a few minutes and leads to the development of a transitory brown color during exposure to UV and visible radiation (320 nm to 400 nm). Immediate tanning results from changes in existing melanosomes or melanin and is a passive chemical process rather than an active biological process. During this process, colorless melanin precursors are thought to be oxidized by UV radiation to dark-colored melanin. Since this oxidation is reversible, the resulting skin tanning is of brief duration.

Long-term tanning or delayed tanning is commonly known as melanogenesis. In response to UV radiation, keratinocytes release α-MSH that binds to specific MCR1 receptors at the surface of the melanocytes. This binding triggers the production of melanin and its transfer to the surrounding keratinocytes. Melanosomes collect melanin granules entering the cell and form a dark, protective cap over the cell nucleus, shielding it from damaging UV rays. Delayed tanning also involves an increase in the number of melanosomes, in the activity of tyrosinase, and in the synthesis of new melanin. Since the process is elaborate, delayed tanning has gradual onset— it may occur after 48 hr with exposure to extreme amounts of UV radiation; modest exposure results in more gradual tanning. UVB radiation induces a more delayed tanning than does UVA.

Protective role of melanin: The skin's protective responses to UV radiation include thickening of the SC and epidermis and the production of melanin. Melanin acts as a protective biological shield against UV radiation. It has the ability to absorb and disperse UV light and acts as a free radical scavenger, thus reducing the penetration of UV radiation. Melanin protects against UV-induced mutations in skin cells, which may cause skin cancers. The more melanin is synthesized in the skin, the more UV is absorbed to protect DNA from mutation and skin cancer.

Dark-skinned individuals, who also tend to tan well, are up to 500 times less likely to develop skin cancer than fair-skinned individuals. However, the ability to tan alone confers protection, researchers say, regardless of the skin's level of pigmentation. This is due in part to the UV-shielding effect of melanin and perhaps in part to an acceleration of DNA repair mechanisms that are activated during tanning.[9]

UV light and skin aging: Up to 90% of the visible skin changes attributed to aging are caused by sun exposure. UV radiation of sunlight has a damaging effect on the skin. Acute damage leads to sunburn, or erythema. It occurs when too much UV light reaches the skin and disrupts the tiny blood vessels near the skin's surface. Besides immediate acute damage, long-term damage occurs; such as the increased incidence of skin cancer, which results from excessive irradiation to light from the UVB region (280–320 nm). In addition, excessive exposure to UVB and UVA radiation (320–400 nm) results in a weakening of the elastic and collagen fibers of the connective tissue.[10] Sunlight exposure may also cause numerous phototoxic and photoallergic reactions and contribute to premature aging. The cumulative effects of sun exposure are wrinkling, blotchy pigmentation and roughness (see **Figure 1**).

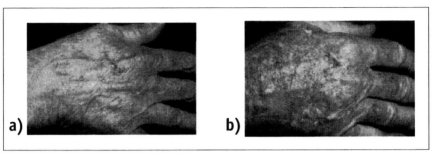

Figure 1. a) Chronologically aged skin versus b) sun-aged skin

Moreover, skin aging is related to a decrease in metabolism and cellular activity. With aging, pigment cells are less active; in turn, the skin tans less easily. These findings suggest that maintaining the natural protective mechanisms in mature skin could provide an approach to tanning and sun protection.[11] Thus, a safer alternative to artificial tanning would be maintaining or increasing skin's physiological tanning to promote melanin's natural UV-shielding effect to limit damage, and decrease the onset of premature aging.

Innovations in Sunless Tanning

Cosmetic companies have experimented with skin darkening agents for decades and as of today, only self-tanning agents that dye the skin without engaging the natural tanning process are on the market.[12] Of more importance is the need to increase skin's natural protection. Indeed, preparing the skin for sun exposure and increasing the natural protection is of particular interest to avoid repeated UV exposure and excessive use of self-tanning products.[1, 13]

One strategy could be to develop active ingredients that target different biological pathways within the physiological skin-tanning process to obtain a synergistic effect on skin tone and protection. With the market push for natural products, research focused on botanical actives has identified a spectrum of protein and peptide profiles of interest, particularly for their potential role in the melanin formation process since they are involved in various signal transduction networks. These materials could provide skin benefits such as evening out skin tone, reducing the appearance of age spots, and protecting against UV-induced damage and photo-aging.

After screening various botanical extracts, research led to the selection of a *Pisum sativum* (pea) extract for the development of a safe active tanning ingredient. The efficacy of *Pisum sativum* results from its origin and a synergy of the molecules present in the extract's composition. Besides the well-documented antioxidant and antiaging properties of *Pisum sativum*,[14] this natural botanical extract holds the capacity to reinforce the cell's natural protection against UV irradiation, as will be shown. This extract was tested under various conditions by several methods to evaluate its properties on tan prolongation and skin protection.

Evaluation of *Pisum sativum* Extract

In vitro and ex vivo tests were performed as follows, then confirmed by a clinical study. The effects of *Pisum sativum* extract in vitro were studied on melanocytes (B16 cell line) by evaluation of tyrosinase activity on normal human fibroblasts (dosage of IL-1 by ELISA). The treatment was applied once at two different concentrations in the culture medium (0.5% and 1.5% *Pisum sativum* extract) for 24 hr. A significant decrease in IL1 beta level was observed, -31% and -39% (see **Figure 2**), respectively, without any significant increase in the tyrosinase activity (data not shown). Evaluations were carried out on melanin production as well. Results of the in vitro evaluation showed a 10% increase in melanin production.

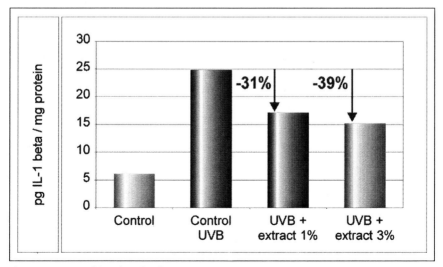

Figure 2. Dosage of IL-1 beta level

Following the in vitro tests, ex vivo studies were conducted on fresh human skin biopsies. *Pisum sativum* extract was applied on top of the epidermis at different concentrations for different lengths of time (0.5%, 1% or 1.5% for 24 hr, 48 hr and 72 hr). Evaluation of the active ingredient properties on skin pigmentation was performed by Fontana-Masson staining. An alternative version of this protocol was used to measure the effects of the active ingredient properties on UV-induced skin pigmentation. In this case, fresh human skin biopsies were irradiated by UVB at 100 mJ/cm^2 and 0.5% *Pisum sativum* extract was applied twice—once 24 hr prior to UVB exposure and once after UVB exposure. Finally, a quantitative evaluation of the melanin content of biopsies treated with the extract versus control biopsies was performed by histogram analysis of the Fontana-Masson staining after several image processing steps. Measurements of the length of skin were also taken so that all data was normalized.

The evaluation of the active ingredient's properties on the basal pigmentation by Fontana-Masson staining of human skin biopsies showed a time- and dose-dependent increase in skin tone (see **Figure 3**). Quantitative analysis of Fontana-Masson pictures showed that the treatment with *Pisum sativum* extract at 0.5% for 72 hr increased the melanin content by 543.8% (see **Figure 4**), compared with the control skin biopsies exposed to UV radiation for the same length of time. The results suggest an additive and synergistic effect of *Pisum sativum* extract on UV-induced skin tanning (see **Figure 5**). The histograms analysis of the results obtained by Fontana-Masson staining allowed the quantification of this additive and synergistic effect: *Pisum sativum* extract was found to increase UV-induced skin tanning by 156.20% in the tested conditions (see **Table 1**).

Finally, a four-week double-blind clinical study was conducted on 17 healthy volunteers of both sexes. A cream formula containing either 1.5% of *Pisum sativum* extract or the placebo cream was applied on the forearm twice daily for 28 days. The study was performed under a three-step dermatologist evaluation prior to the treatment (day 0), during the treatment (day 7) and at the end of the treatment (day 28). Photographs, customer self-evaluation and measurements of the melanin index were carried out during the study. The evolution of skin tone was evaluated by a dermatologist at the beginning and end of the study by comparing the active ingredient-treated side to the placebo-treated side (see **Figure 6**).

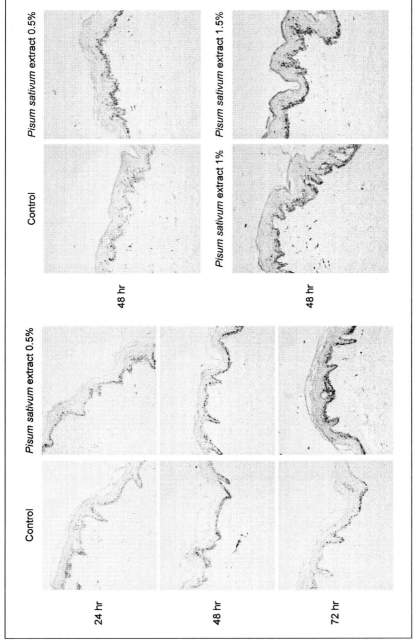

Figure 3. Ex vivo evaluation of *Pisum sativum* extract properties on basal pigmentation by Fontana-Masson staining

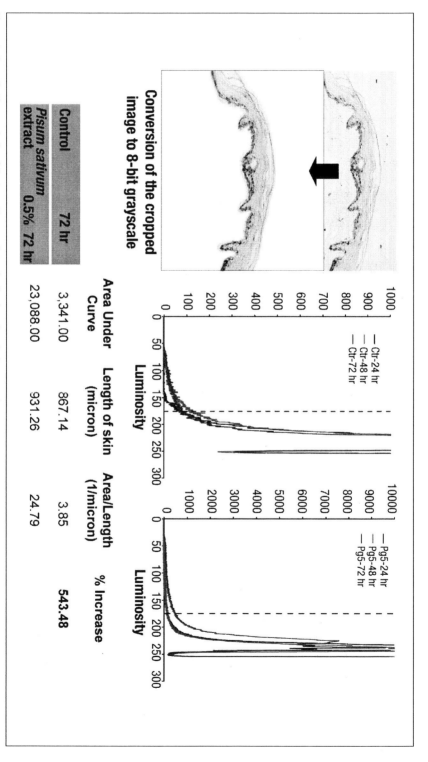

Figure 4. Quantitative analysis of Fontana-Masson data obtained on basal pigmentation

		Area Under Curve	Length of skin (micron)	Area/Length (1/micron)	% Increase
Control	72 hr	3,341.00	867.14	3.85	
Pisum sativum extract	0.5% 72 hr	23,088.00	931.26	24.79	**543.48**

Results of the clinical study demonstrated that *Pisum sativum* extract enhanced skin tone in short term and long-term conditions (see **Figure 7**). After 4 weeks of use under normal exposure, the differences in skin tone between the treated and placebo sides were highly significant—results revealed an increase in skin tone of 137.4% on the *Pisum sativum* extract-treated side. The evolution profiles of skin pigmentation during the treatment confirmed the potential of *Pisum sativum* extract to maintain skin tanning over time (see **Figure 8**).

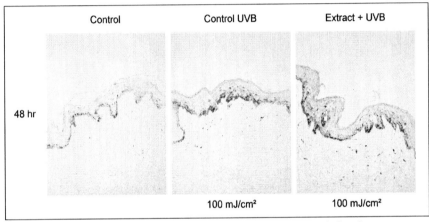

Figure 5. Ex vivo evaluation of *Pisum sativum* extract properties on UVB-induced pigmentation by Fontana-Masson staining

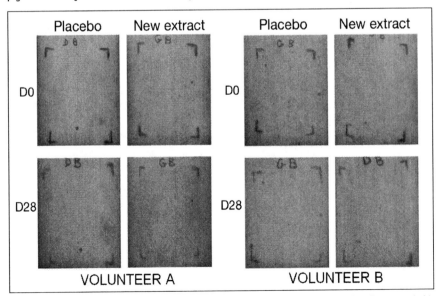

Figure 6. Clinical evaluation of *Pisum sativum* extract-treated skin versus the placebo-treated skin

Table 1. Quantitative Analysis of Fontana-Masson Data Obtained on UV-induced Pigmentation

	Area Under Curve	Length of skin (microns)	Area/Length (l/micron)	% Increase
Control 48 hr	3,029.00	925.27	3.27	---
Control + UVB 48 hr	10,935.00	812.24	13.46	311.29
Pea extract 0.5% + UVB 48 hr	20,033.00	1,078.34	18.58	467.49

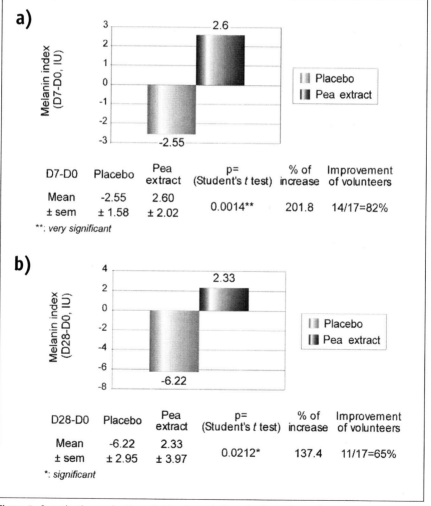

D7-D0	Placebo	Pea extract	p= (Student's t test)	% of increase	Improvement of volunteers
Mean	-2.55	2.60	0.0014**	201.8	14/17=82%
± sem	± 1.58	± 2.02			

**: very significant

D28-D0	Placebo	Pea extract	p= (Student's t test)	% of increase	Improvement of volunteers
Mean	-6.22	2.33	0.0212*	137.4	11/17=65%
± sem	± 2.95	± 3.97			

*: significant

Figure 7. Quantitative evaluation of skin pigmentation a) after 7 days of treatment and b) after 28 days of treatment

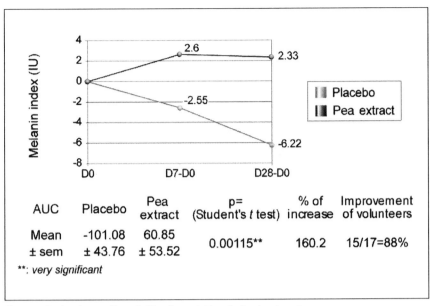

Figure 8. Evaluation profiles of skin pigmentation during treatment

Conclusions

Pisum sativum extract provides a new approach as a safe tanning active. Designed to optimize natural melanin production during exposure to sunlight, the material can protect skin from UV damage while maintaining a homogeneous skin tone. *Pisum sativum* extract naturally increases the skin's melanin production and thus prepares the skin for a healthy tan.

The material has not been shown to induce irritation and in fact tends to reduce inflammatory mediators produced during sunburn while providing a healthier, more radiant and youthful look. It is also botanical in nature and can be produced via eco-friendly means, thus complying with Ecocert guidelines. *Pisum sativum* extract would be of interest for skin care, sun care, and self-tanning formulations.

The research and development of products that offer natural, gradual tanning while providing photo-protective benefits is progressively changing the landscape of sunless tanning. This new approach is gaining considerable interest since sun care is undergoing a period of increased affinity with skin care, as both cosmetic segments look for additional claims and long-lasting benefits. The use of new silky textures together with the incorporation of safe tanning ingredients in sun care formulations is a key way to encourage product application and reach a healthy glowing tan.

Published August 2009 *Cosmetics and Toiletries* magazine

References

1. JE Stryker, AL Yaroch, RP Moser, A Atienza and K Glanz, Prevalence of sunless tanning product use and related behaviors among adults in the United States: Results from a national survey, *J Am Acad Dermatol* 56(3) 387–390 (2007)
2. K Ezzedine et al, Artificial and natural UV radiation exposure: Beliefs and behavior of 7200 French adults, *J Eur Acad Dermatol Venereol* 22(2) 186–94 (Feb 2008)
3. NG Jablonski and G Chaplin, The evolution of human skin coloration, *J Hum Evol* 39(1) 57–106 (Jul 2000)
4. TB Fitzpatrick, The validity and practicality of sun-reactive skin types I through VI, *Arch Dermatol* 124(6) 869–71 (Jun 1988)
5. AJ Thody, EM Higgins, K Wakamatsu, S Ito, SA Burchill and JM Marks, Pheomelanin as well as eumelanin is present in human epidermis, *J Invest Dermatol* 97(2) 340–44 (Aug 1991)
6. HL Norton et al, Genetic evidence for the convergent evolution of light skin in Europeans and East Asians, *Mol Biol Evol* 24(3) 710–22 (Mar 2007)
7. RM Harding et al, Evidence for variable selective pressures at MC1R, *Amer J of Human Genetics* 66 1351–1361 (2000)
8. RL Lamason et al, SLC24A5, a putative cation exchanger, affects pigmentation in zebrafish and humans, *Science* 310 (5755) 1782–86 (2005)
9. I Wickelgren, Skin biology. A healthy tan? *Science* 315(5816) 1214–16 (Mar 2, 2007)
10. R Cui et al, Central role of p53 in the suntan response and pathologic hyperpigmentation, *Cell* 128(5) 853–64 (Mar 9, 2007)
11. JP Ortonne, Pigmentary changes of the aging skin, *Br J Dermatol* 122 suppl 35 21–28 (Apr 1990)
12. C Robb-Nicholson, By the way, doctor. I'd like to keep the tanned look I got during summer vacation. Are self-tanning lotions and sprays a good idea? Are they safe to use? *Harv Womens Health Watch* 14(2) 8 (Oct 2006)
13. S Freeman, S Francis, K Lundahl, T Bowland and RP Dellavalle RP, UV tanning advertisements in high school newspapers, *Arch Dermatol* 142(4) 460 (Apr 2006)
14. A Huang, B Wang, DH Eaves, JM Shikany and RD Pace, Total phenolics and antioxidant capacity of indigenous vegetables in the southeast United States: Alabama Collaboration for Cardiovascular Equality Project *Int J Food Sci Nutr* 18 1–9 (Sep 2007)

CHAPTER 34

Therapeutic Peptides in Aged Skin

**Mike Farwick, Urusula Maczkiewitz, Peter Lersch,
Evonik Goldschmidt GMBH, Tim Falla**
Helix Biomedix, Inc.

Susanne Grether-Bech, Jean Krutmann
Heinrich-Heine University

KEY WORDS: *peptides, skin, aging, topical skin treatments, antiaging, antiwrinkle, HGH, keratin, proteins*

ABSTRACT: *Some peptides have notable effects on chronologically aged and/or photodamaged skin. Large high quality, randomized, double blind, active-controlled trials are required to calculate the exact effect of molecule size in this regard. Results from such trials will lead to an understanding of the best peptide for antiaging treatments.*

In the year 2000, individuals over the age of 65 represented 13% of the US population, and this number is expected to increase to 20% by 2030. This increase in the number of older individuals over younger individuals will transform the shape of age distribution from what currently is graphed as a pyramid into a rectangle.[1] This demographic shift calls for increased efforts to prevent the aging process and to develop safe and effective drugs for the elderly.

In cosmetic dermatology, experts are exploring better anti-solar, antiaging, antiwrinkle and firming products. Pharmaceutical companies frequently use peptides as active ingredients in creams prescribed at medical and dermatology offices. Peptides can have different effects on the skin, especially for cosmetics purposes, but the most important concern regarding their topical use is their ability to penetrate skin.

Ideally, topical drugs have: a molecular weight less than 500 daltons; a moderate log of partition coefficient octanol/water between 1 and 3; a melting point of less than 200°C; a reasonable aqueous solubility (> 1 mg/mL); and few or no polar centers.[2,3] The diffusivity of molecules into the stratum corneum (SC) is related to the number of hydrogen-bonding groups on a molecule; maximal diffusivity is achieved with small non-hydrogen-bonding molecules while minimal diffusivity occurs with molecules containing four hydrogen-bonding groups.[4]

Peptides and proteins contain many amide bonds as hydrogen-bond donor and acceptor groups. Due to their large molecular size, they have low diffusivity in skin. Furthermore, they are often charged at a physiological pH, making them intrinsically hydrophilic and hence, the lipophilic SC is a significant barrier to their penetration.[5]

Overall, topical peptides and proteins have successfully and widely been used. However, note that in the only published systematic review[6] on interventions for photodamaged skin, no peptide therapy was included. Here, published work on peptides and proteins, their characteristics, and randomized efficacy data are examined.

Material and Methods

In an effort to examine different types of peptides and their efficacy in topical skin treatments, *PubMed*, *Embase* and *Scopus* were systematically searched within a date range of 1974 to June 15, 2008. Different search terms were used to locate peptides or proteins, to find all possible topical therapies, to locate all cosmeceutical-related papers, and to rule out irrelevant papers. All references of relevant articles were screened to find other eligible resources. In addition, some in vitro and in vivo data was collected from pharmaceutical company Web sites. For efficacy data, only randomized trials were included.

Results and Discussion

Surprisingly, scarce data regarding the permeation abilities of topical peptides was found. Only the permeation coefficients for three widely used topical cosmeceutical peptides—copper tripeptide-1 (GHK)[7], glutathione (GSH)[7] and melanocyte-stimulating hormone (MSH)[8,9]; some mono-peptides[10,11] and their copper complexes were reported. **Table 1** summarizes the randomized trials referenced.

GHK: Glycyl-L-histadyl-L-lysine or GHK is primarily known as a carrier peptide but it also acts as a signal peptide mainly to help stabilize and deliver copper. Signal peptides refer to all peptides that stimulate matrix protein production in general, specifically collagen synthesis. These peptides may be produced by growth and stimulation of different skin cells such as human skin fibroblasts. Signal peptides can also increase elastin, proteoglycan, glycosaminoglycans and fibronectin. By increasing matrix cell activities and therefore collagen production, the peptides make skin look firmer and younger.

In a randomized, double blind, placebo-controlled study of 67 volunteers, GHK-Cu and a placebo were applied twice daily for 12 weeks on facial skin.[12] GHK-Cu improved skin laxity, clarity and appearance; reduced fine lines, coarse wrinkles and mottled hyperpigmentation; and increased skin density and thickness.

Pal-KTTKS: Palmitoyl pentapeptide-4 (Pal-KTTKS) is a synthetic signal peptide from pro-collagen I fragments. It stimulates collagen I, III and VI, in addition to fibronectin, elastin and glycosaminoglycan production.[13] These effects have made it a popular ingredient in antiaging and antiwrinkle products.

In a study[14] of 93 Caucasian females, Pal-KTTKS performed significantly better than a placebo, as assessed by expert graders and subjective observations, for the treatment of hyperpigmented age spots. Osborne et al. also showed a robust result for this peptide in reducing bumpy texture and fine wrinkles.[15]

Kinetin: Kinetin is another signal peptide that is derived naturally from plants. It exhibits antioxidant properties, delaying the onset of aging characteristics in human fibroblasts, and inhibits keratinocyte growth.[16] Its cosmeceutical indication is mainly limited to antiaging, antiwrinkle and anti-solar purposes.

In a randomized, double-blind study, Chiu et al. compared topical kinetin with niacinamide to niacinamide alone and found significant reductions in spot, pore, wrinkle and erythema index and evenness counts in the kinetin with niacinamide group. Furthermore, significant increases in corneal hydration status were found in the same group.[17] Several growth factors and cytokines have been applied to treat skin problems in elderly individuals.

Table 1. Randomized peptide trials

Peptides	Indication of use	Study design	Characteristics of subjects	Treatment arm(s)	Treatment protocol	Results
GHK-Cu	Antiaging	Randomized, double-blind trial	67 females ages 50–59	GHK-Cu cream vs. placebo cream	Twice daily for 12 weeks on the face	Improved all major tested parameters
Lipopentapeptide	Antiaging	Randomized, active-controlled trial	9 volunteers (2 men and 7 women) ages 42–79	6% vs. 2% total active complex cream vs. tretinoin	Patch test to extensor forearm; patch tests were removed on day 12	Tretinoin and 6% complex was the best trigger for fibrilin-1 and procollagen I deposition
Pal-KTTKS	Antiaging	Randomized, double-blind, placebo-controlled trial	93 females ages 35–55	Pal-KTTKS o/w moisturizer vs. placebo o/w moisturizer	Half-face application twice daily for 12 weeks	Significantly better scores for pal-KTTKS in age-related spots
	Antiaging	Randomized, double-blind, controlled trial	180 females ages 35–65	Pal-KTTKS facial moisturizer vs. Boswellia serrata extract vs. moisturizer base (vehicle)	Applied to half-face skin twice daily for 8 weeks	Significant reduction in fine lines/wrinkles compared to other groups
Soy extract	Antiaging	Randomized, double-blind controlled trial	21 females (55 ± 6 years)	2% soy extract cream vs. placebo cream	Each was applied to volar forearm twice daily for 2 weeks	Papillae index was increased more by soy extract than by the placebo
Silk protein vs. bovine serum albumin (BSA)	Antiaging and anti-tumor	Randomized, controlled trial	30 four-week-old female Hos:HR-1 UVB-exposed hairless mice	Single doses of 5 mg silk protein in 0.2 mL ethanol vs. 5 mg BSA in 0.2 mL ethanol vs. 0.2 mL ethanol	Treatment groups received the solutions immediately after single application of 180 mJ/cm^2 UVB treatment	Silk protein inhibited UVB-induced elevated expression of COX-2 protein significantly more than other materials

Peptide	Type	Study design	Subjects	Comparison	Application	Results
Keratin peptide	Skin moisturizer	Randomized, controlled trial	6 females ages 24–36	5 mg silk protein in 0.2 mL ethanol vs. 5 mg BSA in 0.2 mL ethanol vs. 0.2mL ethanol	Each group received the solutions immediately after 180 mJ/cm² of UVB treatment daily for 7 days	Significant differences of skin capacitance and elasticity in keratin samples; best results for IWL liposomal keratin peptide
		Randomized, controlled trial	16 females ages 24–50	Aqueous vs. liposome vs. IWL liposomes keratin peptide solutions vs. water vs. 0.9% NaCl solution	Creams were applied onto 9 cm²-marked areas once daily for 4 days	Better elasticity and hydration results for keratin cream
		Randomized, controlled trial	9 females ages 24–50	3% keratin peptide vs. 3% water in base cream vs. untreated	Creams were applied to 9cm²-areas of hands daily for 12 days	Significant smaller decrease in hydration for keratin peptide cream (capacitance and TEWL)
				3% keratin peptide vs. 3% deionized water in base cream vs. untreated	Exposure of 2% sodium lauryl sulphate on 9 cm²-areas of the hands for 2 hr	
TGF-β1 serum	Antiaging	Randomized, controlled, assessor-blind study	12 females ages 42–74	TGF-β1 serum vs. the same serum without TGF-β1	Serums were applied twice daily for 3 months	Significant improvement for TGF-β1 serum
TGF-β1 serum vs. TNS cream	Antiaging	Randomized, controlled, assessor-blind study	20 females ages 29–74	TGF-β1 serum vs. TNS cream	Applied twice daily for 3 months	Both were significant compared to baseline
PSP	Antiaging	Randomized, double-blind, controlled trial	20 females ages 35–65	PSP cream vs. a physically identical placebo cream	Creams were applied to the half-face skin twice daily for 2 months	Roughness parameters were significantly better in PSP group; no difference between groups
Kinetin (cytokine) plus niacinamide	Antiaging	Randomized, double-blind, controlled trial	52 female and male subjects (ages 30–60)	Serum containing kinetin 0.03% plus niacinamide 4% vs. serum containing niacinamide 4%	Creams were applied to one side of the face daily for 12 weeks	Significant improvement in major parameters for kinetin group

ᵇProcessed skin-cell proteins (PSP) is a product of Neocutis, San Francisco, Calif., USA.

Human growth factor: An antioxidant serum containing liposome-encapsulated transforming growth factor beta (TGF-β1), ascorbic acid and *Cimicifuga racemosa* extract in a silicone base was developed[a], applied to the arms of test subjects, and compared with a placebo serum omitting the TGF-β1.[18] The skin of subjects treated with TGF-β1 revealed a significant mean improvement (21.7%) in physician-rated wrinkle scores while the placebo-treated skin recorded a slight improvement (6.2%) over the baseline.

The trial then continued with a comparison of the test serum to a tissue nutrient solution (TNS) cream in 20 test subjects.[18] TNS contains growth factors including vascular endothelial growth factor, platelet-derived growth factor A, granulocyte colony-stimulating factor, hepatocyte growth factor, interleukin-6, interleukin-8, and TGF-β1 without vitamin C. Both creams were found to significantly improve wrinkle scores.

Growth factor and cytokine mixture: A bio-restorative skin cream was developed containing a proprietary growth factor and cytokine mixture extracted from cultured, first trimester fetal human dermal fibroblasts. In a placebo-controlled trial, Gold and colleagues concluded that some skin roughness parameters were significantly better in the group treated with the cream but that no statistical difference between two groups was detected.[19]

Soybean proteins: Soybean proteins or peptides are enzyme inhibitor peptides extracted from soybean seeds. Soy proteins inhibit the formation of proteinases and increase trichoblast and atrichoblast numbers without changing their localization pattern;[20] they are used as antiaging, skin moisturizer, anti-solar and hair-promoting agents.

In a randomized double blind placebo-controlled study, soy extract and placebo creams were applied to the forearms of 21 healthy women[21] and overall, the papillae index increased greater with the application of the soy extract than with the placebo (p < 0.05).

Sericin: Another enzyme inhibitor protein, sericin or silk worm secretion, is extracted from the middle silk gland of the *Bombyx mori* silkworm. Sericin exhibits antioxidant properties and has a high affinity for chelating with copper. In addition, it inhibits lipid peroxidation, tyrosinase activity and keratinocyte apoptosis. In another

---

[a]Citrix Cell Rejuvenation Serum is a product of Topix Pharmaceuticals Inc., West Babylon, N.Y., USA.

study, silk protein was compared with bovine serum albumin in a vehicle found to better reduce UVB-induced symptoms in both short-term and chronic treatment courses.[22]

Lipopentapeptide: Another peptide, lipopentapeptide, in combination with white lupin peptide and antioxidants, significantly increased fibrillin-1 and procollagen I deposition at a 6% w/w concentration when compared with 2% tretinoin and the control.[23]

Keratin: Keratin is a major protein in the structure of hair and skin that can be extracted from human hair or sheep's wool. It improves the hydration and elasticity of skin and hair when applied topically and thus is commonly used in moisturizers, firming agents and hair shine enhancers. Barba et al.[24] conducted a randomized trial comparing 3% keratin peptides to water and a control in 16 healthy females and found the keratin peptide to be effective on disturbed but not undisturbed skin.

In another recent trial, significant improvements were achieved for elasticity parameters and especially skin capacitance with the application of the keratin samples.[25] Among all the keratin creams tested, a combination of a keratin peptide with internal wool lipid liposomes provided the most significant benefits, compared with the aqueous solution.[25]

Conclusions

Some peptides have notable effects on chronologically aged and/or photodamaged skin. According to the current evidence, GHK-Cu, Pal-KTTKS, soybean protein and keratin peptides exhibit the best results among the peptides. There is a large gap in data regarding the permeability coefficient of cosmeceutical peptides and proteins, and researchers should focus on this ambiguity to identify substances with better permeability. Large high quality, randomized, double blind, active-controlled trials are required to calculate the exact effect of molecule size in this regard. Results from such trials will lead to an understanding of the best peptide for antiaging treatments.

Published September 2009 *Cosmetics and Toiletries* magazine

References

1. MG Kosmadaki and BA Gilchrest, The demographics of aging in the United States: implications for dermatology, *Arch Dermatol*, 138(11) 1427–8 (2002)

2. RH Guy, Current status and future prospects of transdermal drug delivery, *Pharm Res*, 13(12) 1765–9 (1996)

3. BE Vecchia and AL Bunge, Evaluating the transdermal permeability of chemicals, in *Transdermal drug delivery* (electronic resource), RH Guy and J Hadgraft, eds. Dekker: New York (2003)

4. MS Roberts, SE Cross and MA Pellett, Skin Transport, in *Dermatological and transdermal formulations*, AW Walters, ed. Dekker: New York (2002) p 121

5. C Cullander and RH Guy, Routes of delivery: Case studies (6). Trasdermal delivery of peptides and proteins, *Adv Drug Deliv Rev* 8 291–329 (1992)

6. M Samuel et al, Interventions for photodamaged skin, *Cochrane Database Syst Rev* 1 (2005) p CD001782

7. L Mazurowska and M Mojski, Biological activities of selected peptides: Skin penetration ability of copper complexes with peptides, *J Cosmet Sci* 59 1 59–69 (2008)

8. A Ruland, J Kreuter and JH Rytting, Transdermal delivery of the tetrapeptide hisetal (melanotropin (6-9)): II. Effect of various penetration enhancers, In vitro study across human skin, *Intl J Pharmaceutics* 103 1 77–80 (1994)

9. A Ruland, J Kreuter and JH Rytting, Transdermal delivery of the tetrapeptide hisetal (melanotropin (6-9)). I. Effect of various penetration enhancers: In vitro study across hairless mouse skin, *International J Pharmaceutics*, 101(1–2) 57–61 (1994)

10. L Mazurowska, K Nowak-Buciak and M Mojski, ESI-MS method for in vitro investigation of skin penetration by copper-amino acid complexes: From an emulsion through a model membrane, *Analsis Bioanalasis Chem* 388(5–6) 1157–63 (2007)

11. A Ruland and J Kreuter, Transdermal permeability and skin accumulation of amino acids, *Intl J Pharm* 72(2) 149–151 (1991)

12. MB Finkey, Y Appa and S Bhandarkar, Copper peptide and skin, in *Cosmeceuticals and active cosmetics*, P Elsner and HI Maibach, eds, Marcel Dekker: New York (2005) pp 549–564

13. K Lintner, Promoting production in the extracellular matrix without compromising barrier, *Cutis*, 70 (6 suppl) pp 13-6, discussion 21-3 (2002)

14. LR Robinson et al, Topical palmitoyl pentapeptide provides improvement in photoaged human facial skin, *Int J Cosmet Sci*, 27(3) 155–60 (2005)

15. R Osborne et al, Use of a facial moisturizer containing palmitoyl pentapeptide improves the appreance of aging skin, *J Am Acad Dermatol* 52 (3 suppl 1) 96 (2005)

16. U Berge, P Kristensen and SI Rattan, Kinetin-induced differentiation of normal human keratinocytes undergoing aging in vitro, *Ann NY Acad Sci*, 1067 332–6 (2006)

17. PC Chiu et al, The clinical antiaging effects of topical kinetin and niacinamide, in Asians: A randomized, double-blind, placebo-controlled, split-face comparative trial, *J Cosmet Dermatol* 6(4) 243–9 (2007)

18. M Ehrlich et al, Improvement in the appearance of wrinkles with topical transforming growth factor beta(1) and l-ascorbic acid, *Dermatol Surg* 32(5) 618–25 (2006)

19. MH Gold, MP Goldman and J Biron, Efficacy of novel skin cream containing mixture of human growth factors and cytokines for skin rejuvenation, *J Drugs Dermatol* 6(2) 197–201 (2007)

20. Preregen, Centerchem, available at *www.centerchem.com/PDFs/PREREGEN%20Fact%20 Sheet%206004.pdf* (accessed Jul 9, 2009)

21. KM Sudel et al, Novel aspects of intrinsic and extrinsic aging of human skin: Beneficial effects of soy extract, *Photochem Photobiol* 81(3) 581–7 (2005)

22. S Zhaorigetu, Inhibitory effects of silk protein, sericin on UVB-induced acute damage and tumor promotion by reducing oxidative stress in the skin of hairless mouse, *J Photochem and Photobiology Biol* 71(1–3) 11–17 (2003)

23. RE Watson et al, Repair of photo-aged dermal matrix by topical application of a cosmetic 'antiaging' product, *Br J Dermatol* 158(3) 472–7 (2008)

24. C Barba et al, Wool peptide derivatives for hand care, *J Cosmet Sci* 58(2) 99–107 (2007)

25. C Barba et al, Cosmetic effectiveness of topically applied hydrolyzed keratin peptides and lipids derived from wool, *Skin Res Technol* 14(2) 243–8 (2008)

CHAPTER 35

Chitin Nanofibrils: A Natural Compound for Innovative Cosmeceuticals

Pierfrancesco Morganti and Gianluca Morganti
Mavi Sud, Aprilia (LT), Italy

Riccardo A.A. Muzzarelli and Corrado Muzzarelli
Polytechnic University, Ancona, Italy

KEY WORDS: *chitin nanofibrils, skin hydration, cutaneous aging, biofilm, corneocyte cohesion*

ABSTRACT: *Compared to larger-sized chitin particles, chitin nanofibrils can be hydrolyzed more easily by cutaneous enzymes, leading to applications such as rehydrating dry skin, augmenting cohesion of cells in the stratum corneum, and forming a protective biofilm that supports wound healing.*

Recent improvements in methods to isolate chitin nanofibrils from crustacean chitin suggest cutaneous applications in areas such as skin rehydration, wound healing and maintenance of cutaneous homeostasis.

Chitin (from the Greek χιτων for "protective coat") represents the most important compound of the crustacean and insect cuticle, but it also occurs in the fungal cell wall.

Chemically, chitin is a polysaccharide formed by glucosamine and N-acetylglucosamine units having β-$(1\rightarrow4)$ bonds. These same bonds are found in cellulose. They also are found in the hyaluronic acid of human skin and in other mammalian organs.

Although cellulose is a neutral polysaccharide, chitin is weakly cationic and chitosan is strongly cationic because of the glucosamine effect. On the other hand, hyaluronic acid is an anionic polysaccharide made of d-glucuronic acid and N-acetyl glucosamine. The structural similarity among chitin, cellulose and hyaluronic acid suggests that plants, insects and mammals evolved from a single primordial bacterium.[1]

Crystalline Chitin Nanofibrils

Microstructural hierarchy: Crystalline chitin nanofibrils have a microstructure typical of crustacean and insect cuticles. In the chitin structures present in nature, native chitin crystallizes following crystallographic patterns, giving origin to polysaccharide chains assembled precisely one after another by hydrogen bonds, as in the two edges of a zipper.

The resulting rigid substance is immersed in a matrix of proteins and calcium carbonate, which forms microfibers. The microfibers form layers of a few grades on one another. These staggered layers form a structure like plywood (**Figure 1**). Remarkable is the fact that the crystalline microfibers contain nanofibrils approximately 300 nm long and 10 nm in diameter with high structural and crystalline precision.[2,3]

Recently, chitin nanofibrils have been studied in view of elucidating their structure, but only now it is possible to isolate them in large quantity and make them useful for practical applications. In acidic environments both beta- and gamma-crystalline conformations transform rapidly into the most stable alpha form. This alpha-nanocrystalline form is extracted from crustacean chitin according to a recently patented industrial process[4] developed by the Mavi Sud company (**Figure 2**).

General characteristics: Nanofibrils are extremely small objects, observable only under the transmission electronic microscope; each of them is made of less than 20 polysaccharide chains that recognize each other. Their specific surface area is large: one gram of nanofibrils develops a surface of 180 m^2. Upon slow evaporation of their suspensions, they align side by side to form a film, as on a desktop covered entirely by well-aligned pencils. These films over a certain thickness are opaque, but when the thickness is less than 1 mg/cm^2, they are transparent.

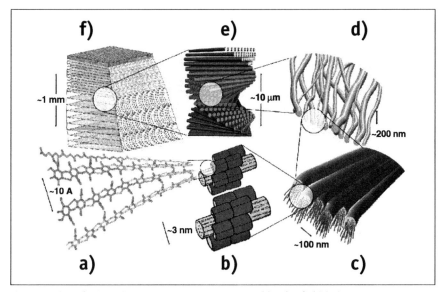

Figure 1. Hierarchy organization comprising six structural levels of chitin in crustaceans (from Reference 2)
a) assembly of the chitin chains to form alpha crystals;
b) nanofibrils (clear cylinders) surrounded by proteins (dark);
c) settlement of nanofibrils in microfibers of chitin and proteins;
d) lamina of a net of fibers of chitin and proteins; calcite crystallizes in the openings;
e) disposition of laminas with a rotating orientation visible under the optical microscope;
f) structure of the cuticle (exo and endo) whose plane section shows the typical arched pattern as a consequence of the grades of rotation of the laminas.

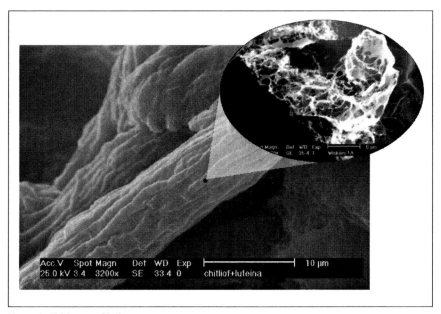

Figure 2. Chitin nanofibrils

Because of their small dimensions and of the large surface area, these nanocrystals are recognized by the enzymes as a more easily attackable material than solid substrates. In other words, an ubiquitary enzyme, such as human lysozyme, can hydrolyze chitin nanofibrils, but it is less active on the same chitin in flake form.

Applications: From a biological point of view, the crystalline nanofibrils applied on a wounded skin are able to form a protective biofilm, thin and elastic, capable of favoring tissue healing. In fact, they stimulate keratinocytes to grow fast and fibroblasts to produce the right amount and quality of collagen fibrils.[5]

For these reasons, chitin nanofibrils used in aesthetic surgery or in cosmetic formulations or to heal wounds can be considered N-acetyl glucosamine reservoirs able to release progressively due to the hydrolytic enzymes active on chitin.

Moreover, it should be recalled that during the last 10 years, human chitinases deemed not to exist in human tissues have been discovered: it has been observed that the defenses of the human organism include the ability to secrete chitinases called chitotriosidases.[6]

Chitin nanofibrils consist of a single substance; therefore, they are pure and organized and disposed in a regular way. This fact enables proteins to recognize chitin easily, as is amply demonstrated by the use of fluorescent lectins.

From a pharmaceutical or cosmetic point of view, nanofibrils represent a carrier able to favor the transcutaneous penetration of many active principles.

Because of the chemical bonds that can be established with many molecules, these nanofibrils are able to carry linked molecules in the different skin areas and at different times according to their typology and the formulation studied. For instance, coenzyme Q10 can be carried as on amorphous compound that can be easily assimilated by tissues.

An important evidence of this phenomenon of superficial adsorption is the capacity of chitin (and chitosan) to induce a fast blood coagulation following adsorption of some enzymes and blood platelets on its surface. This accelerated blood coagulation explains chitin's interesting surgical use in operations performed on varices, lungs, the esophagus and spleen.

The induction mechanism of hemostasis by chitin is redundant because it exploits simultaneously different biological phenomena, such as the interaction of blood platelets with chitin, a catalytic surface favoring the production of thrombin, and the accelerated formation of a fibrin coagulation.[7] Moreover, nanofibrils induce the agglutination of the erythrocytes.[8,9] Approximately 10 years ago the intravenous administration of fagocitable chitin particles of sizes 1–10 micron was suggested for the stimulation of alveolar macrophages, while chitin nanofibrils seemed advisable to obtain the production of interferon and a consequent improvement of the immune defenses.[10]

In veterinary practice, the positive clinical results obtained in the healing of animal wounds by the use of chitin in the form of sponges, flakes and powders, could be improved by the use of the more active chitin nanofibrils.[11]

The metabolic activity of stratum corneum: The skin barrier, localized mainly at the level of the stratum corneum (SC), is formed by a particular tissue composed by corneocytes embedded into the extracellular matrix organized in lipidic unities with a lamellar nature (**Figure 3**).

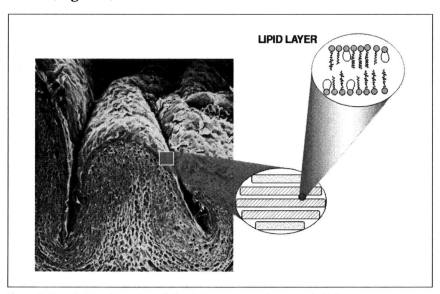

Figure 3. Organizational structure of the stratum corneum (composed skin)

By now, it is known that the SC is active metabolically in the production of hydrolase, proteases and other enzymes. These enzymes convert phospholipids, glycosphingolipids and other polar lipids into a nonpolar mixture of ceramides, cholesterol and free fatty acids that are necessary for the desquamating process (**Figure 4**).[12]

These biochemical transformations cause such skin structural changes to lead to the formation of well-organized lipidic lamellae necessary to protect against an outer hostile environment (**Figure 5**).[13–15] Any barrier alterations linked to the outer environmental modifications induced for example by cutaneous aggressions can cause a prompt response aimed to normalize this important function in hours or days.[16]

The initial response of the first 30 min is linked to the secretion of a pool of preformed lipidic lamellae followed within hours by the synthesis of cholesterol and fatty acids.[17–19] If this physiological process is opposed by changes in stress or environmental humidity, the formation of keloids or hypertrophic scars may occur.[20.]

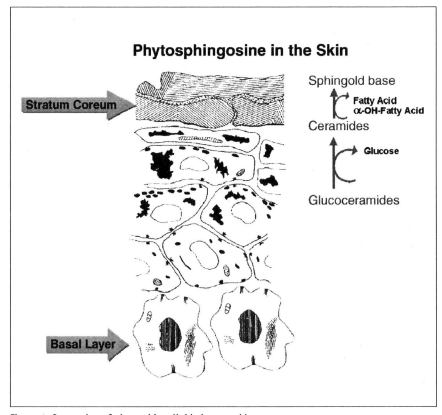

Figure 4. Conversion of glycosphingolipids in ceramides

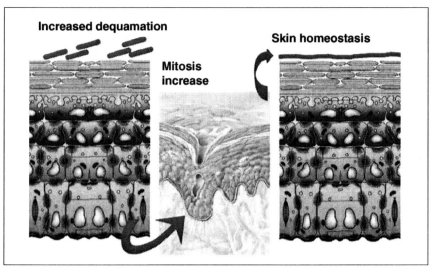

Figure 5. Skin turnover

Mechanism of Action

Chitin is recognized easily by the cutaneous enzymes and hydrolyzed. In this way, N-acetylglucosamine is able to regulate the collagen synthesis at the level of fibroblasts, facilitating also the granulation and the repair of the altered skin tissues.[21,22]

On the other hand, glucosamine diffuses easily through all the biological membranes and enters into the cellular metabolism, working also as a molecule that is able to retain water at the level of the dermal extracellular matrix.[23-25] In fact, some water present in the dermis is strongly linked to GAGs (glycosaminoglycans), which form the supporting gel for both the collagen fibers and the elastic ones.

Interestingly, the crystalline nanofibrils can be used to rehydrate the skin affected by more or less intense forms of xerosis (dry skin).

Moreover, as previously mentioned, these nanofibrils have the ability to connect cells such as corneocytes. In this way, nanofibrils augment the cohesion at the SC level, regulating perspiration. It is known that when the skin structure is damaged, the skin transpiration increases with a possible consequent appearance of psoriasis, atopic dermatitis and other signs of pathological dryness. Mavi's studies showed that the artificial barrier disruption induces or increases the expression of several cytokines in the skin at the levels of mRNA and protein.

Thus the chitin nanofibrils' activity can be useful also in the presence of inflammatory processes caused, for example, by an excessive production of cytokines.

On the other hand the biological functions of cytokines involve the regulation of cell proliferation and function but can be both stimulatory and inhibitory. Therefore it now seems that the homeostatic control mechanism in the skin is a complex network of cytokines mediating interactions between resident cells (keratinocytes, Langerhans cells, endothelial cell and fibroblast) and T-lymphocytes, neutrophils and macrophages.

Their biological activity is, in fact, pleiotropic and flowery (**Figure 6**) and can be represented as a series of cascades in which the production of a cytokine stimulates the secretion of many cytokines that can interact among them in a synergic or antagonistic way.

Chitin nanofibrils act on the cells by modulating their production. Hence they have an interesting anti-inflammatory activity[26] and regulate at the same time the production of both collagen and cutaneous lipids present at the intercorneocitary lamellae level.[27]

Healthy Aging

Effect of aging on cells: The aging process is not so much linked to the passage of time as to the overstock of negative events that deteriorate the body, mind and appearance.[28]

Aging reduces the number of healthy cells of the body. The most destructive event in aging is represented by the loss of the reservoirs due to the reduction of number and functions of the cells of any organ, such as the skin. For example, the level of sugar in the blood remains almost constant during the entire lifetime, but the glucose tolerance decreases. Glucose tolerance measures the ability of human organisms to oppose the numerous stress phenomena.

With aging, the body loses the ability to maintain global homeostasis. This decadence is caused by the accumulation of free radicals that with their reactivity give rise to cellular death and accelerate the general and cutaneous aging process. In fact, they link to the skin proteins, collagen and elastin, damaging the walls of blood capillaries and altering the immune system.

Reintegration of cellular function: It is known that one of the negative effects of free radicals is to interfere at the level of the cellular membrane. The membrane alteration causes damage throughout the cell, compromising hundreds of biochemical reactions taking place continuously in its inner part.

Chitin nanofibrils, protecting both corneocytes and intercorneocitary lamellae, help to maintain the cutaneous homeostasis, neutralize the activity of free radicals and entrap them in their structure, and regularize the correct cellular turnover (**Figure 7**).

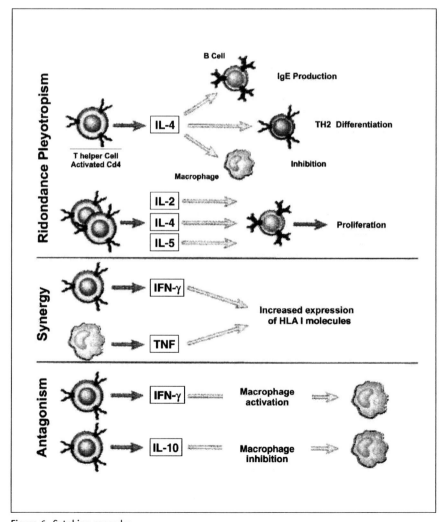

Figure 6. Cytokine cascades

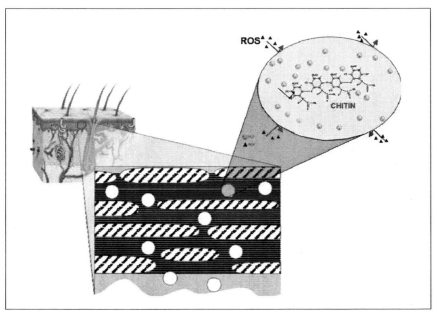

Figure 7. Protective activity of chitin

Summary

Seventy percent of the human body is water, an essential ingredient for performing all the body's functions. Water is everywhere. To appear healthy and beautiful, the skin must be always well-hydrated. A good hydration favors cellular metabolism and helps to give the skin firmness and suppleness.[29,30]

Water as a natural element is necessary for the production of cosmetics, drugs and dietary products. Water as a basic health element is indispensable for cutaneous metabolism. A beautiful skin is also a healthy skin.

Chitin nanofibrils are useful as natural active principles able to promote health and beauty. Their inclusion in cosmetic and/or pharmaceutical solutions or emulsions generates the formation of a hygroscopic molecular film that slows down water evaporation and contributes to keep the skin perfectly hydrated as well. Soon-to-be-published studies[5] on cell cultures and humans also demonstrate the safety and efficacy of formulations based on the use of chitin nanofibrils.

Their mechanism of action can be considered *active* because they repair the intercorneocitary cement that joins the ceramides and joins the phospholipids to form of the lipidic lamellae. Moreover, they seem to help to protect the molecules of the natural moisturizing factor (NMF) present at the level of the corneocytes' membrane, forming a film around their membranes.

The use of the chitin nanofibrils as components of cosmetic or pharmaceutical carriers helps to restore the integrity of the skin barrier and to increase the capacity to link and retain the corneocytes' own water. In this way it is possible to obtain two results:

- A passive strategy linked to the formation of a film able to retard perspiration.
- An active strategy that reinforces the skin capacities to fix water and to protect itself against environmental assaults.

Finally, these nanofibrils have interesting applications in the production of special textiles to which chitin imparts peculiar characteristics of biocompatibility. These yarns can be largely used in the production of hypoallergenic clothing but also for manufacturing innovative bandages and gauzes to be used in the field of advanced medications.[30]

It is of fundamental importance to use these nanofibrils appropriately, including them in carriers that maximize both the physicochemical properties and the biological properties in the setting of the cutaneous ecosystem.

Published April 2007 *Cosmetics and Toiletries* magazine

References
1. BA Neudecker, AB Csóka, K Mio, HI Maibach and R Stern, In *Cosmeceutical: Drugs vs Cosmetics,* P Elsner and HI Maibach, eds, New York: Marcel Dekker (2000) pp 319–355
2. D Raabe, P Romano, C Sachs, A Al-Sawalmih, H-G Brokmeier, S-B Yi, G Servos and HG Hartwig, Discovery of a honeycomb structure in the twisted plywood patterns of fibrous biological nanocomposite tissue, *J Crystal Growth* 283 1–7 (2005)
3. D Raabe, P Romano, C Sachs, H Fabritius, A Al-Sawalmih, S-B Yi, G Servos and HG Hartwig, Microstructure and crystallographic texture of the chitin-protein network in the biological composite material of the exoskeleton of the lobster, *Homarus americanus*. *Materials Science and Engineering A* 421 143–153 (2006)
4. Patent Pending, Mavi (2006)
5. RAA Muzzarelli, P Morganti, P Palombo, M Palombo, G Bigini, M Mattioli-Belminte, F Giantomassi and C Muzzarelli, Wound care preparations based on chitin nanofibrils and chiosa, In print: *Biomaterials* (2007)
6. A Erikson, H Forsberg, M Nilsson, M Astrom and JE Mansson, Ten years' experience of enzyme infusion therapy of Norrbottnian (type 3) Gaucher disease. *Acta Paediatrica* 95(3) 312–317 (2006)

7. TK Fischer, HS Thatte, TC Nichols, DE Bender-Neal, DA Bellinger and JN Vournakis, Synergistic platelet integrin signaling and factor XII activation in poly-N-acetyl glucosamine fiber-mediated hemostasis *Biomat* 27 543 (2005)

8. D Kulling, JN Vournakis, S Woo, MV Demcheva, DU Tagge, G Rios, S Finkielsztein and RH Hawes, Endoscopic injection of bleeding esophageal varices with a poly-N-acetyl glucosamine gel formulation in the canine portal hypertension model, *Gastroint Endos* 49 764–771 (1999)

9. MW Chan, SD Schwaitzberg, M Demcheva, J Vournakis, S Finkielsztein and RJ Connolly, Comparison of poly-N-acetyl glucosamine with absorbable collagen (Actifoam), and fibrin sealant (Bolheal) for achieving hemostasis in a swine model of splenic hemorrhage, *J Trauma* 48 454–457 (2000)

10. Y Shibata, LA Foster, WJ Metzger and QN Myrvik, Alveolar macrophage priming by intravenous administration of chitin particles, polymers of N-acetyl-D-glucosamine, in mice. *Infection and Immunity* 65 1734–1741 (1997)

11. Okamoto, S Minami, A Matsuhashi, H Sashiwa, H Saimoto, Y Shigemasa, T Tanigawa, Y Tanaka and S Tokura, Application of polymeric N-acetyl-D-glucosamine (chitin) to veterinary practice, *J Vet Med Sci* 55 743–747 (1997)

12. L Williams, Lipid in normal and patho, In *Advances in Lipid Research: Skin Lipids*, PM Elias, ed, New York: Academic Press (1991) pp 211–252

13. PM Elias and GK Menon, Structural and lipid biochemical correlates of the epidermal permeability barrier, In *Advances in Lipid Research: Skin Lipids*, PM Elias, ed, New York: Academic Press (1991) pp 1–26

14. WM Holleran, Y Takagi, KR Feingold et al, Processing of epidermal glucosylceramide is required for optimal mammalian permeability barrier function, *J Clin Invest* 91 1656–1664 (1993)

15. M Mao-Qiang, M Jain, KR Feingold and PM Elias, Secretory phospholipase A2 activity is required for permeability barrier homeostasis, *J Clin Invest* 106 57–63 (1996)

16. T Mauro, WM Holleran, S Greyson et al, Barrier recovery is impeded at neutral pH, independent of ionic effects: implications for extracellular lipid processing. *Arch Dermatol Res* 290 215–222 (1998)

17. M Elias and R Ghadially, Geriatric dermatology, Part II: The aged epidermal permeability barrier: Basis for functional abnormalities, *Clin Geriatr Med* 18(1) 103–120 (2002)

18. PM Elias, Stratum corneum architecture, metabolic activity, and interactivity with subjacent cell layers, *Exp Dermatol* 5 191–201 (1996)

19. GK Menon, KR Feingold and PM Elias, The lamellar body secretory response to barrier disruption, *J Invest Dermatol* 98 279–289 (1992)

20. M Denda, T Tsuchiya, T Hirao et al, Stress alters cutaneous permeability barrier homeostasis, *Am J Physiol Regul Integr Comp Physiol* 278 R367–R372 (2000)

21. KR Feingold, BE Brown, SR Lear et al, Effect of essential fatty acid deficiency on cutaneous sterol synthesis, *J Invest Dermatol* 87 588–591 (1986)

22. KR Middleton and D Seal, Sugar as an aid to wound healing, *Pharm J* 235 757–759 (1985)

23. J Kössi, M Vähä-Kreula, S Peltonen, J Risteli and M Laato, Effect of sucrose on collagene metabolism in keloid, hypertrophic scar, and granulation tissue fibroblast cultures, *World J Surgery* 25(2) 142–146 (2001)

24. M Adams, About glucosamine, *Lancet* 354 353–354 (1999)

25. B Berra, Glucosamina, In *Nutraceuticals*, C Rapport and B Lockwood, eds, Milan: MDM Medical Media (2003) pp 17–29

26. Mavi, data on file (2006)

27. M Mao-Qiang, L Wood, PM Elias and KR Feingold, Cutaneous barrier repair and pathophysiology following barrier disruption in Il-I and TNF Type 1 receptor deficient mice, *Exp Dermatol* 6 98–104 (1997)

28. B Gilchrest and J Krutmann, *Skin Aging*, Berlin: Springer Verlag (2006)

29. JJ Leyden and AV Rawlings, *Skin Moisturization*, New York: Marcel Dekker (2002)

30. P Morganti, RAA Muzzarelli and C Muzzarelli, Multifunctional use of innovative chitin derivatives for skin care, *Proceedings: Tessile & Salute, Biella, 4–5 May 2006* (2006)

CHAPTER 36

Metabolism of Vitamin D in Skin: Benefits for Skin Care Applications

Françoise Arnold
MMP Sarl

Michel Mercier and My Trinh Luu
MMP Inc.

KEY WORDS: *7-dehydrocholesterol, vitamin D receptor, barrier function, cathelicidin, skin protection*

ABSTRACT: *The skin innately possesses metabolic pathways and receptors to protect against external assaults. Here, one protective component, 7-dehydrocholesterol or provitamin D, naturally present in the skin, is described, which serves as the precursor for active metabolites that influence the formation and maintenance of barrier function, the activation of antimicrobial peptides, photoprotective activities, and protection against senescence.*

Although known since 1922, vitamin D3 or cholecalciferol was identified only as recently as the late 1960s as the precursor of the active steroid 1,25-dihydroxyvitamin D3 or calcitriol, and this active steroid was known for its involvement in the metabolism of calcium—i.e., for its effects on bone mineralization. For this reason, children were administered fish oils, which are highly concentrated in vitamin D3. Food supplementation with vitamin D is common today and benefits the entire population.

Initially, the metabolism of vitamin D3 to calcitriol was thought to occur only in the liver and kidneys. However, the vitamin D receptor (VDR) for 1,25-dihydroxyvitamin D3 was more recently discovered in more than 30 tissues or organs including the skin, thus initiating new studies and reports on the activities of vitamin D metabolites and their regulation of important cellular skin functions.

Metabolism in Skin

The metabolism of vitamin D in the skin is a multi-step process that starts from 7-dehydrocholesterol.[1-3] This is an important molecule in the synthesis of cholesterol and is present mainly in the stratum spinosum and stratum basale of the epidermis. 7-Dehydrocholesterol is a strong UV absorber with 3 λ max around 270 nm, 280 nm and 295 nm, and under UV irradiation, it is partly photolyzed to create previtamin D3 (see **Figure 1**). During prolonged exposure to the sun, the synthesis of previtamin D3 reaches a plateau at a concentration of about 10–15% of the original 7-dehydrocholesterol concentration.

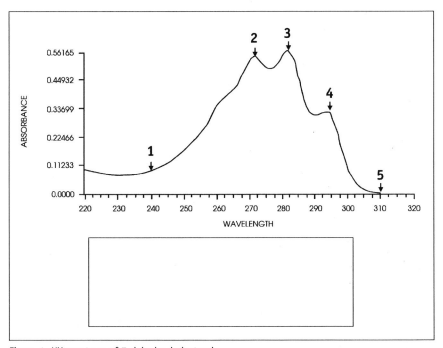

Figure 1. UV spectrum of 7-dehydrocholesterol

In turn, previtamin D3 is rapidly isomerized into inactive vitamin D3, which then undergoes enzymatic hydroxylation in epidermal keratinocytes with the production of 1,25-dihydroxyvitamin D3. This calcitriol is an active steroid and mediates its effects by binding to the VDR. Under irradiation, other previtamin D3 derivatives also are formed, lumisterol and tachysterol, as well as other hydroxyl metabolites of vitamin D3, which are formed by the action of various hydrolases (see **Figure 2**).[4]

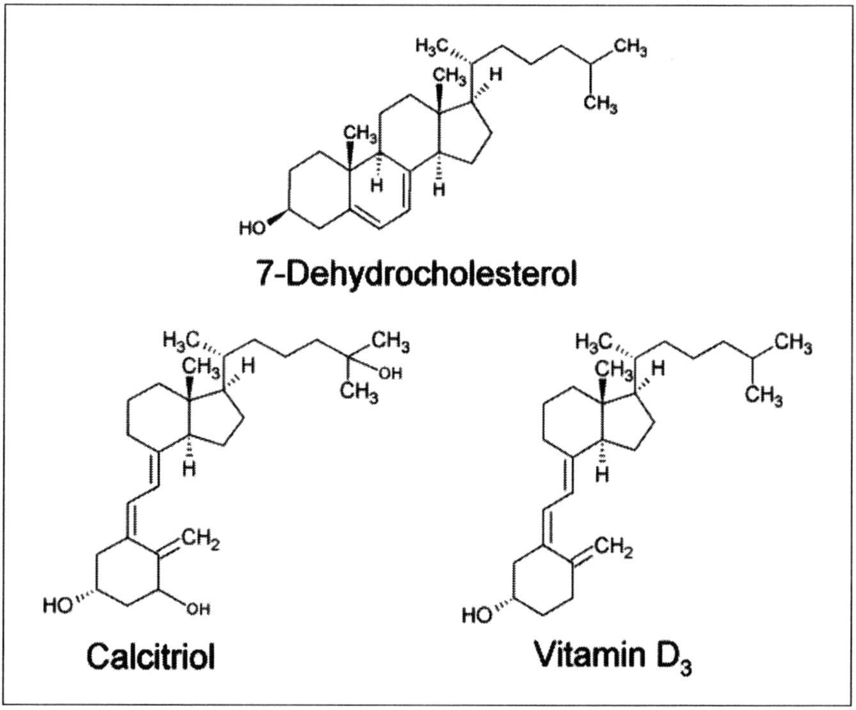

Figure 2. Chemical structures of 7-dehydrocholesterol, calcitriol and vitamin D

Therefore, it is obvious that UV exposure is a key factor in the production of vitamin D3 in the skin and that conditions affecting or limiting skin exposure to UV or skin absorption of UV may affect the formation of the vitamin D3 active metabolite—i.e., overuse of sunscreens or clothing; nursing home residents who remain indoors; seasonal and regional factors including latitude and altitude; time of the day; and skin pigmentation.[5-7] The generation of calcitriol also is reported to be wavelength and UV dose dependent.[2]

Skin Cell Differentiation

Calcitriol is known to be involved in the differentiation and regulation of growth of keratinocytes.[8] As such, analogues of 1,25-dihydroxyvitamin D3 are used topically to treat hyperproliferation in skin diseases such as psoriasis to provide anti-proliferative and pro-differentiating effects; the effectiveness of a specific wavelength to optimally generate calcitriol has been studied for this purpose.[9]

Similarly it is well-known that the production of 1,25-dihydroxyvitamin D3 influences the formation of the epidermal calcium gradient, which is involved in skin cell differentiation and in the formation of the envelope barrier.[10-11] Calcium levels in the epidermis are the lowest in the stratum basale and the highest in the stratum granulosum, and calcium and calcitriol together regulate keratinocyte differentiation and induce involucrin, a protein important for the formation of the cornified envelope and for skin barrier function.[12]

Chronic low dose UV irradiation also stimulates the enzymes responsible for lipid synthesis in the skin—i.e., fatty acid synthase, serine palmitoyl transferase and HMG-CoA reductase—as well as the expression of filagrin and involucrin, in parallel with changes in vitamin D3 metabolism.[13] Calcitriol and other hydroxylated derivatives of vitamin D exhibit this stimulating effect on keratinocyte differentiation and enhance the expression of proteins involved in barrier function.[14] Obviously the stimulation of vitamin D production in the skin by suberythemal UV irradiation has an effect on the skin's function.

Another recent report showed that 7-dehydrocholesterol by itself plays an important role in the formation of the cornified envelope of the skin, and on the maturation of the corneocytes.[15]

Protection from Microbial Attack

Interestingly, calcitriol also regulates immunocompetent cells. Skin is constantly exposed to microbes and constitutes an active barrier against pathogen attacks. The cutaneous production of antimicrobial peptides, such as defensins and cathelicidins, provides protection against infections[16] as well as activates Toll-like receptors (TLRs), which trigger antimicrobial activity.

Low dose UV irradiation stimulates the expression of cathelicidin LL-37 and β-defensin 2 in the skin in parallel with an up-regulation of the cutaneous vitamin D3 system.[13] Recent studies have demonstrated that the vitamin D3 metabolite is a major factor in the regulation of cathelicidin expression in keratinocytes through the induction of its precursor, hCAP18, by 1,25-dihydroxyvitamin D3.17 This molecule is also able to increase TLR-2 expression in keratinocytes.

Several skin diseases are associated with cathelicidin dysfunction. For instance, in atopic dermatitis and eczema, cathelicidin expression is reduced. In other diseases, cathelicidin expression is induced such as in rosacea or psoriasis, both with increased skin inflammation. Obviously, a sophisticated system operates between innate immunity and the vitamin D system. It is also interesting that the formation of 1,25-dihydroxyvitamin D3 in wound healing processes is regulated to amplify the antimicrobial response.[16,18-20] Sebaceous glands also express cathelicidin, where it is inducible by 1,25-dihydroxyvitamin D3, suggesting a possible role of vitamin D metabolite in the defense of the follicle and in acne.[21]

UV Irradiation and Skin Damage

The contribution of vitamin D to protect keratinocytes against cell death induced by various stimuli and against senescence has been demonstrated on various models. Keratinocytes irradiated by ionizing radiation to simulate radiotherapy were treated with calcitriol, and an inhibition of caspase-dependent and independent programmed cell death was observed.[22]

Enhancement of the survival of cells under exposure to aggressive conditions has also been observed in vitro with the stimulation of protective Heat Shock Proteins by 7-dehydrocholesterol, the vitamin D3 precursor.[23] In addition, protection brought by 1,25-dihydroxyvitamin D3 on skin survival under stressed conditions was also obtained in vitro with 7-dehydrocholesterol, which is active on the tumor suppressor protein p53 (the "guardian of the genome") and on senescence-associated β-galactosidase, therefore contributing to the slowing of senescence in the keratinocytes.[24]

Calcitriol protects human skin cells from UV irradiation-induced apoptosis and from DNA damage by decreasing sunburn cells and cyclobutane pyrimidine dimers in surviving cells. In parallel, an increase in p53 expression and a reduction in the formation of nitric oxide and its derivatives were obtained with 1,25-dihydroxyvitamin D3 treatment in UV irradiated keratinocytes. This photoprotective effect of calcitriol has been observed in vitro and in vivo.[25] It was also found that topically applied 7-dehydrocholesterol increases the minimal dose of UVB required to induce erythema.[23] **Formulas 1** and **2** illustrate the use of 7-dehydrocholesterol in applications.

Skin Pigmentation

Besides psoriasis, vitamin D analogs are used to treat another severe skin condition, vitiligo—a pigmentary disorder characterized by the loss of functional melanocytes in the epidermis.[26] A number of studies have reported that topical treatment with vitamin D compounds or their combination with UV light or corticosteroids enhances re-pigmentation in vitiligo.

For instance, 1,25-dihydroxyvitamin D3 was shown to increase the tyrosinase content and melanin formation in B16 mouse melanoma cells.[27] Findings indicate that calcitriol promotes the advanced stage development of melanosomes and expression of endothelins in melanocyte precursors. Human keratinocytes produce endothelin-1, which is increased after UVB irradiation, and the endothelins secreted play an essential role in the maintenance of melanocyte proliferation and differentiation and pigmentation in the epidermis.[28,29] Calcium regulation in melanocytes also regulates the supply of tyrosine for melanogenesis, and vitamin D analogs have been shown to restore calcium homeostasis and calcium flux in the melanocytes.[30]

Hair Follicles

Hair follicles are composed of epidermal keratinocytes and underlying dermal papilla cells, and these cells express the VDR. The VDR also is essential for hair follicle integrity, and the absence, loss or inactivation of the VDR leads to hair loss and the development of alopecia.[31] In mice, the VDR is expressed throughout the basal layer of the interfollicular epidermis, the outer root sheath of the hair follicle, and at the periphery of sebaceous glands. During the murine hair cycle, the VDR expression in the hair follicle is stronger in anagen IV-VI and catagen phases than during telogen and early anagen phases, correlating with decreased proliferation and increased differentiation of the keratinocytes.[32]

Formula 1. Protective moisturizing cream

A. Water (*aqua*)	74.42% w/w
B. Beta-sitosterol (and) sucrose stearate (and) sucrose distearate (and) cetyl alcohol (and) stearyl alcohol (Crystalcast MM, MMP)	4.00
C. Tetrasodium EDTA	0.05
Hydroxypropyl Bispalmitamide MEA (Vegeceramide PC-104, MMP)	1.00
D. Scleroglucan (Clearogel CS 11D, MMP)	0.20
Polyglycerin-3 (Polycast 3, MMP)	5.00
E. Isododecane (and) isononyl isononanoate (Clearocast 550, MMP)	5.00
Dimethicone (and) dimethicone/vinyl dimethicone (Clearocast 200, MMP)	5.00
Zea mays (corn) oil (and) 7-dehydrocholesterol (7-DHC, 1% in corn oil, MMP)	5.00
F. Preservative	0.30
Lavandula angustifolia (lavender) oil	0.03
	100.00

Procedure: Add A to a main vessel and heat to 80–85°C. At 80–85°C, add B to A, mixing with propeller agitation and holding the temp. for 30 min. Add C to AB and mix batch. Add premixed D to ABC and mix for 15 min; homogenize for 5 min. Start cooling to 60–65°C. In a separate vessel, combine E and start heating to 60–65°C. Add E to main batch and homogenize for 15 min. Start cooling to 45–50°C and add F to batch. Switch to a sweep blade, continue mixing and homogenize for 5 min at 34°C; pH = 6.2–7.2; viscosity, LV4 @ 12 rpm = 30,000–40,000 cps.

Formula 2. After-sun repair

A. Water (*aqua*)	94.60% w/w
B. Beta-sitosterol (and) sucrose stearate (and) sucrose distearate (and) cetyl alcohol (and) stearyl alcohol (Crystalcast MM, MMP)	2.00
C. Tetrasodium EDTA	0.05
D. Xanthan gum	0.15
Polyglycerin-3 (Polycast 3, MMP)	2.00
E. Caprylyl glycol (Sodiol ON-D, MMP)	0.70
Zea mays (corn) oil (and) 7-dehydrocholesterol (7-DHC, 1% in corn oil, MMP)	0.50
	100.00

Procedure: Add A to a main vessel and heat to 80–85°C. Add B to A and mix with propeller agitation, holding the temp. for 30 min. Add C to AB and continue mixing. Add premixed D to batch and continue mixing. Homogenize for 5 min and begin cooling. At 40–45°C, add E to batch and mix for 15 min. Homogenize for 5 min at 34°C.

Cytotoxic agents used in chemotherapy induce apoptosis of anagen hair bulbs in mice, and while pretreatment of the mice with topical 1,25-dihydroxyvitamin D3 did not prevent the chemotherapy-induced alopecia, the degree of apoptosis on follicle keratinocytes was reduced. In addition, hair shaft regrowth was improved as compared to non-pretreated mice.[33-35]

Mode of Action

The ability of calcitriol to generate biological responses is mediated through binding to the vitamin D3 receptor. Initially it was thought that the VDR was located in the cell nuclei like other steroid hormone receptors and was therefore involved in selective gene transcriptions for long-term genomic biological responses. However, rapid biological responses mediated by 1-25-dihydroxyvitamin D3 have also been obtained in minutes, which cannot be explained by nuclear VDR-regulating gene transcription. It appears that VDR is present not only in the cell nuclei, but also in the caveolae-enriched plasma membranes where it can generate rapid and direct responses through non-genomic mechanisms.[36]

An interesting approach to explain the various kinds of response is related to the chemical conformation of calcitriol, which provides exceptional flexibility and exhibits various structural shapes that can bind the receptor for either VDR-mediated nuclear responses or for rapid responses.[37]

Conclusion

7-Dehydrocholesterol, vitamin D3 and calcitriol—these molecules are involved in complex processes to protect and influence mechanisms in the skin such as: the skin envelope and barrier function, through cell differentiation; antimicrobial activation of antimicrobial peptides; protection against damage from UV irradiation; action on melanocytes and melanogenesis; and protection of the hair follicle. These benefits start with the 7-dehydrocholesterol naturally present in the epidermis—a natural precursor in vitamin D3 metabolism. Supplying 7-dehydrocholesterol to the skin in topical formulations is therefore an easy way to take advantage of these multiple activities.

References

1. MF Holick, The cutaneous photosynthesis of previtamin D3: A unique photoendocrine system, *J Invest Dermatol* 76 51–58 (1981)
2. B Lehman, P Knuschke and M Meurer, UVB-induced conversion of 7-dehydrocholesterol to 1 alpha,25-dihydroxyvitamin D3 (calcitriol) in the human keratinocyte line HACaT, *Photochem Photobiol* 72 803–809 (2000)
3. B Lehmann, T Genehr, P Knuschke, J Pietzsch and M Meurer, UVB-Induced conversion of 7-dehydrocholesterol to 1α,25-dihydroxyvitamin D3 in an in vitro human skin equivalent model, *J Invest Dermatol* 117 1179–1185 (2001)
4. O Guryev, RA Carvalho, S Usanov, A Gilep and RW Estabrook, A pathway for the metabolism of vitamin D3: Unique hydroxylated metabolites formed during catalysis with cytochrome P450scc (CYP11A1), *Proc Natl Acad Sci USA* 100 14754–14759 (2003)
5. MF Holick, JA MacLaughlin and SH Doppelt, Regulation of cutaneous previtamin D3 photosynthesis in man: Skin pigment is not an essential regulator, *Science* 211 590–593 (1981)
6. AW Norman Sunlight, Season, skin pigmentation, vitaminD and 25-hydroxyvitamin D: Integral components of the vitamin D endocrine system, *Am J Clin Nutr* 67 1108–1110 (1998)
7. MF Holick, TC Chen, Z Lu and E Sauter, Vitamin D and skin physiology: A D-lightful story, *J Bone Miner Res*, 22 suppl 2 28–33 (2007)
8. J Hosomi, J Hosoi, E Abe, T Suda and T Kuroki, Regulation of terminal differentiation of cultured mouse epidermal cell by 1 alpha,25-dihydroxyvitamin D3, *Endocrinology* 113 6 1950–1957 (1983)
9. B Lehman, P Knuschke and M Meurer, The UVB-induced synthesis of vitamin D3 and 1alpha,25-dihydroxyvitamin D3 (calcitriol) in organotypic cultures of keratinocytes: Effectiveness of the narrowband Philips TL-01 lamp (311 nm), *J Steroid Biochem Mol Biol* 103 682–685 (2007)
10. DD Bikle, Y Oda and Z Xie, Calcium and 1,25(OH)2D: Interacting drivers of epidermal differentiation, *J Steroid Biochem Mol Biol* 89-90 355–360 (2004)
11. DD Bikle, Vitamin D regulated keratinocyte differentiation, *J Cell Biochem* 1 436–444 (2004)
12. DD Bikle, D Ng, Y Oda, K Hanley, K Feingold and Z Xie, The vitamin D response element of the involucrin gene mediates its regulation by 1,25-dihydroxyvitamin D3, *J Invest Dermatol* 119 1109–1113 (2002)
13. SP Hong et al, Biopositive effects of low-dose UVB on epidermis: Coordinate up-regulation of antimicrobial peptides and permeability barrier reinforcement, *J Invest Dermatol* 128 2880–2887
14. B Zbytek et al, 20-hydroxyvitamin D3, a product of vitamin D3 hydroxylation by cytochrome P450scc, stimulates keratinocyte differentiation, *J Invest Dermatol*, 128 2271–2280 (2008)
15. D Maes, L Van Overloop, H Corstjens and L Declercq, The maturation index, the ultimate differentiation marker, *IFSCC Barcelona* (Oct 2008)
16. J Schauber, RL Gallo, Antimicrobial peptides and the skin immune defense system, *J Allergy Clin Immunol* 122 2 261–266 (2008)
17. G Weber, JD Heilborn, CI Chamorro Jimenez, A Hammarsjö, H Törmä and M Stahle, Vitamin D induces the antimicrobial protein hCAP18 in human skin, *J Invest Dermatol* 124 1080–1082 (2005)
18. M Peric et al, IL-17A enhances vitamin D3-induced expression of cathelicidin antimicrobial peptide in human keratinocytes, *J Immunol* 181 8504–8512 (2008)
19. S Segaert, Vitamin D regulation of cathelicidin in the skin: Toward a renaissance of vitamin D in dermatology? *J Invest Dermatol* 128 773–775 (2008)
20. J Schauber et al, Histone acetylation in keratinocytes enables control of the expression of cathelicidin and CD14 by 1,25-dihydroxyvitamin D3, *J Invest Dermatol* 128 816–824 (2008)
21. DY Lee et al, Sebocytes express functional cathelidin antimicrobial peptides and can act to kill Propionebacterium acnes, *J Invest Dermatol* 128 1863–1866 (2008)

22. M Langberg, C Rotem, E Fenig, R Koren, A Ravid, Vitamin D protects keratinocytes from deleterious effects of ionizing radiation, *Br J Dermatol* 160 151–161 (2009)

23. T Mammone et al, Normal human epidermal keratinocytes treated with 7-dehydrocholesterol express increased levels of heat shock protein, *J Cosm Sci* 55 149–155 (2004)

24. A Meybeck et al, Certain sterols can lower the incidence of senescent skin fibroblasts, *IFSCC Barcelona* (Oct 2008)

25. R Gupta et al, Photo-protection by 1,25 dihydroxyvitamin D3 is associated with an increase in p53 and a decrease in nitric oxide products, *J Invest Dermatol* 124 707–715 (2007)

26. SA Birlea, GE Costin and DA Norris, Cellular and molecular mechanism involved in the action of vitamin D analogs targeting vitiligo depigmentation, *Curr Drug Targets* 9 4 345–359 (2008)

27. J Hosoi, E Abe, T Suda and T Kuroki, Regulation of melanin synthesis of B16 mouse melanoma cells by 1 alpha,25-dihydroxyvitamin D3 and retinoic acid, *Cancer Res* 45 1474–1478 (1985)

28. G Imokawa, Y Yada and M Miyagishi, Endothelins secreted from human keratinocytes are intrinsic mitogens for human melanocytes, *J Biol Chem* 267 24675–24680 (1992)

29. H Watabe et al, Differentiation of murine melanocytes precursors induced by 1,25-dihydroxyvitamin D3 is associated with the stimulation of endothelin B receptor expression, *J Invest Dermatol* 118 583–589 (2002)

30. WD Bush and JD Simon, Quantification of Ca (2+) binding to melanin supports the hypothesis that melanosomes serve a functional role in regulating calcium homeostasis, *Pigment Cell Res* 20 134–139 (2007)

31. MB Demay, PN MacDonald, K Skorija, DR Dowd, L Cianferotti and M Cox, Role of the vitamin D receptor in hair follicle biology, *J Steroid Biochem Mol Biol*, 103 3-5 344–346 (2007)

32. J Reichrath, M Schilli, A Kerber, FA Bahmer, BM Czarnetzki and R Paus, Hair follicle expression of 1,25-dihydroxyvitamin D3 receptors during the murine hair cycle, *Br J Dermatol* 131 477–482 (1994)

33. MB Schilli, R Paus and A Menrad, Reduction of intrafollicular apoptosis in chemotherapy-induced alopecia by topical calcitriol analogs, *J Invest Dermatol* 111 598–604 (1998)

34. R Paus, MB Schilli, B Handjiski, A Menrad, BM Henz and P Plonka, Topical calcitriol enhances normal hair regrowth but does not prevent chemotherapy-induced alopecia in mice, *Cancer Res* 56 4438–4443 (1996)

35. J Siderov, Calcitriol and alopecia—Is it the hair apparent? *J Clin Oncol* 21 2044–2045 (2003)

36. KM Dixon, SS Deo, AW Norman, JE Bishop, GM Halliday, VE Reeve and RS Mason, In vivo relevance for photo-protection by the vitamin D rapid response pathway, *J Steroid Biochem Mol Biol* 103 451–456 (2007)

37. AW Norman, Mini-review: Vitamin D receptor: New assignments for an already busy receptor, *Endocrinology* 147 5542–5548 (2006)

CHAPTER 37

Hair and Amino Acids

Eiko Oshimura, PhD

Ajinomoto Co., Inc., Kawasaki, Japan

KEY WORDS: *amino acid, hair, interaction, damage care, luster*

ABSTRACT: *Amino acids are taken up by hair and assist in improving hair surface hydrophobicity, tensile strength and luster. This chapter discusses interactions between amino acids and hair.*

According to a rigid definition, an amino acid is an organic acid that possesses at least one amino group.[1] Almost a limitless number of molecules with various functional groups fall under this definition, but in more general terms, the definition limits the number of choices to the small group of natural L-α-amino acids that make up proteins and some other naturally occurring compounds.

Most proteins are composed of approximately 20 types of amino acids in varying proportions. Some additional amino acids are only found in special proteins; for example, hydroxyproline occurs in collagen and gelatin. All amino acid constituents of proteins are α-amino acids, referring to their molecular structure wherein the amino group is attached to the same carbon atom as the carboxyl group. Amino acids with a β-, *g*- and δ- structure, or even with a sulfonate acid group instead of a carboxyl group, are found in living organisms in forms of small peptides or as free amino acids. The term *free* here is used to describe the amino acids that are not embedded in proteins.[2]

For most consumers, the term *amino acid* is still not as familiar as protein or vitamin, yet amino acids have been used in cosmetics for a long time. Among the various applications, the most significant is the use of natural moisturizing factor (NMF) amino acids and hydrolyzed proteins, and the latter has been used in hair care applications for nearly 50 years.[3] Several moisturizers for cosmetic applications containing amino acids were reported as early as 1983.[4]

NMF is a complex mixture of free amino acids and other low molecular weight, water-soluble compounds found in corneocytes.[5] It is known to contribute to the maintenance of water balance in the stratum corneum. The main components of NMF are pyrollidone carboxylic acid (PCA), lactic acid and amino acids, and it is used mainly in skin care as a powerful moisturizer.

Hydrolyzed proteins often contain free amino acids, to some extent. They are used in skin care and also are known to contribute to conditioning and protection of hair. Hydrolyzed collagen and hydrolyzed keratin are well-known, although various hydrolyzed proteins of vegetable origin have been introduced in recent years.

The properties of hydrolyzed proteins are determined by their average molecular weight and amino acid composition. Thus, it should be quite useful to understand the properties of amino acids before applying them in hair care. In this paper, the interaction and benefits of amino acids for hair are discussed.

Amino Acids and Hair Interaction

Fundamentals: Two fundamental factors can be involved in the interaction of hair and amino acids in simple aqueous solutions: diffusion and electrical charge of the molecules.

Given the small molecular size of amino acids and their hydrophilicity, diffusion is considered to play a major role in the uptake of amino acids but the hydrophobic nature of human hair is apparently a barrier for the diffusion process. Thus it is supposed that damaged hair shows higher affinity for amino acids than the natural hair due to its lower hydrophobicity. In addition, the increased number of ionic groups on the damaged hair protein will also contribute to the higher affinity. **Figure 1** shows the comparison of arginine uptake by natural and damaged hair. The damaged hair takes up more arginine than the natural hair.

Amino acids that possess additional carboxylic groups on their carbon backbone are called acidic amino acids, and those with additional basic groups are called basic amino acids. This classification is useful to understand the nature of the interaction. Arginine is a basic amino acid that possesses a guanidinium group. The acid dissociation constant of the guanidunium group is 9.04, so it bears a cationic charge at a pH below 9. Therefore, arginine has strong affinity for hair in a pH range of 4–9. Acidic or neutral amino acids have a negative or neutral net charge in a pH range of 3–7, thus they are hardly taken up by hair (see **Figure 2**).

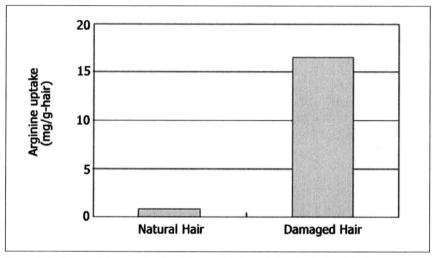

Figure 1. Arginine uptake by natural and damaged hair; arginine: $5.74\mu M$, pH 6, 1 min immersion @40°C; damaged hair was treated with a thioglycolic acid waving lotion and a sodium bromate neutralizer

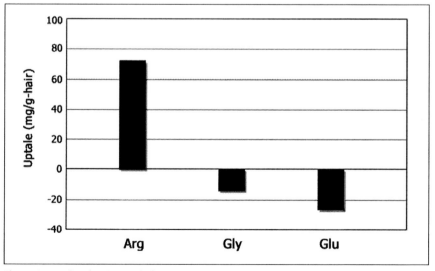

Figure 2. Uptake of amino acids from the aqueous solutions by waved hair; amino acid: $11.5\mu M$, 30 min immersion @25°C.

Above all, the guanidinium group of arginine is known to have quite a high affinity for hair protein.[6] **Figure 3** shows the amount of arginine recovered from hair either by water or by acidic buffer solution (pH 3.5).

The arginine recovery differed between the two conditions, shown by the errors, and the difference increased as the pH of the arginine solution was increased. This difference represents the existence of a strong interaction between acidic groups on hair and arginine.

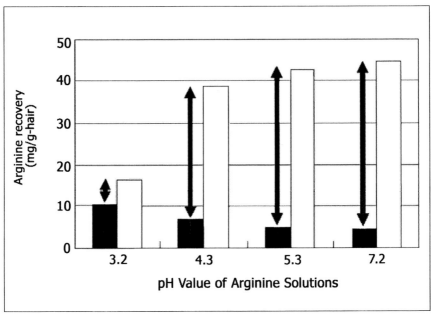

Figure 3. The amount of arginine recovered from intensively bleached hair by water (■) or by buffer solution (❏); note how the difference of the two columns (arrows) changes depending on the pH of arginine treatment. Arginine treatment: 30 min immersion, 20 sec rinse @25°C; recovery: 30 min immersion @25°C

Applications: Understanding the interaction of hair and amino acids in cosmetics is much more complicated than the above described cases because cosmetic formulations are complex mixtures of chemicals. Consequently, the chemical interaction between amino acids and other ingredients has to be taken into consideration. For example, neutral glycine and acidic glutamic acid present in conditioner are also taken up by hair.

Figure 4 shows the amount of each amino acid taken up by hair from solutions containing different concentrations of a mixture of amino acids[a].

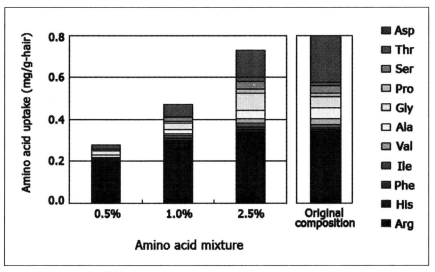

Figure 4. Uptake of amino acids from solutions containing a mixture of the amino acids; original mixture including amino acid composition is shown on the right; amino acid treatment: 10 min immersion, 1 min rinse, pH 5 @35°C; recovery: 30 min immersion in a buffer solution (pH 3.5) @25°C

At lower concentrations, arginine uptake predominates, and at higher concentrations, the uptake of the other amino acids increases. This hints at the possibility of arginine being used as an anchor for the deposition of other ingredients having weaker affinity to hair. One example is illustrated in **Figure 5**.

When PCA is applied to hair as an arginine salt, the uptake is larger than that of sodium, lysine and histidine salts.

Benefits of Amino Acids

Arginine is employed as an alkalizer in oxidative coloring agents and bleaching agents to reduce the irritative odor of ammonia and to develop milder products for the hair and scalp.[6] Arginine prevents the decrease of tensile strength and hair surface hydrophobicity that are caused by oxidative coloring. It is also reported to prevent undesirable effects of hydrogen peroxide on hair proteins and hair

[a] Prodew 500 (INCI: Sodium PCA (and) sodium lactate (and) arginine (and) aspartic acid (and) PCA (and) glycine (and) alanine (and) serine (and) valine (and) proline (and) threonine (and) isoleucine (and) histidine (and) lhenylalanine) is a product of Ajinomoto Co., Inc., Tokyo, Japan.

surface lipids.[7] During the coloring process, a considerable amount of the arginine contained in coloring agents is taken up by hair. This residual arginine confers a moist feel to hair and prevents color loss during the shampooing process.

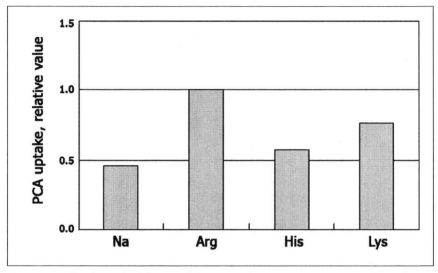

Figure 5. Uptake of PCA–the influence of the counter ion; PCA treatment: 0.2% w/w as the PCA salt, 30 min immersion, pH 5.4 @25°C; recovery: 30 min immersion in a buffer solution (pH 3.5) @25°C; the amounts of PCA uptake are described as the relative value against that of arginine salt

Damage Care

A layer of fatty acids covalently linked to the surface of hair cuticle is responsible for the hydrophobic nature of natural hair. It also provides some benefits such as the low friction, smoothness and combability to the hair.[8] Oxidative processes cause a decrease in hair surface hydrophobicity, resulting in the lack of smoothness. Cationic surfactants and silicones are often employed to improve the hydrophobicity.

Figure 6 shows surface hydrophobicity of bleached hair treated with hair conditioners. The average contact angle for natural hair was 100 degrees and a four-time bleaching treatment brought it down to 65 degrees. After treatment with a steartrimonium chloride conditioner (STAC), the contact angle increased slightly. The addition of 1.5% w/w of L-alanine resulted in a significant increase of the contact angle to a value, similar to that obtained with a distearyldimonium chloride conditioner (DSDAC).

Several amino acids have been reported to increase the tensile strength of hair in a dry state.[9] This reinforcement is mainly achieved by ionic and hydrogen bonds, so the effect should diminish in a wet state; however, some amino acids have proven to be effective even in a wet state. **Figure 7** shows the tensile strength of bleached hair measured in water. A significant increase was observed when phenylalanine and histidine were applied.

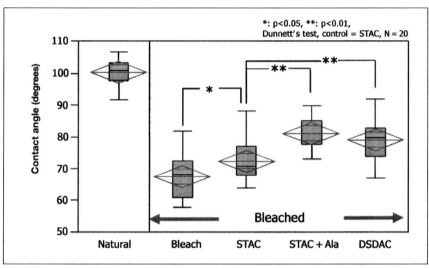

Figure 6. Improvement of surface hydrophobiciy by alanine; conditioner formulations: cationic surfactant 0.6% w/w active, cetyl alcohol 3.0% w/w. A hair fiber was fixed in a horizontal position and 1 µL of deionized water was mounted on the point 10 cm from the hair tip end. A contact angle on which a water droplet on the fiber surface was formed was measured microscopically 20 sec later.

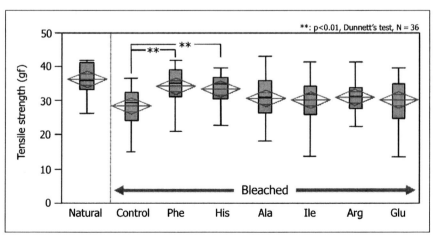

Figure 7. Effects of amino acids on the tensile strength measured in water; amino acid treatment: 2.0% w/w, 10 min immersion, pH 5.3 @35°C; rinse: 1 min immersion in deionized water @35°C

Improvement of Luster

Formation of *medulla*, or air-filled structures sometimes found at the center of hair shafts, and *voids*, hollow structures formed among cuticlar or cortical cells, by chemical treatment and grooming is known to result in a lusterless appearance in Asian hair.[10] This finding is interesting because it indicates that not only the hair surface but also its internal structure is responsible for luster. Hair luster improved by treating bleached Asian hair with an amino acid mixture (see **Figure 8**).

A decrease of the light scattering lacunal structure is observed under a microscope, suggesting the amino acids penetrate and fill the void spaces to make hair shine from the inside. The moisturizing effect of amino acids is hypothesized to complement this function.

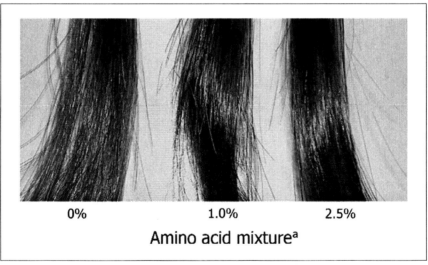

0%   1.0%   2.5%

Amino acid mixture[a]

Figure 8. Appearance of hair tresses treated with solutions of a mixture of amino acids; treatment: 10 min immersion, 1 min rinse, pH 5 @35°C

Conclusion

As mentioned, understanding the chemistry and interaction between amino acids and hair can provide a base for the development of hair care formulations containing hydrolyzed protein. However, it also should be noted that using specifically chosen, purified amino acids instead of hydrolyzed protein apparently has some advantages, such as: the possibility of avoiding odor and color problems; formation of stable products of high quality; minimizing the risk of allergic reactions; and the possibility of designing custom blends. Amino acids have been known and used as moisturizers for a long time, but because of their diverse chemical structure, they have the potential to exert a variety of functions in hair care preparations. This paper provides only a quick introduction for the novice formulator.

Published March 2008 *Cosmetics and Toiletries* magazine

References
1. SH Pine, JB Hendrickson, DJ Cram and
   GS Hammond, Amino Acids, Peptides and Proteins, in *Organic Chemistry* 4th edition, London: McGraw-Hill (1981) ch 16–1
2. JP Greenstein and M Winitz, Nomenclature, Structure, and Occurrence of Amino Acids, in *Chemistry of the Amino Acids*, New York: John Wiley & Sons. Inc. (1961), ch 1
3. I Bonadeo and GL Variati, Affinity of hair for protein derivatives, *Cosmet Toil* 92 45–51 (1977)
4. M Takehara, Recent applications of amino acids for cosmetics: Interactions and synergistic effects of amino acids, *Cosmet Toil* 98 51–56 (1983)
5. CR Harding et al, Effect of Natural Moisturizing Factor and Lactic acid Isomers in Skin Function, in *Dry Skin and Moisturizers: Chemistry and Function*, M. Lodén and HI Maibach, eds, New York: CRC press (2000) ch 19, pp 229–267
6. M Arai, T Suzuki, Y Kaneko and M Miyake, Properties of aggregates of amide guanidine type cationic surfactant with 1-hexadecanol absorbed on hair, *Proc Int Conference on Colloid Surface Sci.* (2000)
7. E Oshimura and M Ino, Effects of arginine on hair damage via oxidative coloring process, *J Cosmet Sci* 55 suppl S155–S170 (2004)
8. JA Swift, Human hair cuticle: Biologically conspired to the owner's advantage, *J Cosmet Sci* 50 23–47(1999)
9. K Hashimoto and Y Nakama, The features of recent damage hair in Japanese and development of shampoos and conditioners for the damaged hair, *Fragrance J* 10 29–36 (2003) (in Japanese)
10. S Nagase, S Shibuichi, K Ando, E Kariya and N Satoh, Influence of internal structures of hair fiber on hair appearance. I. Light scattering from the porous structure of the medulla of human hair, *J Cosmet Sci* 53 89–100 (2002)

CHAPTER 38

Polyelectrolyte Complex for Mending Damaged Hair

Ray Rigoletto and Yan Zhou

International Specialty Products, Wayne, NJ, USA

KEY WORDS: *polyelectrolyte complex, synergism, hair repair, split ends, phase behavior, complexity theory*

ABSTRACT: *Complexity theory is used here to explain the formation and properties of polyelectrolyte complexes, whereby organized structures built through self-association exhibit synergistic properties. These materials can create new compounds and offer new benefits, as shown by the present work in which a complex based on PVM/MA copolymer and polyquaternium-28 is used to treat damaged hair.*

A molecular complex is formed by the association of two or more molecules or ions. More specifically, a polyelectrolyte complex (PEC) is made up of differing macromolecules bound together by noncovalent bonds, which include primarily coulombic interactions.[1] PECs often are referred to in the patent and technical literature as polymer-polymer complexes, interpolyelectrolyte complexes, or complex coacervates; these terms all are based on the interaction of large macromolecules. Regarding the formation and application of PECs, the authors propose they instead be characterized by the term *complex system*, as defined by complexity theory.

In this paper, PECs will be described in some detail, including their basic chemistry and formation process. Also, a mechanism will be proposed to explain how a microgel cross-linking structure formed from a PEC consisting of the two polymers PVM/MA copolymer and polyquaternium-28 repairs damaged hair. The potential benefit of this PEC for hair treatments illustrates how this complex system can produce results beyond what could be predicted from the characteristics of its individual polymers. As defined by complexity theory, a complex system contains multiple parts that have local relationships to each other. From the interaction of these parts, a new property of behavior emerges that could not have been predicted from a study of its individual parts alone.[2]

Although some may view complexes as insoluble species that form when something goes awry during formulating or processing a formula, they do have a functionality that has been demonstrated in various industries. Some examples include microencapsulation, separation membranes, controlled and sustained release of drugs, flocculation of colloidal dispersions, bioadhesion and, less frequently, personal care.

The Chemistry Behind The Complex

Figure 1 shows the basic reaction in which mixing an anionic polyelectrolyte with a cationic polyelectrolyte produces a PEC. Magnifying one section shows the localized ionic interaction of the two oppositely charged macromolecules.[3] Complexes also can be based on hydrogen bonding and/or hydrophobic bonding through Van Der Waals forces acting between the hydrophobic grafted side chains on the molecule. Usually all three types of bonds are involved in the complex; however, the predominant bond is electrostatic. A typical PEC is based on a polyacrylic acid and a cationic polyelectrolyte consisting of multiple quaternary groups (see **Figure 2**).[4] Besides synthetic polymers, PECs also can be made from naturally derived polymers.[5]

The degree of interaction depends on the charge density of each polymer. For the cationic polyelectrolyte, this would be the level of cationic substitution; for the anionic polymer, the level of substitution with carboxylate groups and pH. Increasing the pH ionizes the anionic polymer so that a greater interaction with the cationic polymer is obtained.

Sometimes creating PECs can prove challenging; for example, if an incorrect order of addition is used to make a simple clear hair gel, a complex will form if a fixative resin like PVP is added to an unneutralized anionic polyacrylate gellant such as carbomer. In its acidic form, the polyacrylate donates a proton to the tertiary amine of the PVP. This will cause a differential charge in the two polymers, which is responsible for forming the complex. Therefore, to produce a clear, uniform system, it is recommended to add the neutralizer either first to the gellant, or to the fixative resin before adding the fixative resin to the gellant.

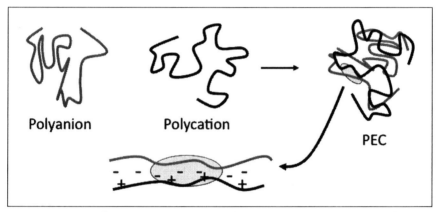

Figure 1. Schematic of the polyelectrolyte complex formation process; adapted from Reference 3

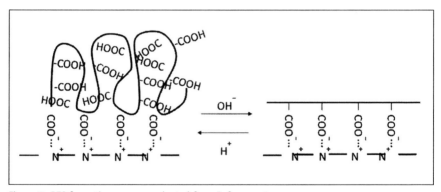

Figure 2. PEC formation process; adapted from Reference 4

The Complex Nature of PECs

There are several variables to consider when designing PECs, many of which can be controlled by the chemist, but there also are uncontrollable variables such as those found in typical synthesis reactions involving covalent bonds. There are three types of controllable independent variables: intrinsic polymer variables, formulation variables and processing variables. Intrinsic variables include polymer molecular weights, charge densities and distribution, and functional groups that provide a specific chemistry to the molecule. Formulation variables include solvent type, electrolyte content, weight ratios of the polymers, total polymer solids, and pH. Processing variables include order of addition, viscosity/concentration of pre-phases, rate of addition, mixing time/speed/type, and temperature. To determine the effect of these variables would take a multitude of experiments.

Consideration of this overabundance of variables leads to the realization that a world of opportunity exists not only for the number of PECs that can be made, but also for potential applications as yet undiscovered. Finding these correct polymer ratios through the production of phase diagrams would be tedious; fortunately, other experimental strategies can be utilized to help the discovery process.

Design of experiment: One strategy is Design of Experiment, commonly termed DoE. Here, a computer generates design points in the factor space. Regression analysis of the measured response variables produces a response surface. Phase regions can be identified and the region of maximum complexation can be predicted, which may dictate the optimal weight ratio of polymers to use.

Stoichiometry calculations: Another technique to reduce the number of experiments required is calculating the stoichiometry of charge neutralization. Maximum complexation usually occurs when anionic and cationic charges are equal on a molar basis. The weight ratio of the polymers can then be determined based on these stoichiometric calculations.

Combinatorial high-throughput methods: Although not employed here, a third possibility to increase the efficiency of experimentation is combinatorial methods for high-throughput techniques utilizing automated workstations. This type of equipment is currently being used to explore polymer-surfactant complexes, the study of which is providing an increased understanding of polymer molecular weight, charge density, electrolyte content and order of addition on coacervate formation.[6,7]

Uncontrollable Variables

Having a number of interacting variables does not make PECs complex from a complexity theory point of view. Their complexity lies in their uncontrollable variables. Small molecules tend to react in a random fashion. When the orientation and the threshold in the energy of activation are correct, new covalent bonds are formed. When polymers associate through electrostatic bonds, the process is also random. **Figure 3** illustrates the process.[8]

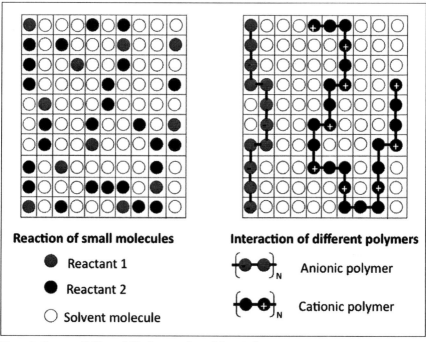

Figure 3. Uncontrollable variable factor; adapted from Reference 8

The reacting species in polymers, however, are tied to each other since they are part of the polymer chain. Due to the conformation of the polymer in solution, there is an incomplete reaction between polymers of unlike charge. Some parts of each chain remain unassociated. Dautzenberg designated this as the scrambled egg structure, as illustrated in **Figure 4**.[9] The complex formed between the two polymers, although it may have a net zero charge on a stoichiometric basis, may still have a residual charge on the surface based on the dangling parts of each of the unassociated chains.

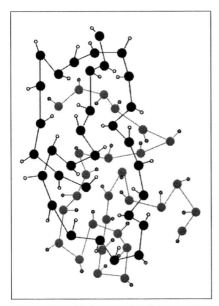

Figure 4. Scrambled egg model of the complex formation process; adapted from Reference 9

In the formation of polymer complexes, there is no way to hook one monomer with a cationic charge precisely with a specific monomer of another polymer with an anionic charge; interaction is completely governed by local interactions of the two types of polymers in a random fashion. This self-association illustrates one of the uncontrollable factors that make the system complex.

A Synergistic Effect

Another factor leading to the complexity of PECs is synergism. Granted, there are mixtures that are synergistic in behavior without forming a complex—for example, two discrete ingredients intimately mixed with a solvent to form a mixed solution. This can be represented as:

$$\text{Mixture: A + B = [A + B]} \quad \textbf{Eq. 1}$$

If a dependent response variable such as viscosity is higher than the additive effects of the two ingredients by themselves, then synergism has occurred. However, when two polymers join together to form a complex, the result is not just a mixture of two polymers, but the formation of a new species, which can be represented as:

$$\text{Synergy: A + B = C} \quad \textbf{Eq. 2}$$

R. B. Fuller defined this new species (C) as synergistic because its properties could not be predicted from its component parts. To illustrate synergy, Fuller cited the use of alloys to increase the tensile strength of metals. Combining chrome, nickel and steel alloys achieves a tensile strength of 350,000 pounds per square inch (psi). Yet the tensile strength of the individual components ranges from 60,000 to 80,000 psi. This significant disparity can be explained by the spatial arrangement of each of the individual types of atoms in space. This increased packing due to the arrangement of atoms provides for greater interatomic attractions and results in an increase in tensile strength. In this case, the behavior of the whole is unpredictable by the behavior of its parts.[10]

PVM/MA Copolymer and Polyquaternium-28

The factors necessary to make a system complex, namely self-association and synergism as defined by Fuller, can be exhibited by combining anionic and cationic polymers together. A complex is formed when the copolymer of methyl vinyl ether-maleic anhydride (INCI: PVM/MA Copolymer), the anionic portion of the complex, is combined at certain ratios with different types of cationic poly-electrolytes. Examples of the cationic polyelectrolytes explored include polyquaternium-7, -10, -28 and -55. Also, complexes have been made using the hydrophobically modified anionic polymer VP/acrylates/lauryl methacrylate copolymer, in order to interact with the polymers containing the cationic quaternary group.[11]

The complexation of many other polymers can be envisioned based on the disparity of charge between two or more polymers. The complex described in the present paper for hair mending benefits is formed between PVM/MA copolymer and polyquaternium-28. Their structures are represented in **Figure 5**. PVM/MA copolymer acts as the anionic component containing the ionizable carboxylate groups, and polyquaternium-28 is the cationic component containing multiple quaternized nitrogens.

Figure 6 shows a phase diagram constructed to determine the region of maximum complexation[a]. The phase diagram was constructed by combining various weight ratios of the two polymers together keeping various formulation variables constant. The response surface was built by quantifying the macroscopic character of the combination of the two polymers on a weight basis; see **Figure 6** legend for a description of each of the phase regions. The area desig-nated as "1" represents the weight ratios where the resultant products exhibited a milky appearance. This was initially judged from a macroscopic point of view as the region of maximum complexation.

---

[a] Design Expert 6, used here, is a product of Stat-Ease Inc., Minneapolis, Minn., USA. (2003)

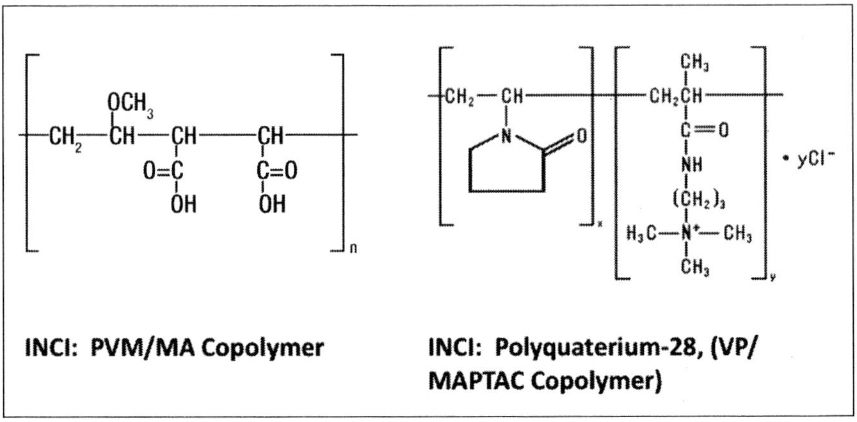

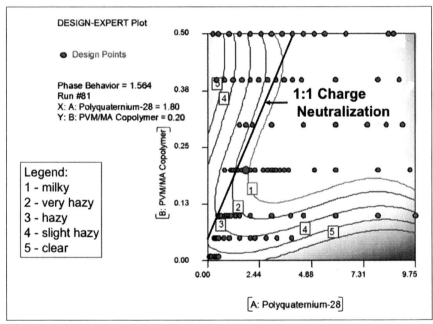

Figure 5. Structure of component polymers of tested complex

INCI: PVM/MA Copolymer

INCI: Polyquaterium-28, (VP/ MAPTAC Copolymer)

Figure 6. Phase diagram of PVM/MA copolymer and polyquaternium-28 constructed from different weight ratios of the two polymers

The controllable variables in making each of the formulations for this phase diagram included such things as polymer-weight ratios, order of addition, temperature, solvent type, and pH of the PVM/ MA copolymer, which controls the level of anionic charge of this polymer. However, it is when the uncontrollable variables are considered that complexity is revealed. These uncontrollable variables are responsible for the self-association of the two polymers into polyelectrolyte complexes. The nature of these self-associating species is shown upon closer analysis. This was accomplished through optical microscopy and measuring the viscosity of the mixtures of the two polymers. These techniques proved to be more revealing of the nature of the PEC system compared to simply observing the macroscopic character of their solutions.

Viscosities were measured on a series of combinations of poly-quaternium-28 and PVM/MA copolymer, keeping the PVM/MA copolymer constant at 0.20%. Viscosity was then plotted against the molar ratio of the reacting species of each polymer. As **Figure 7** shows, there was a trend found in the unit mole ratio of the two polymers with viscosity, as portrayed by the concave response curve. Stoichiometric calculations further revealed that this minimal level was the result of a one-to-one charge neutralization ratio of each of the polymers identifying the point of maximum complexation. On either side of this ratio, an excess of uncomplexed polyanion or polycation was responsible for increasing solution viscosity. This property has been reported in other systems as typical of PECs.[12] The 1:1 charge neutralization line is drawn in **Figure 6** to show other polymer concentrations, which theoretically shows the points of minimum viscosity and maximum complexation.

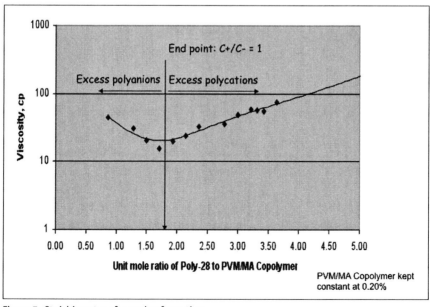

Figure 7. Stoichiometry of complex formation

The systems produced to build the phase diagram of **Figure 6,** when observed microscopically, except for the clear systems, contained small dispersed particles, or microgels. The morphology of these microgels, illustrated in **Figure 8**, is characterized as translucent, odd-shaped, free-flowing particles with an average measured particle size of 5 to 10 microns. The microgel structure explains why systems that have a 1:1 charge neutralization produce a low-viscosity response: this is the condition for maximum complex formation. These microgel particles are not produced by any variable controlled by the researcher, but result from the way that the polyelectrolytes self-assemble. The microgels produced from PVM/ MA copolymer and polyquaternium-28 result in properties that exemplify their synergistic behavior, again that cannot be fully explained by considering its component parts.

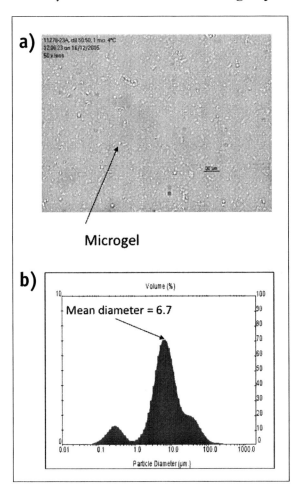

Figure 8. a) Optical microscope image of microgel structure; b) particle size distribution of microgels in water

From Synergy to Split Ends

Concurrent to exploring the nature of PECs, research efforts were under way to design a test method to identify an ingredient or composition to repair damaged hair. These efforts tested the efficacy of a leave-in treatment product to mend the split ends that form during aggressive hair styling processes such as brushing and blow drying.[13] The method consisted of evaluating split-end fibers under a stereomicroscope to assess the degree of mending, then confirming via scanning electron microscopy (SEM).

The procedure included tagging the split-end fibers at their root end in a tress, which allows their assessment during the different steps of the experimental protocol. Durability of the mend can be assessed in a realistic fashion since the treated fibers are part of the tress. In this case, durability is tested by shear forces induced by combing. The mending as well as cuticular smoothing is also observed at higher resolution by SEM, as shown in **Figure 9**.

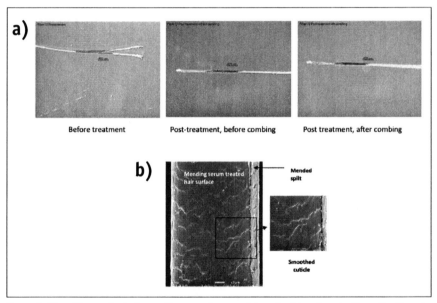

Figure 9. The efficacy of a hair mending complex was determined by a) evaluation of split-end fibers under a stereomicroscope, and b) confirmation via SEM.

If a complex were to be considered as efficacious for hair mending, it was conjectured that it would be in the region of maximum complexation, as judged from the character of the composition. This was shown by testing a complex in the region designated as "1" in **Figure 6** and achieving positive results. The exact composition tested is shown with the largest dot in that region.

This result initiated a flurry of activity to investigate the nature of these microgels and their ability to mend damaged hair. The series of experiments revealed that the highest efficacy was found when the polymers were complexed such that their charge neutralization was at a 1:1 ratio of anionic to cationic charge. Complexes formed at charge neutralization ratios deviating from this, as well as testing the polymers alone, had lower efficacy; the 1:1 charge neutralization line is depicted in **Figure 6**.

These microgels represent a new species of material even though they are not formed through the breaking and making of covalent bonds; that is, without the use of chemical transformation. The proposed mechanism consists of their ability to form cross-linking structures that bind and mend the broken subassemblies of the fibers.

The first step begins with the interaction of the microgels with the damaged components of the hair fiber through adhesive ionic interactions. During application, the microgels infiltrate the subassemblies of the broken fiber and form cross-linking structures to bind these components together. During drying, the microgels contract, pulling the subassemblies together as well as sealing the cuticle, thus helping to increase mending durability. The mechanism is illustrated in **Figure 10**. The mend based on PVM/MA copolymer and polyquaternium-28 is semi-permanent in nature in that reapplication is necessary after shampooing.

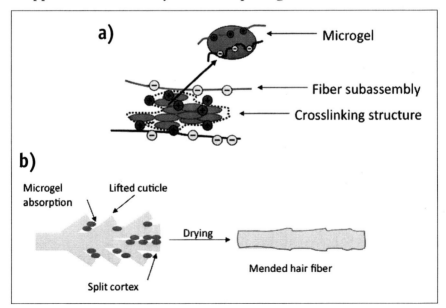

Figure 10. Proposed mechanism of hair repair with PEC cross-linking structure of microgels: a) microgels attach to subassemblies of the fiber through cationic bridging and adhesion; and b) microgels infiltrate subassemblies of the fiber and bind them together during drying.

Besides hair mending, there are many examples of complexes formed between two polymers having properties that are not apparent simply by considering the mere blending of their component parts. The interest in PECs is evident from the extent of the references available in patent and technical literature. Although applications are not prevalent in the personal care industry, examples exist, such as rheological effects for suspensions applied in surfactant-free formulations,[14, 15] moisture delivery,[16] and facial-wrinkle masking.[17]

Conclusion

Complexity theory teaches that viewing systems as a whole and not just as simple mixtures of their component parts will provide researchers with a new paradigm for scientific inquiry.[18, 19] Considering all the factors in the formation of PECs, and the fact that their resultant novel application properties cannot be predicted by the properties of their component parts alone, the case can be made that PECs are indeed complex systems. A good example of an emergent property of this system is the complex formed between PVM/MA copolymer and polyquaternium-28, which can be used in a treatment product for mending damaged hair. Numerous examples of PECs containing synergistic properties abound in many industries, which hopefully will encourage chemists to consider them as another avenue in the discovery of new compounds to achieve new performance benefits.

Published March 2009 *Cosmetics and Toiletries* magazine

References

1. H Dautzenberg et al, Structure formation in polyelectrolyte systems, ch 6 in *Polelectrolytes—Formation, Characterization and Application*, Cincinnati, OH: Hanser Publishers (1994)
2. Complex Systems, *Science* 284 (Apr 2, 1999)
3. N Karibyants et al, Characterization of PSS/PDADMAC-co-AA polyelectrolyte complexes and their stoichiometry using analytical ultracentrifugation, *Macromolecules* 30 7803–7809 (1997)
4. E Tsuchida et al, Formation of polyion complexes between polycarboxylic acids and polycations carrying charges in the chain backbone, *Die Makromolekulare Chemie* 175 583–592 (1974)
5. FM Goycoolea et al, Stoichiometry and conformation of xanthan in synergistic gelation with locust bean gum or konjac glucomannan: Evidence for heterotypic binding, *Macromolecules* 28(24) (1995)

6. RY Lochhead et al, Deposition from conditioning shampoo: Optimizing coacervate formation, *Cosm &Toil* 121(3) (Mar 2006)

7. RY Lochhead and LR Huisinga, Revolutionary trends in the advancement and integration of cosmetic science: Combinatorial formulation, *IFSCC* 10(3) (2007)

8. FM Winnick, Elements of polymer science, in *Principles of Polymer Science and Technology in Cosmetics and Personal Care*, ED Goddard and JV Gruber, eds, Boca Raton, FL: Marcel Dekker Inc. (1999)

9. H Dautzenberg, Polyelectrolyte complex formation in highly aggregating systems: Methodical aspects and general tendencies, ch 20 in *Physical Chemistry of Polyelectrolytes*, v 99, Surfactant Science Series

10. RB Fuller, *Synergetics, Explorations in the Geometry of Thinking*, New York: Macmillan Publishing Co., Inc. (1975)

11. US Patent 2006/0251603 A1, R Rigoletto and Y Zhou (Nov 9, 2006)

12. F Bian and M Liu, Complexation between poly(N,N-diethylacrylamide) and poly (acrylic acid) in aqueous solution, *European Polymer Journal* 39 1867–1874 (2003)

13. R Rigoletto et al, Semi-permanent split end mending with a polyelectrolyte complex, *J Cosmet Sci* 58 451–476 (Jul/Aug 2007)

14. JV Gruber and PN Konish, Aqueous viscosity enhancement through helical inclusion complex cross-linking of a hydrophobically modified, water-soluble, cationic cellulose ether by amylose, *Macromolecules* 30(18) 5361–5366 (1997)

15. PN Konish and JV Gruber, Surfactant-free formulations employing a synergistic complex between a hydrophobically modified, cationic cellulose ether and amylase, *J Cosmet Sci* 49 335–342 (Sept/Oct 1998)

16. US Patent 4,767,463, GL Brode et al (Aug 30, 1988)

17. JP Pavlichko, Polymer interactions to enhance the function of hyaluronic acid, *Drug & Cosmetic Industry* (Sept 1990)

18. F Heylighen, Complexity and self-organization, *Encyclopedia of Library and Information Sciences*, MJ Bates and MN Maack, eds, London, UK: Taylor and Francis (2008)

19. M Mitchell Waldrop, *Complexity—The Emerging Science at the Edge of Order and Chaos*, New York: Simon and Schuster (1992)

CHAPTER 39

Natural Preservation from Concepts in Nature

Fernando Ibarra, PhD

Dr. Straetmans GmbH, Hamburg, Germany

Christopher H. Johnson

Kinetik Technologies Inc., Hazlet, New Jersey, USA

KEY WORDS: *preservation, natural antimicrobials, organic acids, glyceryl monoesters*

ABSTRACT: *Chemical defense mechanisms used in the plant kingdom are the basis of natural antimicrobials with multifunctionality for preservation of cosmetic formulations. Two examples are organic acids and glyceryl monoesters.*

Nature demonstrates various protective strategies in the animal and plant kingdom. At the macroscopic scale, mobility (i.e., the ability to run) is the first and most obvious example, but slow or immobile creatures have evolved other fascinating ways to protect themselves. Chemical strategies can play an important role in this context. Strong odors and bright colors are often employed to point out that an attack may bring more harm to the aggressor than to the prey. This strategy depends on the large variety of naturally toxic materials produced by animals and plants in their "natural laboratories" in which some of the world's most effective poisons are developed. **Figure 1** gives the structures of some exemplary natural poisons.

Somewhat more hidden and therefore less known are the activities in the microscopic world. The strategy for chemical defense against microorganisms will normally differ from that against larger invaders due, in part, to differences in the metabolism. While large alkaloids

or polypeptides may successfully harm animals, it is sometimes small
and simple molecules that are effective against bacteria or fungi.
Chemical defense against microbes is normally found in plants
or other competing microorganisms, while animals rely on their
biological immune response.

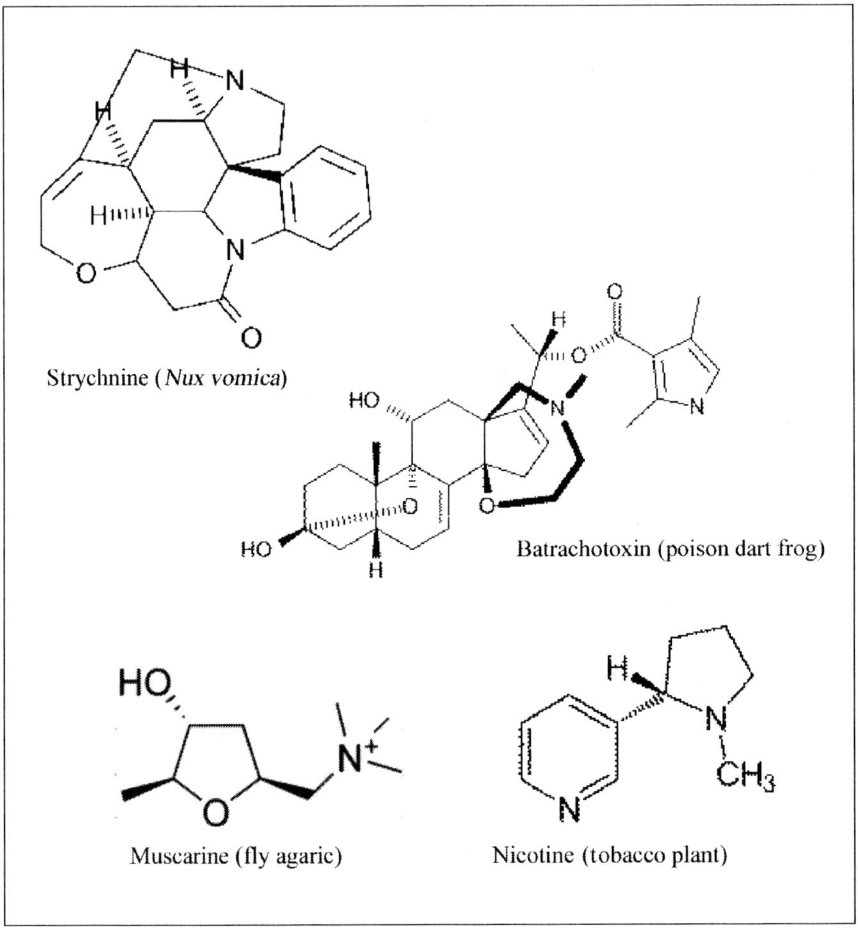

Figure 1. Structures of some exemplary naturally occurring poisons

The following discussion will focus solely on the chemical
defenses against microorganisms. It will define some general principles that can be exploited to determine metabolic weaknesses for
the control of target organisms. It also will point out how natural
systems protect themselvesi.e., which chemical compounds are best
against the permanent pressures of harmful microbes. Finally, it will

demonstrate the concepts that currently are available to the industry to achieve natural and sustainable—yet efficient—preservation of cosmetic products.

Throughout this discussion, the term *natural* is used to describe preservatives and will have a meaning as clarified by the relevant European certification bodies—BDIH (the Federation of German Industries and Trading), EcoCert (France) and the Organic Soil Association (UK) (see **Petrochemical Preservatives and the Term** *Natural*).

Petrochemical Preservatives and The Term *Natural*

There is no official legal definition of the term *natural* as it applies to cosmetic ingredients in the United States or Europe. However, Ecocert, BDIH and the Soil Association agree that the term implies restricted use of petrochemical-derived ingredients, silicones, ethoxylated raw materials and halogenorganic compounds.

In regard to preservation, some exemptions are allowed in the general rule to ban petrochemical-based raw materials. Benzoic acid, sorbic acid and benzyl alcohol may be used as preservatives in certified natural cosmetic products. In addition, salicylic acid (Ecocert, BDIH), propionic acid, formic acid (Ecocert) and phenoxyethanol (Soil Association) are permitted as additional petrochemical preservatives. In most cases, certified natural cosmetic products utilizing those preservatives must carry the information "preserved with ... " on the package.

It is of course permitted to use alternative multifunctional antimicrobial actives to avoid the "preserved with ... " statement on the package. For example, antimicrobial actives that also have activity for fragrance, refatting or moisturizing can be listed on the package under their alternative function. Those ingredients still have to comply with the general requirements of the *natural* standards in terms of the source and manufacturing method of the raw material. Therefore only materials extracted from nature with permitted solvents/methods or raw materials assembled from natural building blocks by accepted chemical conversionse.g., hydrolysis, condensation (esterification), hydration, oxidation and fermentationare suitable. Petrochemical-derived antimicrobials, e.g., glycols and ethylhexylglycerine, are not an option for certified natural cosmetic products.

These definitions have no legal character. The above-mentioned organizations have created them as a self-imposed commitment for those companies that want to be granted the respective label. The compliance of raw materials and cosmetics with the criteria is thoroughly assessed by authorized certification bodies.

Natural Strategies Against Microorganisms

With the discovery of penicillin in 1928, the Scottish biologist Alexander Fleming identified one of the most prominent examples of a potent biologically active agent. This historic event has served as the foundation from which to consider different concepts in the control of microorganisms. Penicillin is an antibiotic agent and must be distinguished from active compounds for use in preservation or disinfection. The major difference is the selectivity against the target organism and as a result thereof, the possibility for the bacteria to build up a resistance. Because of their selectivity, antibiotics can be used within the human body to fight bacteria.

Active compounds for preservation are not selective, nor should they be. Ideally their mission is to fight all microbes present—bacteria, yeasts and fungi.

The desired antimicrobial effect is directed by some general principles:

- denaturization of membrane proteins and enzymes (alcohols);
- chemical alteration of enzymes and DNA (aldehydes);
- oxidation of membrane proteins and enzymes (ozone, H_2O_2, halogen compounds);
- disturbance of membrane function (organic acids); and
- disruption of the cell membrane (surfactants, alcohols).

Plants, animals and microorganisms employ these principles and produce the respective compounds to combat microbes. Often, mixtures or synergistic systems are in place to fight the imminent invasion.

Phytoalexins are antimicrobial phytochemicals produced by plants under attack by bacteria and fungi. Numerous phytoalexins have been identified, including hydrogen peroxide, terpenoids, aromatic acids, oxygenated fatty acids, aliphatic alcohols and polyols. Many of these compounds are not suitable for use in cosmetics. Therefore, the question remains: *Can natural systems be used to gently, safely and effectively preserve cosmetics?*

Among the decisive criteria for the use of natural preservative concepts in cosmetics are the availability, effectiveness and the toxicological profile of the actives. Another factor to consider is whether the conversion of naturally occurring building blocks offers a possibility to produce either nature-identical compounds or even more effective analogues thereof. Here is where a thorough understanding of natural concepts becomes decisive for the development of active agents that are new and potent, yet mild and sustainable.

The consumer's perception that natural raw materials are often better tolerated than non-naturally occurring ones in cosmetic applications follows a simple, comprehendible philosophy: the human organism is the product of an evolutionary process lasting millions of years. As is true for all other creatures on earth, human metabolism has adapted to the surrounding chemical environment. As a consequence it is concluded by many consumers that the human body is far more adapted to cope with naturally occurring compounds than with synthetic ones. For example, although both mineral oils and oils of plant origin may be excellent sources of energy if burned, the human body is able to metabolize only oils of plant origin.[1,2]

This philosophy about the link between human metabolism and the chemical environment is the basis for the trend for *natural* cosmetics, but for preserving agents it has to be judged very carefully. It would be misleading or even dangerous to assume that antimicrobials from nature are free from any risks to the consumers. Because an intrinsic property of antimicrobial structures is that they can affect living cells, the toxicological evaluation of antimicrobial substances from nature has to be as thorough as for synthetic ones. However, there is little dispute that raw materials from natural origin have significant benefits over synthetic materials with respect to their impact on the environment and the maintenance of resources.

Identifying preserving agents derived from nature is a complex task. Efficacy and safety have to be the first priority because microbiological contamination of cosmetic products can pose substantial threat to the consumer's health. It is the art of the researcher to identify adequate structures in nature or build them from natural building blocks.

The same may be true for cosmetic applications: although both synthetic and naturally occurring ingredients may have an excellent cosmetic performance, the synthetic ones often exhibiting a better performancethe skin will more easily deal with naturally occurring compounds than with synthetic compounds that cannot be degraded or built into biological structures. Although the biochemical inertness of mineral oils is well known and most of these compounds will not enter the human metabolism, the intake and accumulation of hydrocarbons are regarded as undesirable.[1,2] Natural oil components that are identical to the constituents of human cell membranes can be integrated into living cells. Mineral oils, although having a cosmetic function, preferably will be washed away with the next shower.

For the illustration of antimicrobial actives for natural preservation, two examples from organic acids and glyceryl monoesters will show how these concepts apply to cosmetic formulations.

Organic Acids

The widely accepted principle of antimicrobial action of organic acids is illustrated in **Figure 2** and explained here. The cell incorporates molecules of the protonated acid through the membrane. Within the cell plasma the acid dissociates and thus changes the pH within the cell.[3] The bacterium has to pump out protons permanently and take in sodium ions to maintain the physiological pH of the cell. This energy-consuming process as well as the decreased pH level inside the cell will lead to a decreased rate of reproduction. Because it also lowers the pH outside the cell to a favorable acidic level, the cell makes things worse by favoring the protonated acid side of the acid-base-equilibrium, enabling the membrane to be penetrated by the protonated acid, which is the active species. Finally the process will end with the death of the microorganism.

The nature of the acid is of utmost importance to end up with an efficient active compound. The right compound will be one that ensures biological availability, penetrates the cell membrane and deprotonates within the cell.

If suitable organic acids are available in sufficient amount they will effectively control the growth of microbes in the product. The chosen active compounds should have the following properties:

- Sufficient solubility in the water phase;
- Availability in the protonated form at a given pH in a formulation;

- A structure that permits passage through the membrane; and
- Ready dissociation of the acid within the cell plasma.

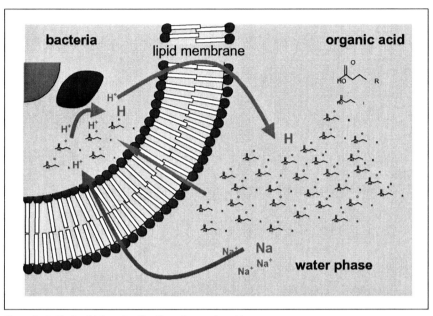

Figure 2. Antimicrobial mode of action of organic acids

For use in self-preserving formulations or in cosmetics making *natural* claims, there are various compounds, also found in nature, that are in accordance with the requirements of the BDIH, EcoCert and the Organic Soil Association. One commercial product line[a] of multifunctional additives has, alone or in combination with others, a demonstrated performance against bacteria, yeast and fungi.[4] Among the active species within this product line are levulinic acid and anisic acid, which are well-known for their antimicrobial activity and are found in many natural sources.[5,6] According to their primary function as very light perfumes they are declared as "fragrance (*parfum*)" on the ingredients list shown in **Formula 1,** an exemplary formulation with biological stabilization by organic acids. The function of the glyceryl caprylate, the only other ingredient with an antimicrobial function in **Formula 1,** will be described next.

---

[a] Dermosoft is a product line and registered trade name of Dr. Straetmans Chemische Produkte GmbH, Germany.

Figure 3 shows the results of a challenge test on **Formula 1** conducted according to the European Pharmacopoeia (EP). The EP's criteria regarding the death rate are somewhat stricter than those of the US Pharmacopoeia and the Personal Care Products Council (formerly the Cosmetic, Toiletry, and Fragrance Association).[7]

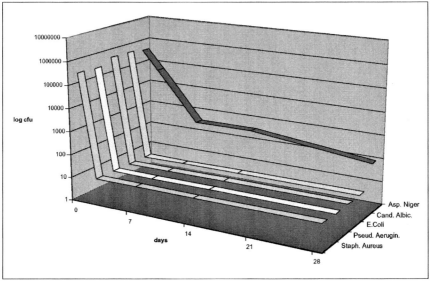

Figure 3. Results of challenge test on the moisture cream in Formula 1. Preservation is based solely on glyceryl caprylate, anisic acid and levulinic acid.

Glyceryl Monoesters

A different mode of action is found in another prominent group of multifunctional molecules, the glyceryl monoesters. Some of these multifunctional surfactants have amphiphilic properties and an excellent microbiological performance. The design of the molecules is optimized to bring them into the cell membrane of microbes and destabilize that membrane because of the presence of an incompatible structure such as an incompatible chain length (**Figure 4**).[8,9]

The key is to find molecules with suitable structures.[10] In addition, the molecules must be soluble and therefore available in the water phase or in the interface between water and oil, and they must be able to penetrate the outer layer of the membrane. Once there, the molecules will deteriorate the stability of the membrane and finally disrupt it completely.[11] To enhance the activity against fungi, a faster-acting agent like certain organic acids can be added.

Formula 1. Moisture cream preserved with organic acids

A. Water (*aqua*)	73.30% w/w
Sodium phytate and water (*aqua*) (Dermofeel PA-3, Dr. Straetmans)	0.10
Glycerin	3.00
Glyceryl caprylate (Dermosoft GMCY, Dr. Straetmans)	0.50
Fragrance (*parfum*) (Dermosoft 700 B, Dr. Straetmans)	0.30
Fragrance (*parfum*) (Dermosoft 688, Dr. Straetmans)	0.20
Sodium hydroxide, 10%	0.75
B. Xanthan gum (Keltrol RD, Kelco)	0.20
Galactoarabinan (Lara Care, Rahn)	0.50
C. Glyceryl stearate citrate (Dermofeel GSC, Dr. Straetmans)	3.50
Decyl cocoate (Tegosoft DC, Goldschmidt)	3.00
Olea europaea (olive) fruit oil	2.00
Squalane (Phytosqualan, NRC/Sophim)	6.00
Cetearyl alcohol (Lanette O, Cognis)	2.00
Caprylic/capric triglyceride (Miglyol 812, Sasol)	4.00
Tocopherol (and) *Helianthus annuus* (sunflower) seed oil	
(Dermofeel Toco 70 non-GMO, Dr. Straetmans)	0.15
D. Fragrance (*parfum*) (Parfum Baby Cotton 449264, Symrise)	0.20
	100.00

Procedure: Heat A and B to 78°C. Disperse B in A. Heat C to 78°C. Emulsify C to AB under stirring. Homogenize for 1–2 min using a homogenizer-disperser. Start to cool to 30°C under stirring. Add D and adjust pH. *Specification values:* Appearance: Soft white emulsion; pH: 5.0–5.4; Viscosity (Brookfield: Helipath TF; Speed 10):

~ 40,000 mPas; Centrifuge (15 min, 4000 rpm): No separation; *Stability:* More than 3 months stable at 20°C, 40°C, 4°C; *Microbiological stability:* Proven.

The primary function of these glyceryl monoesters is moisturizing and refatting of the skin. To avoid the need for altering an existing basic formulation, the formulator and the supplier should discuss the additional functions of these raw materials and their possible impact on the formulation.

Formulations for cosmetics making *natural* claims can be preserved effectively with glyceryl monoesters. As long as they are produced from naturally occurring, sustainable sources, they are in accordance with the requirements of the relevant European certification bodies (BDIH, EcoCert and Organic Soil Association).

These active compounds are not declared as preservatives due to their primary function as moisturizing and refatting agents. With optimum activity is in the pH range of 4.5 to 7, the field of application is very broad. **Formula 2** shows a body spray with biological stabilization using glycerol monoesters as the only antimicrobial agent for preservation in the formula. **Figure 5** shows the results of a challenge test on this formulation.

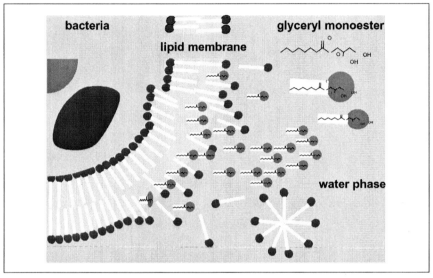

Figure 4. Disruption of the cell membrane of a bacterium by the action of glyceryl monoesters. The stability of the membrane is corrupted by the incompatible chain length and finally destroyed.

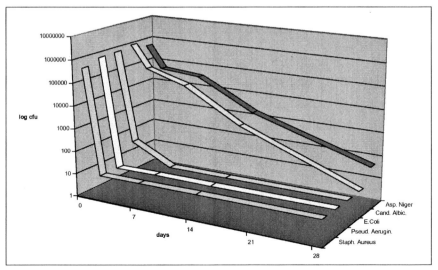

Figure 5. Results of challenge test on the body spray in Formula 2. Preservation is based solely on glyceryl caprylate.

Formula 2. Body spray preserved with glyceryl monoesters

A. Water (*aqua*)	80.05% w/w
Rosa centifolia flower water (Rose Flower Water, Sanoflore)	3.00
Glycerin	3.00
Glyceryl caprylate (Dermosoft GMCY, Dr. Straetmans)	1.00
B. Sclerotium gum (Amigel Granulat, Alban Muller)	0.25
C. Tocopheryl acetate (and) *Helianthus annuus* (sunflower) seed oil	
(Dermofeel E 74 A non-GMO, Dr. Straetmans)	0.50
Prunus armeniaca (apricot) kernel oil	
(Apricot Kernel Oil, Henry Lamotte)	1.00
Tricaprylin (Dermofeel MCT, Dr. Straetmans)	4.00
Lecithin (and) glycerin (and) alcohol (Pro-Lipo Duo, Lucas Meyer)	7.00
Fragrance (*parfum*) (Parfum Baby Cotton 449264, Symrise)	<u>0.20</u>
	100.00

Procedures: Mix A and B under stirring until B dissolves. Mix C at RT and add to AB while stirring. Homogenize ABC at medium speed for ~3 min using a homogenizer-disperser. Adjust pH if necessary. *Specification Values:* Appearance: Creamy sprayable lotion; pH: 5.5–6.5; Viscosity (Brookfield: LV 4; 10 rpm): ~ 2,000–3,000 mPas; Centrifugation (4000 rpm, 20 min): No separation; *Microbiological stability:* Proven.

Evaluation of Preservatives

For the formulator it is sometimes difficult to determine which preservative system will work best. There are dozens of antimicrobial actives and hundreds of commercial products. There are single compounds and more or less complex blends. The formulator should select from among the ones that are efficient antimicrobials, toxicologically unobjectionable and accepted by consumers.

If certain traditional preservatives cannot be used, there are many alternative and natural antimicrobial compounds. A closer look into microbiological data and challenge tests will reveal the usefulness or unreliability of alternative preservatives. The evaluation and comparison of, for example, MIC data can only be a first and rather unreliable step, because this generalized approach takes into account neither the influence of the various raw materials present in a formulation nor chemo-physical hurdles such as solubility and migration of preservatives into the oil phase. The MIC values of some exemplary traditional products are compared to a multifunctional microbial agent in **Table 1**. Even after studying the MIC or other generalized data, the formulator still must test the preservative system in the targeted cosmetic formulation.

Table 1. Comparison of MIC values of different commercial products. All data is taken from technical information provided by the manufacturers.

Preservative	P. aeruginusa	S. aureus	A. niger
Glyceryl caprylate (Dermosoft GMCY, Dr. Straetmans)	0.05%	0.03%	0.1%
Methylparaben (Nipagin M, Clariant/Nipa)	0.2	0.15	0.1
Phenoxyethanol (and) methylparaben (and) ethylparaben (and) butylparaben (and) propylparaben (and) isobutylparaben (Phenonip, Clariant/Nipa)	0.225	0.2	0.125
Benzyl alcohol (and) methylchloroisothiazolinone (and) methylthiazolinone (Euxyl K 100, Schülke & Mayr)	0.06	0.25	0.03
Methyldibromo glutaronitrile (Euxyl K 135, Schülke & Mayr)	0.5	0.13	0.25

Summary

To meet the growing demand for alternative preservation concepts in cosmetic products making "natural" claims, there is a broad range of active compounds already available to the cosmetic industry. Examples from among organic acids and glyceryl monoesters were described here.

Due to the compounds' primary properties there is no need to declare them as preservatives, although results of microbiological testing indicate that they provide excellent biological stability. They also allow for a new set of benefits and marketing claims, such as "reduced allergenic load" and "ingredients from sustainable resources." Indeed, it is difficult to ignore the fact that certain preservatives have suffered from bad press, and more and more cosmetic manufacturers are introducing alternative and natural preservatives in their formulations.[12]

Natural, sustainable and efficient preservation of cosmetic products can be achieved from the chemical defense mechanisms of nature.

Published March 2008 *Cosmetics and Toiletries* magazine

References

1. *Seventeenth Report of the Joint FAO/WHO Expert Committee on Food Additives*, World Health Organization Technical Report Series, No 539 (1974)
2. FAO Nutrition Meetings Report Series, No 53 (1974)
3. JJ Kabara, Fatty acids and esters as multifunctional components, In *Preservative-Free and Self-Preserving Cosmetics and Drugs*, JJ Kabara and DS Orth, eds, New York: Marcel Dekker (1997) p 131
4. JC Meng et al, New antimicrobial mono- and sesquiterpenes from *Soroseris hookeriana* subsp *Erysimoides, Planta Med* 66 541–544 (2000)
5. AC Dweck, Natural preservatives, *Cosmet Toil* 118(8) 45–50 (2003)
6. AC Dweck, An update on natural preservatives, *Personal Care* 6(4) 11–15 (2005)
7. DS Orth and DC Steinberg, The safety factor in preservative efficacy testing, *Cosmet Toil* 118(4) 51–58 (2003)
8. G Bergsson et al, In vitro inactivation of *Chlamydia trachomatis* by fatty acids and monoglycerides, *Antimicrob Agents Chemother* 42 2290–2294 (1998)
9. DS Orth and JJ Kabara, Preservative-free and self-preserving cosmetics and drugs, *Cosmet Toil* 113(4) 51–58 (1998)
10. D Smith and W Petersen, The self-preserving challenge, *Cosmet Toil* 115(5) 67–74 (2000)
11. O Cozzoli, The role of surfactants in self-preserving cosmetic formulas, In *Preservative-free and Self-preserving Cosmetics and Drugs*, JJ Kabara and DS Orth, eds, New York: Marcel Dekker (1997) pp 110–111
12. J Woodruff, Getting the balance right, SPC (9) 51–54 (2006)

CHAPTER 40

Antibacterial and Anti-inflammatory Effects of a Magnolia Extract

Jongsung Lee, Eunsun Jung, Sungran Hur and Deokhoon Park
Biospectrum Life Science Institute, Gyunggi-do, Korea

Anthony Ansaldi and Roy Heckl
DKSH North America Inc., Baltimore, USA

KEY WORDS: *magnolia, antibacterial, P. acnes, anti-inflammatory, antimicrobial, irritation, acne*

ABSTRACT: P. acnes *can exacerbate acne as a result of the inflammatory properties of the cell wall short chain fatty acids and chemotactic factors. Here, researchers investigate the effectiveness of a magnolia extract as an acne treatment, based on the known anti-inflammatory and antimicrobial effects from magnolol and honokiol within the material.*

Acne, an inflammatory disease of the sebaceous glands, is a common skin disease that induces inflammation at the skin surface of the face, neck, chest or back. Adolescents and young adults are most often afflicted, with estimates of 85–100% of 12- to 24-year-olds being affected, at least intermittently, during those years.[1]

The likelihood of developing acne is greatest during adolescence because hormone levels become elevated. Elevated hormones stimulate the sebaceous glands, which are attached to hair follicles, to produce greater amounts of sebum. An acne lesion such as a whitehead, blackhead or pimple occurs when a hair follicle becomes plugged with the sebum and dead cells. The etiology of acne lies in a confluence of several factors, including: hormonal imbalance, bacterial infection, stress, diet and the application of cosmetic products.

Propionibacterium acnes (P. acnes), one of the major organisms isolated from the skin's surface,[2] specifically induces an inflammation in the sebaceous glands or hair pores.[3] *P. acnes* secretes lipase and degrades sebum oils into free fatty acids (FFA), which are potent acne stimuli. FFA are major irritative components of skin surface lipids. Intracutaneous injection of small amounts of FFA, as compared with other surface lipids, produces a marked inflammatory response.[4]

P. acnes irritates the hair follicle and forms blackhead-inducing inflammation.[5] These bacteria also secrete leukocyte chemotatic factors, infiltrating leukocytes in the hair follicle; in turn, these leukocytes stimulate and destroy the hair follicle wall. Subsequently, the contents of the hair follicle flow into the dermis.[6] While it does not actually cause the acne, *P. acnes* exacerbates the condition as a result of the inflammatory properties of the cell wall (lipoteichoic acid), short chain fatty acids and chemotactic factors. Therefore, *P. acnes* is considered to play an important role in acne development.

As therapeutic agents for acne, antimicrobials are usually employed to inhibit inflammation or kill the bacteria.[7] Examples include triclosan, benzoyl peroxide, azelaic acid, retinoid, tetracycline, erythromycin, macrolide, and clindamycin.[8] However, these antibiotics have been known to induce side effects.

Benzoyl peroxide and retinoid bring about dry skin and skin irritation if they are used excessively;[9] several reports also suggest that in the case of tetracycline, erythromycin, macrolide and clindamycin, side effects include the appearance of resistant bacteria, organ damage and immunohypersensitivity—if they have been taken for a long time.[10,11]

In addition, triclosan is converted into an environmental hormone when exposed to light, inducing severe environmental pollution. Latch et al. reported that triclosan rapidly photodegrades by direct photolysis and both 2,8-dichlorodibenzo-p-dioxin (2,8-DCDD) and 2,4-dichlorophenol (2,4-DCP) are produced.[12] Dioxin can be highly carcinogenic and can cause health problems as severe as weakening of the immune system, decreased fertility, altered sex hormones, miscarriage, birth defects, and cancer.[13] Therefore, many researchers have sought to develop therapeutic agents for acne that have no side effects yet have high antibacterial activity.[14–17]

In Oriental medicine practices in Korea, China and Japan, the stem bark of magnolia has been used as treatments for cough, diarrhea and allergic rhinitis. Several recent reports have indicated that magnolol and honokiol, major components of the stem bark of magnolia[a], function medicinally as anxiolytic agents and anti-inflammatories;[7, 14, 18, 19] they have been shown to inhibit skin tumor promotion[18, 20] and, in addition, have exhibited high antimicrobial activity against microorganisms such as: *Escherichia coli, Pseudomonas aeruginosa, Trichophyton mentagrophytes, Porphyromonas gingivalis, Epidermophyton floccosum, Aspergillus niger, Cryptococcus neoformans* and *Candida albicans*.[21–24]

Thus, based on the known anti-inflammatory and antimicrobial effects of magnolol and honokiol, components of magnolia stem bark, the effectiveness of magnolia extract as an acne treatment was investigated. The following discussion demonstrates the material's effects against acne-inducing bacteria, as well as examines its potential for irritation in a human skin model. Results suggest the extract may be employed as an effective agent to ameliorate acne.

Magnolia Extract

Magnolia extract obtained from the stem bark of the magnolia tree is a natural extract that has been developed and proven effective against *Propionibacterium sp*. As noted, the active compounds are magnolol and honokiol (see **Figure 1**).

The chemical structure of magnolol and honokiol consists of a biphenyl skeleton with phenolic and allylic functionalities. The chemical structure of magnolol is an ortho, ortho-C–C dimer of 4-allyl-phenol that consists of a biphenyl skeleton with phenolic functionalities and two p-allyl groups as side chains. The structure of honokiol consists of para-allyl-phenol and an ortho-allyl-phenol that link together through ortho, para- C–C coupling.

---

[a] HerbEx Magnolia Extract (INCI: Water (Aqua) (and) Butylene Glycol (and) Magnolia Biondii (Bark) Extract) is a product of Bio-Spectrum Inc.

The magnolia extract is standardized for magnolol and honokiol content. It contains at least 1% of magnolol and honokiol as an analytical index (**Figure 2**).

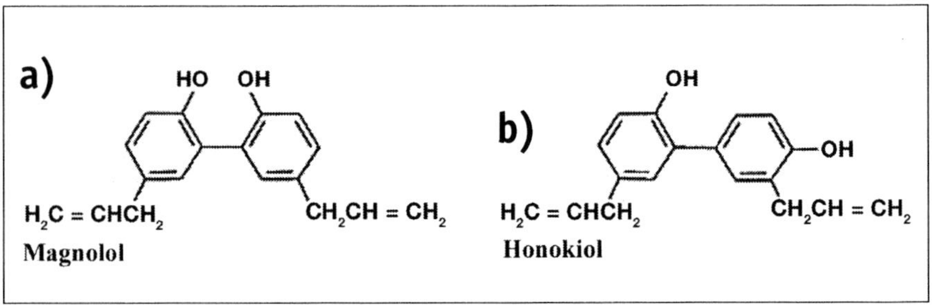

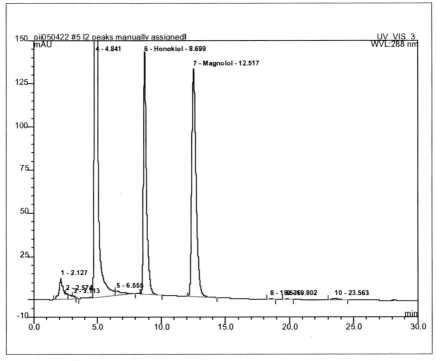

Figure 1: Chemical structures of magnolol and honokiol

Figure 2. Analytical profile of magnolia extract

Materials

The extract: A magnolia solution was prepared by dissolving the 100 mg of magnolia bark extract per milliliter of dimethyl sulphoxide. This solution was used for the efficacy and irritancy studies.

Cells and cell culture: THP-1 cells[b] were cultured in a medium containing 10% heat-inactivated fetal bovine serum, 100 U/mL of penicillin and 100 µg/mL streptomycin.[c] The THP-1 cells were incubated with *P. acnes* in 24-well plates at 1×10^6 cells per mL for 24–72 h. Human keratinocytes HaCaT (epithelial cell line from adult human skin) and human normal fibroblast cells derived from neonatal foreskin were obtained and cultured in a medium containing 10% fetal bovine serum and penicillin-streptomycin at 37° C in a humidified 95% air/5% CO_2 atmosphere.

Bacteria: Two types of acne-exacerbating bacteria were tested: *P. acnes* and *Propionibacterium granulosum*[e]. Both strains were cultured at 37°C for 24 h within a GAM semisolid medium under anaerobic conditions before the assay.

Statistical evaluation: Averages ± S.E.M. of the means were calculated and statistical analysis of the results were performed by students' *t*-test for independent samples. Values of $P < 0.05$ were considered significant.

Tests and Results

Antibacterial test of magnolia extract: To elucidate the antibacterial activity of magnolia extract against *P. acnes* and *P. granulosum*, researchers introduced a disk diffusion method, with which erythromycin was employed as a positive control. Initially, the magnolia extract was found to have significant antibacterial activities against both bacterial cells, although its activity was less potent than erythromycin. The magnolia extract and erythromycin were then added to 10-mm diameter disks with 16, 32, 64 and 128 µm of *P. acnes* and *P. granulosum*.

The magnolia extract produced 11±0.1, 13±0.7, 16±0.4 and 20±1.4 for *P. acnes*, and 13±0.3, 15±0.5, 18±0.8 and 24±2.1 for *P. granulosum*, where $P < 0.05$. Erythromycin produced 40±2.4, 40±3.5, 42±2.8 and 46±6 for *P. acnes*, and 42±4.1, 44±1.5, 46±4.5

---

[b] TIB 202 is a human monocytic THP-1 cell line produced by ATCC.

[c] RPMI 1640 was developed by Moore et al. at the Roswell Park Memorial Institute and is a product of Thermo Fisher Scientific.

[d] Dulbecco's Modified Eagles Medium is a product of Thermo Fisher Scientific

[e] ATCC 6919 (P. Acnes) and ATCC 25564 (*P. granulosum*) are produced by ATCC.

and 50±8.5 for *P. granulosum*. The inhibitory zones indicating the antibacterial activities of magnolia extract against both *P. acnes* and *P. granulosum* were conspicuously detected at over 16 µg/disk of magnolia extract.

Determination of MIC of magnolia extract: The antibacterial activities of the magnolia extract were further evaluated by determining the minimum inhibitory concentration (MIC); i.e., the lowest concentration of the test sample used that yielded no bacterial growth.

The MIC of the magnolia extract was determined using a two-fold serial dilution method. The magnolia extract inhibited the growth of *P. acnes* at 10.25 µg/mL and *P. granulosum* at 7.69 µg/mL. Therefore, the MIC of magnolia extract was determined to be 7.69–10.25 µg/mL.

Cytokine production: Magnolia extract also inhibited *P. acnes*-induced secretion of proinflammatory cytokines such as interleukin-8 and TNF-α.

It is widely accepted that the main pro-inflammatory mediators induced by bacteria and their cell components are cytokines—primarily TNF-α and interleukin-8—and enzymes such as cyclooxygenase-2 (Cox-2). Therefore, to investigate anti-inflammatory effects of magnolia extract, the researchers performed ELISA for interleukin-8, TNF-α, and PGE_2 in THP-1 cells.

As shown in **Figure 3**, *P. acnes*-induced production of TNF-α and interleukin-8 in THP-1 cells were reduced by the magnolia extract. In addition, enzymatic activity of Cox-2 was also inhibited. However, there is the possibility that the reduction of pro-inflammatory cytokines was induced by the cytotoxic effect of the magnolia extract. To confirm this, an MTT assay in THP-1 cells was performed. According to this result, the magnolia extract showed no cytotoxic effect at the tested concentrations (**Figure 4**).

DPPH assay: Magnolol and honokiol have antioxidant activity. In order to examine antioxidant activity of the magnolia extract, in vitro testing for diphenyl-p-picrylhydrazyl (DPPH) scavenging assay was conducted. This test showed the magnolia extract to have radical-scavenging activities (**Figure 5**).

Antibacterial and Anti-inflammatory Effects of a Magnolia Extract

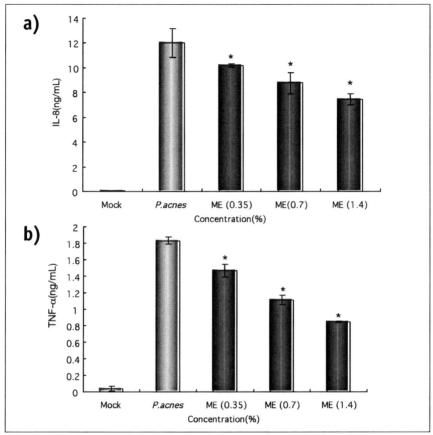

Figure 3. Dose-dependent effect of magnolia extract treatment on: a) **P. acnes**-induced interleukin-8, or b) TNF-α release. Mock: untreated control. (Jongsung Lee et al.)

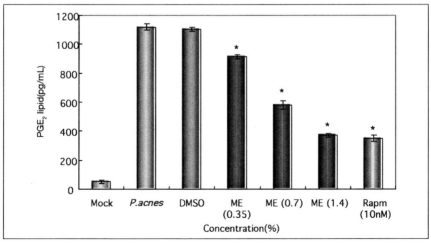

Figure 4. The **P. acnes**-induced increase of PGE_2 lipid was decreased by magnolia extract in THP-1 cells. Mock: untreated control. Rapm (10 nM): rapamycin (10 nM). (Jongsung Lee et al.)

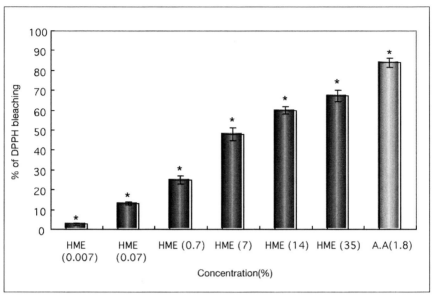

Figure 5. In vitro antioxidant activities of magnolia extract. DPPH assay. AA: ascorbic acid. (Jongsung Lee et al.)

Human skin primary irritation test of magnolia extract: To evaluate the irritation effect of the magnolia extract for clinical applications to human skin, a patch test was performed. In the test, the magnolia extract was applied to the skin at 0.1%, 1.0%, 5.0%, 10.0% and 20.0%, and compared to a control of petrolatum. As a result, not one of the 30 subjects experienced a reaction based on the 30 min reading and 1 day reading. Specifically, researchers did not observe adverse reactions such as erythema, burning or pruritus in the study subjects that was related to the topical treatment of the magnolia extract.

Discussion and Conclusions

As previously described, researchers identified the antibacterial and anti-inflammatory effects of a magnolia extract against acne-inducing bacteria. The MIC of the magnolia extract was examined and determined to be 7.69–10.25 µg/mL. In addition, *P. acnes*-induced production of TNF-α, interleukin-8, and PGE$_2$ in THP-1 cells were reduced by the magnolia extract, indicating an anti-inflammatory effect.

However, the authors noted the potential for the extract to cause cytotoxic effects to human skin cells. Thus, an MTT assay was performed in both human normal fibroblasts and HaCaT cells. Researchers found the extract to have cytotoxic effects, although weak—similar to triclosan (2, 4, 4–trichloro–2–hydroxy–diphenylether), which has been used as an active ingredient for many antibacterial skin care products, owing to its antibacterial and anti-inflammatory properties.[22]

Having relatively low cytotoxic effects, the magnolia extract may be suggested for use as a safe topical therapeutic agent for acne. To further test the safety of the magnolia extract, a patch test was performed and confirmed it to be safe for use on human skin.

Based on these results, the researchers conclude that the magnolia extract may be introduced as a possible therapeutic agent for acne, as well as a soothing agent; although, the mechanisms of action were not determined and its possible inhibition mechanisms of pro-inflammatory cytokines require further study.

Currently, NF-κB (nuclear factor-κB) has been reported as being involved in maximal transcription of many cytokines, including TNF-α, interleukin-1, interleukin-6, and interleukin-8, which are thought to be important in the generation of acute inflammatory responses. Therefore, it is possible that the magnolia extract inhibited NF-κB activation induced by *P. acnes*.

Overall, in the present study, researchers found the magnolia extract collectively exhibited strong antimicrobial and anti-inflammatory activities, indicating its potential introduction as a cosmetic material indicated to soothe irritated skin, or to improve skin diseases such as acne and atopic dermatitis.

Published January 2009 *Cosmetics and Toiletries* magazine

References

1. GM White, Recent findings in the epidemiologic evidence, classification, and subtypes of acne vulgaris, *J Am Acad Dermatol* 39 34–37 (1998)
2. RR Marples, The microflora of the face and acne lesions, *J Invest Dermatol* 62 326-331(1974)
3. GF Webster, JJ Leyden, ME Norman and UR Nilsson, Complement activation in acne vulgaris: in vitro studies with *Propionibacterium acnes* and *Propionibacterium granulosum*, *Infect Immun* 22(2) 523–529 (1978)
4. JS Strauss and AM Kligman, The pathologic dynamics of acne vulgaris, *Arch Derm* 82 779 (1960)

5. DT Downing, ME Stewart, PW Wertz and   JS Strauss,Essential fatty acids and acne, *J Am Acad Dermatol* 14 221–225 (1986)

6. GF Webster, JJ Leyden, CC Tsai, P Baehni and WP McArthur, Neutrophil lysosomal release in response to *Propionibacterium acnes, J Invest Dermatol* 73, 266–268 (1980)

7. J Guin, D Huber, P Gielerak, Antibiotic sensitivity of comedonal Propionibacterium acne *Acta Derm Venereol,* 59(6) 552–554 (1979)

8. AS Breathnach, M Nazzaro-Porro and S Passi, Azelaic acid, *Br J Dermatol* 111(1) 115–120 (1984)

9. A Zesch, Adverse reactions of externally applied drugs and inert substances (benzoyl peroxide/retinoid-skin irritation) *Derm Beruf Umwelt* 36(4) 128–133 (1988)

10. E Eady, Bacrerial resistance in acne, *Dermatology* 196(1) 59–66 (1998)

11. T Fisher and H Maibach, Finn Chamber Patch Test Technique, *Cont Derm* 11 137–140 (1984)

12. DE Latch et al, Aqueous photochemistry of triclosan: formation of 2,4-dichlorophenol, 2,8-dichlorodibenzo-p-dioxin, and oligomerization products, *Environ Toxicol Chem* 24(3) 517–25 (2005)

13. M Wawruch, L Bozekova, S Krcmery, M Kriska, Risks of antibiotic treatment *Bratisl Lek Listy* 103(7–8) 270–275 (2002)

14. CTFA Safety Testing Guideline, the Cosmetic, Toiletry, and Fragrance Association Inc. Washington, D.C. (2003)

15. FN Marzulli and HI Maibach, Dermatotoxicity, fourth edition, Hemisphere Publishing Corp. (1991)

16. C Nam, S Kim, Y Sim and I. Chang, Anti-acne effects of oriental herb extracts: a novel screening method to select anti-acne agents, *Skin Pharmacol Appl Skin Physiol* 16 84–90 (2003)

17. HJ Park, SH Kwon, YN Han, JW Choi, K Miyamoto, SH Lee, and KT Lee, Apoptosis-Inducing costunolide and a novel acyclic monoterpene from the stem bark of *Magnolia sieboldii, Arch Pharm Res* 24(4) 342–348 (2001)

18. H Tan, Antibacterial therapy for acne: a guide to selection and use of systemic agents, *Am J Clin Dermatol* 4(5) 307–314 (2003)

19. TY Shin, DK Kim, BS Chae, and EJ Lee, Antiallergic action of *Magnolia officinalis* on immediate hypersensitivity reaction, *Arch Pharm Res* 24(3) 249–255 (2001)

20. JP Wang, TF Ho, LC Chang and CC Chen, Anti-inflammatory effect of magnolol, isolated from *Magnolia officinalis*, on A23187-induced pleurisy in mice, *J Pharm Pharmacol* 47 857–860 (1995)

21. K Ikeda and H Nagase, Magnolol has the ability to induce apoptosis in tumor cells, *Biol Pharm Bull* 25(12) 1546–1549 (2002)

22. KH Bang, YK Kim, BS Min, MK Na, YH Rhee, JP Lee, and KH Bae, Antifungal activity of magnolol and honokiol, *Arch PharmRes* 23 46–49 (2000)

23. B Chang, Y Lee, Y Ku, K Bae and C Chung, Antimicrobial activity of magnolol and honokiol against periodontopathic microorganisms, *Planta Med* 64 367–369 (1998)

24. A Clark, F El-Feraly, W Li, Antimicrobial activity of phenolic constituents of *Magnolia grandiflora, J Pharm Sci* 70 951–952 (1981)

25. KY Ho, CC Tsai, CP Chen, JS Huang, CC Lin, Antimicrobial activity of honokiol and magnolol isolated from *Magnolia officinalis, Phytother Res* 15 139–141 (2001)

26. H Kuribara, E Kishi, N Hattori, M Okada and Y Maruyama, The anxiolytic effect of two oriental herbal drugs in Japan attributed to honokiol from magnolia bark, *J Pharm Pharmacol* 52(11) 1425–1429 (2000)

CHAPTER 41

Recent Advances in Biopolymers and Biomedical Materials

Robert Y. Lochhead, Stephen F. Foster, Ashley L. Cox, Margaret B. Lochhead, Vipul Padman and Emily A. Hoff

University of Southern Mississippi, Hattiesburg, Miss., USA

KEY WORDS: *filmstrips, aloe vera pectin, hydrogels, mucoadhesive gels, controlled delivery, nanofibers*

ABSTRACT: *This overview of recent literature provides a snapshot of research trends in biopolymers and biomedical polymers. To improve product efficacy, the personal care industry often looks to other sectors for innovative materials and ideas. Here, the authors encourage readers to innovate by technology transfer and by gaining a better understanding of biopolymers.*

In this overview of recently published scientific literature, the authors provide a snapshot of current research trends in biopolymers and biomedical polymers. During experimentation to improve product benefits, the personal care industry eagerly formulates with new and different materials and ideas. Sometimes these new materials are generated within the industry while other times, they are borrowed from other sectors. In reviewing the current scientific literature, the authors hope to encourage readers to innovate by technology transfer and by gaining a better understanding of biopolymers at a time when they are escalating in importance.

Renewable Resources

Rising oil prices and environmental concerns have focused public interest and scientific research on renewable material sources produced from agriculture and biological stock. The drive within the scientific community is to meet the current thermal and mechanical properties of standard petroleum materials with that of materials produced from agricultural sources such as corn or soybeans. With this in mind, a recent scientific publication in biomacromolecules[1] focused on analyzing the material properties as well as phase separation in copolymer blends of poly(3-hydroxybutyrate) (PHB), with poly(L-lactic acid) (PLA), and poly(ε-caprolactone) (PCL).

PHB is a polymer that is synthesized from bacteria and PLA can be obtained from agricultural resources such as corn. The polymers PLA and PCL were blended with PHB in varying weight ratios of 15% to 85%. This publication compared the copolymer blends of PHB/PLA to PHB/PCL in both mechanical properties as well as phase behavior. The mechanical properties were determined by using a miniaturized stretching machine at a 10% strain/min setting. FT-IR imaging was used to detect phase separation in the cast films by using calibration curves.

Both of these copolymer blends have similar mechanical properties with PHB content less than approximately 40%, resulting in elongation to break percentages >100%. It is interesting that for PHB/PCL copolymers, the elongation to break did not result in values of 100% until the PHB content was below 35%. PHB/PLA copolymer possesses higher mechanical deformation properties than PHB/PCL copolymers. Analyzing the copolymers for phase separation behavior reveals that both copolymer systems become phase-separated at weight concentrations of approximately 50/50.

For the PHB/PLA composition range, phase separation occurred from 45% to 65% PHB weight values. The miscibility gap in the PHB/PCL copolymers occurred over a smaller range of approximately 45% to 55% PHB weight values. The mechanical property values measured from the copolymers demonstrated that substitution of a petroleum-based polymer, PCL, with a polymer produced from an agricultural source, can yield similar or better mechanical properties.

Micropackaging of Aroma, Flavor in Filmstrips

Packages for cosmetic products are ideally designed to contain the product and prevent losses due to evaporation; they should also protect the product from degradation by the intrusion of external contaminants such as oxygen or microorganisms. There currently is an emerging trend toward the delivery of fragrance and flavors from filmstrips, which is expected to be boosted by restrictions on liquids and gels by airport security. Edible packaging is used to provide thin, protective layers that keep ingredients such as flavors and fragrances localized and prevent them from intermingling before the point of use. These barrier films can be made from hydrocolloids, i.e., proteins and polysaccharides.

The requirements of a film for this purpose are good film cohesion, good mechanical properties, impermeability to target fragrances and flavors, and good water-barrier properties. The films can also be in the form of a "solid" emulsion in which lipid-encapsulated flavor and fragrance are dispersed in a hydrocolloid film. Crystallization of the lipid waxes in such films decreases water transfer and, if the lipid globules are small, the water permeability deceases when the lipid concentration in the film is close to 30%.[2]

Edible films made of iota(i)-carageenan offer the advantages of good mechanical properties, emulsion stabilization and decreased oxygen permeability; this biopolymer also has recently been evaluated as a hydrocolloid film-former for edible aroma emulsion films[a].[3]

Carrageenans are sulfated polysaccharides obtained by extraction from seaweed (see **Figure 1**).

There are three major classes, namely *kappa*, *iota* and *lambda* carageenan. This classification is based on the number and position of sulfate groups on the disaccharide repeat unit of the polysaccharide with *kappa*, *iota* and *lambda* carageenans being 20%, 33% and 41%, respectively. The ready availability and reasonable cost of the carrageenans has resulted in their wide use in the food industry as thickeners and texturizers. i-Carrageenan is soluble in hot water and gels below 50°C . The gel structure is a network in which the junction zones are aggregated double-helix coils. When cast, carrageenan produces a dense film of helices 1.39 nm apart.

---

[a] The Gelsite polymer is a product and registered trademark of Delsite Biotechnologies, Irving, Tex., USA.

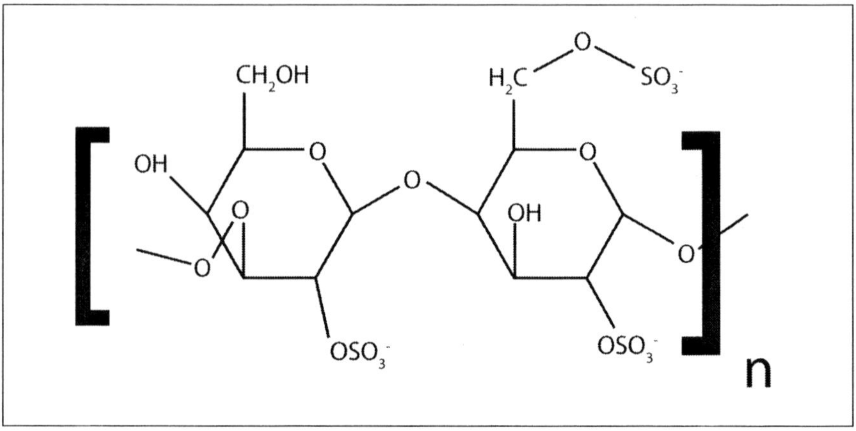

Figure 1. Carrageenan is a sulfated polysaccharide

Emulsion films were prepared by the inventor by solubilizing the fragrance *n*-hexanal in a mixture of glyceryl mono- and di-acetates and beeswax. This aroma fat-blend was homogenized into an *i*-carrageenan solution and the mixture was cast as a film. The aroma compound *n*-hexanal changed the structure of the carrageenan gel, raising the sol-gel transition temperature from 50°C to 85°C, and the water-vapor permeability increased while oxygen permeability was unchanged. These changes were attributed to plasticization of the film by *n*-hexanal, and wavelength shifts in FT-IR of the films indicated that the aldehyde group of the *n*-hexanal interacted with the –OH or sulfate groups of the *i*-carrageenan molecules.

This plasticization by *n*-hexanal apparently increased the mesh-size of the film sufficiently to allow the intrusion of water molecules but not enough to allow permeation of the larger oxygen molecules. Thus, oxidation of the fragrance would be slowed or prevented by the film's gel network, but the ready intrusion of water would favor the release of aroma on demand.

Polysaccharide Gels: Pectin From a New Source

Like carrageenan, pectin is another polysaccharide that is commonly used as a gellant and texturizer in the food industry. The properties of pectin extracted from aloe vera have recently been disclosed.[4]

Pectins are anionic polysaccharides consisting primarily of 1,4 α-D galacturonic acid repeat units with 1,2 rhamnose branch points (see **Figure 2**).

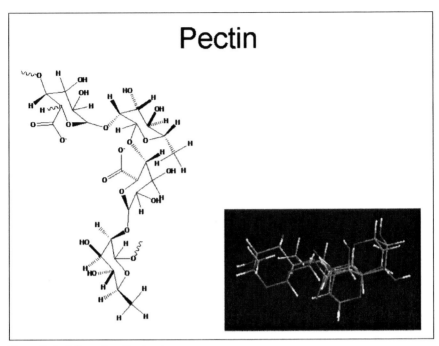

Figure 2. Depiction of pectin structure

Similarly to alginates, pectins gel in the presence of calcium ions. In these gelled structures, the calcium ions are located specifically between the polyelectrolyte chains like eggs in an egg carton.[5-7] By measuring the intrinsic viscosity as a function of ionic strength, it was shown that aloe vera pectin has an inherently stiff polymer backbone; the intrinsic viscosity is an indication of a polymer's molecular hydrodynamic volume in solution.

Zeta potential measurements showed that, in aqueous solution, the potential on the pectin molecule is high and the polymer molecules interact strongly to the water and generally avoid each other. However, above a sodium chloride concentration of only 0.1M, the potential drops to a level that allows the polymer molecules to interact with each other, and if the concentration is above the polymer's critical overlap concentration, a gel network can be established. This is shown by the "scaling" of the electrolyte solution's intrinsic viscosity with pectin concentration.

The exponent of 10.9 is much larger than the theoretical value of 4. In this concentration regime, hydrophobic junction zones between the pectin molecules have been detected by the fluorescent probe 8-anilino naphthalenesulfonic acid, confirming that the gel structure is a hydrophilic polymer network linked by hydrophobic junction zones.

It is interesting though, that, even in the absence of salt and above the critical overlap concentration, the intrinsic viscosity rises faster with concentration than would be predicted (8.6) for a random coil polymer, indicating that even when the polymer molecules effectively repel one another, the flow of the system is constrained. In the presence of calcium the gel had a higher shear storage modulus than loss modulus, indicating that it was more solid-like than liquid-like. Moreover, aloe vera pectin at only 0.20% w/w exhibits almost the same values of elastic modulus as other pectins tested at higher concentrations (2.0% w/w) and higher calcium concentrations (10mM).

Polymers for Tissue Engineering

In medical sciences, tissue engineering has become a highly researched area focusing on the repair of damaged cells and restoration of function to damaged areas of the human body.[8] One key area that has inherent difficulties is that of nerve repair, since nerve damage is notorious for being difficult if not impossible to heal.

Scientists have begun researching new "smart" materials, or materials that perform a specific function upon external stimulus such as light, electric currents, pH, ionic strength and temperature, and have used these stimuli triggers to develop materials that could be useful in tissue engineering.

In a recent article submission,[9] researchers synthesized an electroactive copolymer (PLAAP) using PLA and aniline pentamer (AP) with the goal of creating a copolymer that could be used as a nerve repair scaffold material. The conjugated ring backbone of the AP allows the polymer to be electroactive—a property that has been demonstrated as useful in proliferation or differentiation of various cell types.

This copolymer is soluble in relatively inexpensive solvents such as THF and $CHCl_3$ and is capable of forming films in either. The contact angles of various films formed in these solvents are relatively independent based on film formation in solvents THF and $CHCl_3$. The contact angle of the films are approximately 90 degrees but after the introduction of camphor sulfonic acid to emeraldine PLAAP, the contact angle lowers to almost 50 degrees. This contributes to the copolymer the right surface properties for biocompatibility of rat neuronal pheochromocytoma PC-12 cells, and results in the cells being able to spread across the surface of the PLAAP copolymer.

According to the study, two substrates were seeded with PC-12 cells, a PLAAP substrate and a tissue-culture-treated polystyrene (TCPS), and an electrical stimulus of 0.1V was applied across them using platinum microwire electrodes for 1 hr every day. Two more substrates were seeded, but not electrically stimulated so as to provide a contrasting sample group. It was shown that after four days, neurite extension occurred only in the PLAAP substrate stimulated by electrical stimulus, and demonstrated that the electroactive PLAAP copolymer can accelerate the differentiation of nerve cells through electrical stimulus. This study proved that PLAAP copolymers can be modified so that they are biocompatible with PC-12 cells and then electrically stimulated to differentiate the nerve cells. The copolymer solubility in inexpensive solvents allows relative ease of processing for practical application, and the electroactivity of the copolymer provides the capability for cellular adhesion, growth and proliferation.

Scaffolds are artificial extracellular matrices used in tissue engineering to integrate tissues and organs, and to provide a structure for cells to propagate, migrate and differentiate and become integrated with intrinsic body tissues. Collagen is the most abundant protein in vertebrates and Type I collagen is the most widely used scaffold material because it is abundant, biocompatible, bioabsorbable and it is not antigenic.[10] Monomeric collagen self-assembles to form fibrils in vitro under physiological conditions, the fibrils confer enhanced mechanical properties and biological stability, and the properties are further improved by cross-linking.

Collagen biomaterials are usually produced by sequential processing in which fibrils are allowed to form. They subsequently are cross-linked;[11] however, the mechanical properties of scaffolds formed by this process are inadequate for tissue engineering of hard tissues. Simultaneous processing in which the fibrils are grown and simultaneously cross-linked produces collagen gels with improved mechanical properties.[12]

The structure of these collagen gels, cross-linked with 1-ethyl-3-(3-dimethylaminopropyl)-carbodiimide, was recently studied by scanning electron microscopy and atomic force microscopy and it was discovered that, despite their improved mechanical properties, simultaneously processed collagen gels had fewer fibrils than those that had been sequentially processed. AFM showed that nonfibrous collagen filled the spaces between the fibrils in the simultaneously processed gels. It was postulated that the improved properties resulted from cross-linking of the fibrils with nonfibrous collagen.[13]

Hydrogels are promising scaffolds for cell adhesion, spreading and proliferation, and also for the repair and regeneration of tissues and organs.[14, 15] In order to be used as cell-growth scaffolds for tissue engineering, hydrogels must be biocompatible, must have the correct mechanical properties and pore size, and must be compatible with surrounding living cells.[16] pH sensitive hydrogel copolymers of cross-linked acrylic acid, ε-caprolactone and 2-hydroxyethyl-methacrylate showed good biocompatibility, good biodegradation by the enzyme lipase, and good cell adhesion.[17]

However, natural physiological tissue regeneration during wound healing involves the simultaneous appearance of multiple growth factors in controlled amounts.[18] Conventional inert hydrogels are severely limited in their capability to deliver multiple proteins because these gels cannot distinguish between proteins of similar size, nor can they govern the release rate of a smaller protein and simultaneously maintain a constant rate of release of a larger protein. In order to mimic the natural process, layer-by-layer polymeric composites capable of the simultaneous, but individually controlled, release of two or more proteins have been developed.[19]

Despite many studies, the effect of charge density on multilayer growth is still unclear. For example, very thick films can be prepared from weak polyelectrolytes at high salt concentrations. The exponential growth of these films has been attributed to diffusion of the polyelectrolytes in and out of the multilayer during the B process of layer deposition.[20] This knowledge gap prompted a recent study of the formation of multilayer adsorption of alternating layers of chitosan and pectin as a function of degree of acetylates of pectin. During the process of chitosan deposition, it was discovered that the chitosan diffused in and out of the film, and as the fresh become more charged and more water-soluble, this effect was magnified. Due to the excess of positive charge, the interaction between pectin and chitosan did not lead to 1:1 stoichiometric complexes.[21]

In addition to these fundamental difficulties, the layer-by-layer composites are fabricated by a series of complex steps; thus, a simpler approach is desirable. Ideally this simpler approach would be monolithic inert hydrogels—however, the tuned-free, diffusive delivery of different actives from an inert hydrogel is almost impossible.

As a consequence of these shortcomings of inert hydrogels, polymer networks with specific protein affinity sites have been developed to release target molecules at a rate determined by the association constant of the site-target molecule couple rather than the passive diffusion of the target molecule through a matrix.[22] Recently, a proof of concept study of monolithic affinity hydrogels for controlled protein release was reported.[23]

These hydrogels are prepared by copolymerizing poly(ethylene glycol) diacrylate [PEGDA] with glycidylmethacrylate-iminodiacetic acid [GMIDA]. The metal-binding capabilities of iminodiacetic acid [IDA] have been used extensively for protein purification, and this nondegradable hydrogel uses the ligand of IDA capability to tune the simultaneous delivery of two proteins: histidine-tagged green fluorescent protein and lysozyme.

For example, the affinity-binding of histidine-tagged proteins and GMIDA ligands is mediated by metal ions such as nickel, but nickel at low concentrations does not significantly affect lysozyme release from the hydrogel. Use of this dual-release mechanism allows the release to be tuned for each protein separately. As a corollary, complete and immediate release of the bound protein can be achieved by merely adding a metal chelating agent such as EDTA. Perhaps well-designed hydrogels such as these will someday trickle beneficial agents from topically applied compositions.

It is interesting that Chen et al. reported that bovine fetal aorta endothelial cells could spread and proliferate on poly(acrylic acid) without any cell adhesive protein modification.[24] Another short-coming of in vitro cell growth scaffolds is that they are irreversible physical gels of materials extracted from cells or tissue, chemically cross-linked gels or nanofiber networks, and it is difficult to remove cells from the matrices of these existing gels without damaging the cells in the process. In order to address this issue, thermoresponsive hydrogels have been developed as matrices that would allow facile harvesting of intact cells for implantation.[25]

The advent of living free-radical polymerization has made possible the synthesis of precise molecularly designed block copolymers for this purpose. Amphipathic BAB block copolymers in which the A block is hydrophilic and the B block is thermoresponsively hydrophobic are preferred for this application. A recent study reported that the synthesis and characterization of such amphipathic molecules having a poly(N-isopropylacrylamide) and a hydrophilic inner a block of poly(N,N-dimethylacryamide).[25] Poly(N-isopropylacryl-amide) was chosen because its lower critical solution temperature (LCST) of 32°C is close to the human physiological temperature (37°C); this polymer is soluble in water below 32°C and it phase-separates when the solution temperature is raised above this threshold.

For this block copolymer, the B-blocks become relatively hydrophobic and this causes them to aggregate above the LCST to form the core of polymer micelles. When the concentration is low, the micelles are isolated in solution and the composition is liquid-like; however, above a critical concentration, a network structure forms with the micelle cores becoming junction zones in the gel and the rheology becomes more solid-like; the elastic modulus becomes larger than the loss modulus.

The formation of the gel was shown on a molecular level in this case by measuring the diffusion coefficient of water by pulsed field gradient NMR and by contour microscopy using the fluorescent probe 8-anilino-1-naphthalenesulfonic acid. The apparent diffusion coefficient was high at short times, but it dropped with time of observation and plateaued at 400 milliseconds, indicating that the water was probably being bounded by a gel network. The hypothesis of a gel network was further supported by measurement of the fluorescence observed by confocal microscopy. The fluorescence intensified at elevated temperatures and the image showed large hydrophobic domains separated by tens of micrometers. These are assigned as the micelle core junction zones in the gel. This type of thermoreversible gel could form the basis of a topical treatment that could be removed by merely rinsing with cold water (see **Figure 3**).

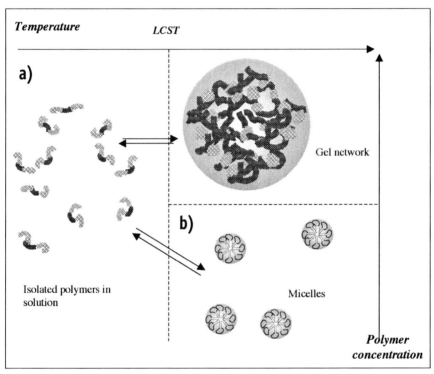

Figure 3. Thermoresponsive block copolymers are a) isolated in solution at low temperatures and b) above the "trigger" temperature, they form micelles at low concentrations and gels at high concentrations. The transitions are reversible.

Mucoadhesive Gels

The emergence of antibiotic-resistant pathogens has the potential of driving civilization back to the pre-penicillin era, when relatively minor infections were life-threatening. In such an environment, even the administration of injections could compromise the body's natural barrier and allow the ingress of undesirable bacteria. In order to meet this challenge, the pharmaceutical industry is directing research attention to more efficient and advanced drug excipients, controlled-release systems and bioadhesives. This is because of lower adminstration and dosage frequencies, longer retention times and the possibility of site specific drug delivery. One attractive route is via the mucus membranes of, for example, the nasal or buccal cavity. Mucus membranes are relatively thin and well served with blood vessels; this makes them attractive targets for penetration of drugs into the vascular system.

The polymer poly(acrylic) acid has been heavily researched for bioadhesion and mucoadhesion application. Poly(acrylic) acid contains a high number of carboxylic groups, providing a criticial characteristic of bioadhesion through hydrogen bonding (see **Figure 4**).

Organogels of a dispersion of poly(acrylic acid), nonaqueous solvent and a model antimicrobial agent have been formed with the application of an antimicrobial implant in the buccal cavity in mind. The proposed mechanism of mucoadhesion for these organogels is initial secondary interactions between the poly(acrylic) acid and the nonaqueous solvent, and once introduced into

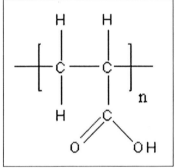

Figure 4. Poly(acrylic) acid

the oral cavity, interactions between poly(acrylic) acid and mucin.

The rheological properties, specifically pseudoplastic flow, of a mucoadhesive gel are critical to the success of drug delivery because of application ease and manufacturing ease. The quick structural recovery of pseudoplastic materials also aids in retention of the gel in the oral cavity. Because of swallowing and a constant flow of saliva, retention time of a mucoadhesive gel in the buccal cavity poses a major challenge. Correlations between viscoelastic properties and mucoadhesion were found in the poly(acrylic) acid organogels where highly structured gels exhibited high mucoadhesion, because of molecular polymer chain entanglements. As the concentration of poly(acrylic) acid increased in the bioactive organogels, loss modulus, storage modulus, dynamic viscosity, compressibility, mucoadhesion and drug release rate also increased. Choice of nonaqueous solvent also affected the physiochemical parameters. The organogel with 5–10% w/w poly(acrylic) acid and the nonaqueous solvent PEG 400 maintained the most potential as an antimicrobial implant.[26]

Controlled Delivery from Micellar Aggregates and Vesicles

While micelle-aggregated gels are being developed for tissue engineering, the need for better chemotherapeutic agents is driving the reach for precise tailoring of the interactions between hydrophilic polymers and vesicles. In this context, it has recently been shown that polyaspartylhydrazide copolymers, containing butyl moieties and/or (carboxypropyl)trimethylammonium moieties, bind to the surface of phosphatidylcholine/cholesterol vesicles, and this causes the vesicles to bind more strongly to cancer cells to increase the effectiveness of chemotherapy.[27]

Since the 1960s it has been known that cholesterol fills the voids in the palisade layer of lecithin monolayers and the scientific community understands that one of the roles of cholesterol in cells is to strengthen the phospholipid structure of the cell membranes. Recently, it has been shown that hydrophobic matching between the cholesterol and fatty acid is required for the formation of lamellar liquid ordered phases.[28]

It has also been demonstrated by nearest neighbor recognition methods that cholesterol-rich fluid bilayers have an ordered bilayer structure in which free cholesterol and longer chain phospholipid homodimer co-exist in equilibrium with a stoichiometric complex composed of one molecule of cholesterol for every two molecules of longer chain phospholipid homodimer.[29] It is not surprising, therefore, that attempts have been made to decorate hydrophilic polymers with cholesterol mesogens to enhance their interaction with lipid membranes and vesicles. Through studies, Langmuir showed that for a homopolymer formed from cholesterol acrylamidobutyrate (CAB), the preferred configuration of the cholesterol rings is to lie flat at the air-water interface (see **Figure 5**).[30]

The inference to be drawn from this finding is that presumably the cholesterol rings of such a homopolymer would also lie flat at the surface of a lipid bilayer. If this happened, the cholesterol rings would be sterically restricted from insertion between the lipid molecules of the bilayer and the resulting polymer-lipid interaction would be weak. A copolymer of CAB and 2-acrylamido-2-methylpropanesulfonic acid AMPS gave a similar surface configuration of the cholesterol when the mole ratio of CAB:AMPS was 15:85. However, a copolymer containing 10 mol% CAB gave a close-packed surface structure with the cholesterol rings being organized side-by-side with a vertical orientation to the surface. The inference in this case is that this copolymer would be ideal for interacting with, and perhaps stabilizing, phospholipid bilayers (see **Figure 6**).

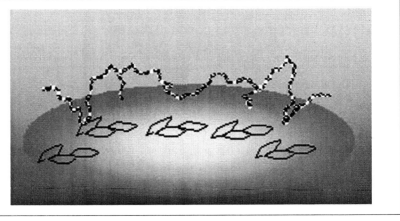

Figure 5. When present in the polymer in excess of 15 mol%, cholesterol side chains lie flat at the air/water interface. This may indicate that they would adopt this conformation at the surface of vesicles.

The precision with which these molecules have to be designed to fit their function is demonstrated by the finding that when the cholesterol mesogens content of the copolymer was reduced to 5 mol%, the polymer tended to form bilayers and micelle assemblies. Similarly, the introduction of cholesterol mesogens to carboxymethylchitosan caused this polymer to form nanomicelles that could function as injectable drug carriers.[31]

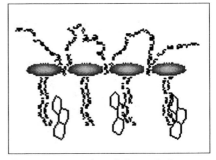

Figure 6. At 10 mole% cholesterol, the cholesterol side groups align in close-packed vertical conformation at the air/water interface. Presumably, these polymers would be structured appropriately to interpenetrate the palisade layers of vesicles.

Nanofiber Materials

Scaffolds for tissue engineering can be formed by the self-assembly of peptides into β-pleated sheets[32–34] and it has been shown that configurational and conformational organization of peptides can lead to self assembly into complex hierarchical structures such as nanotubes,[35] nanofibers[36] and helical fibrils.[37] An interesting development has been the demonstration that β-sheet-forming wheel-like synthetic peptides self assemble into nanofibers in phosphate buffer and rod-like structures in acid and alkaline media.[38] The nanofiber structures were clearly visible in transmission electron micrographs of specimens stained with phosphotungstic acid or uranyl acetate. An emphatic increase of fluorescence on binding with thioflavin T showed that the nanofibers self-assemble as β-pleated sheets and increase in fluorescence upon binding 8-anilino-1-naphthalenesulfonic acid indicated that the outside of the nanofibers were hydrophilic (see **Figures 7** and **8**).

Modified microcrystalline celluloses are used extensively as rheology modifiers in personal care and also in foods. The rheology conferred by these materials is attributed to the formation of composite network structures between cellulose microcrystalline fibrils and soluble polymers.

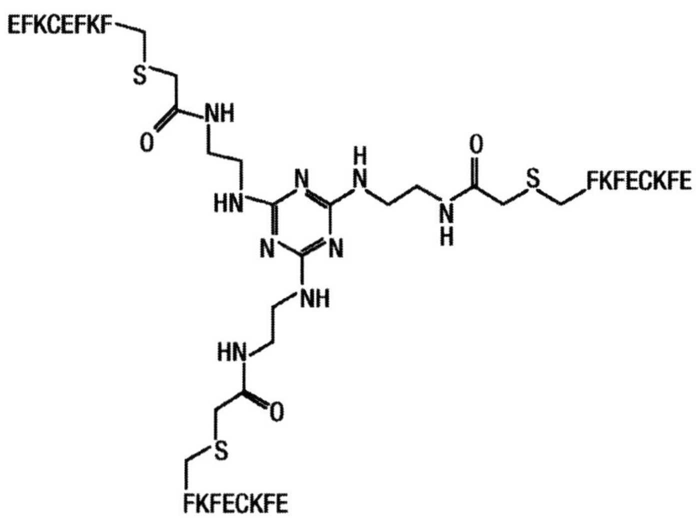

Figure 7. A ß-sheet-forming wheel peptide

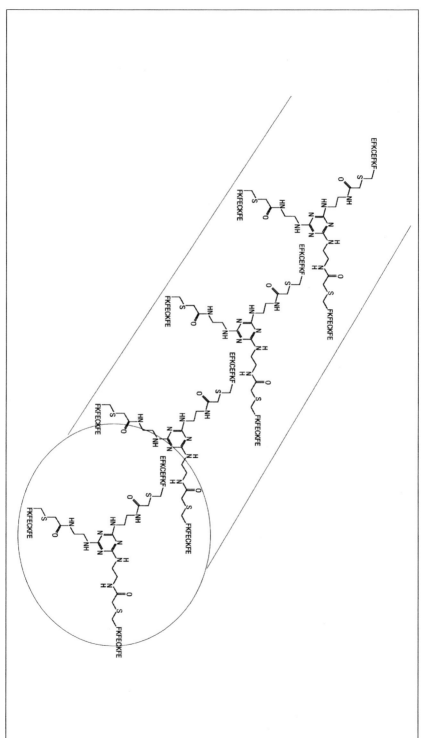

Figure 8. Wheel-like peptides can self-assemble to form nanofibers

A recent study on the interaction between cellulose nanofibers may shed some light on exactly what is happening between the crystalline microfibrils when they form higher order structures.[39] The nature of the surface of cellulose nanocrytals differs depending upon the method of preparation. Thus, hydrolysis with sulfuric acid might be expected to yield surfaces that contain sulfate groups. The effect of surface charge density on the structuring of cellulose nanocrystal films was probed using quartz crystal microbalance with dissipation and atomic force microbalance measurements.

Cellulose nanofibrils were prepared by mechanically disintegrating bleached sulfite pulp by a microfluidizer. Low-charge density nanofibrils were pretreated by enzymatic hydrolysis and mechanical disintegration, whereas high charge density nanofibrils were carboxymethylated. The cellulose nanofibers were spin-coated on a silica wafer. Interestingly, the carboxymethylated anionically charged nanofibrils gave good homogeneous surface coverage that can be attributed to hydrogen-bonding, whereas the low-charge density nanofibrils did not adhere readily to the silica surface.

Surface coverage was improved by treatment with polyvinylamine, titanium dioxide or 3-aminopropyltrimethoxysilane, implying that these low charge density nanofibrils carry a negative charge. Quartz crystal microbalance measurements in aqueous media showed that low-charge density nanofibril films were relatively insensitive to changes in electrolyte concentration and pH, but high change density nanofibril films swelled and de-swelled dramatically under the influence of such changes.

Electrolyte addition caused the films to imbibe water; much more for the high charge density nanofibers. This enhanced swelling was attributed to a Donnan effect; increased electrolyte concentration causes an increase in the pH inside the film, leading to dissociation of more carboxyl groups that in turn causes polyelectrolyte swelling. At high electrolyte concentrations, the water uptake decreases again and this can be explained by electrochemical attraction of counter ions to the nanofibrils being favored over the chemical potential-driven diffusion of counterions into the surrounding aqueous environment. The resulting proximity of the counterions shields the nanofibril charges and causes de-swelling of the film.

Atomic force microscope measurements of the interfibril interaction were conducted by attaching a cellulose sphere to the tip of the probe and then carefully measuring force as a function of distance between the nanofibril film and the cellulose sphere. These measurements in water at pH 8 indicated the presence of electrical double-layer repulsion, consistent with DLVO theory. However, when the ionic strength was increased, the forces did not decay to the extent expected by double-layer repulsion. This indicates that there is steric repulsion, for both low-charge density and high-charge density nanofibrils and this may also indicate the presence of anchored soluble polymers, presumably hemicelluloses, at their surface.

Impurities in polysaccharides often diffuse to the surface, making it difficult to measure the true surface energy. Chitosan and cellulose fall under the same class of materials but they differ chemically since OH groups in the cellulose are replaced by NH_2 groups. The dispersive components of the surface energy are comparable within the two polymers, but the polar component is higher in cellulose than chitosan.[40-42]

In one study, chitosan surface energies were compared with N-acetyl-D-glucosamine (GlcNAc) before and after purification and extraction processes. These processes removed nonpolar impurities present in chitosan; then samples in the form of pellets and films were obtained. Before purification chitosan showed low values of the polar component of surface-free energy compared to GlcNAc, but after purification there was a dramatic increase. For the purified pellets, increase in the polar component confirmed that nonpolar impurities caused the decrease in the polar component of chitosan. The polar component was independent of the degree of deacetylation (DDA).

For films, the polar component was lower compared to GlcNAc, as the residual impurities in films migrated to the surface and caused a decrease in the surface energy. Scratching the film surface spontaneously increased the surface energy. Thus, the impurities present in the commercially available chitosan were responsible for low polar component of surface energies.[43]

These latest findings indicate that the industry's understanding of the interactions between nanofibrils is far from complete and more fundamental studies could yield rich rewards in the design of new, improved rheology modifiers and nanofiber composites.

Published June 2008 *Cosmetics and Toiletries* magazine

References

1. C Vogel, E Wessel and HW Siesler, FT-IR imaging spectroscopy of phase separation in blends of poly(3-hydroxybutyrate) with poly(L-lactic acid) and poly(E-caprolactone), Biomacromolecules 9 523 (2008)
2. T Karbowiak, F Debeaufort, D Champion and A Voilley, Wetting properties at the surface of iota-carrageenan-based edible films, *J Colloid Interface Sci* 294 400 (2006)
3. A Hambleton, F Debeaufort, T Karbowiak and A Voilley, Protection of active aroma compound against moisture and oxygen by encapsulation in biopolymeric emulsion-based edible films, *Biomacromolecules ASAP*, published on the Internet (Feb 8, 2008)
4. SD McConaughy, PA Stroud, B Boudreaux, RD Hester and CL McCormick, Structural characterization and solution properties of a galacturonate polysaccharide derived from aloe vera capable of in situ gelation, *Biomacromolecules* 9 472 (2008)
5. M Gidley, ER Morris, EJ Murray, DA Powell and DA Rees, *Chem Commun* 990–991 (1979)
6. DA Rees, Carbohydr Polym 2 254–263 (1982)
7. DA Powell, ER Morris, MJ Gidley and DA Rees, *J Mol Biol* 155 517–531 (1982)
8. R Langer, JP Vacanti, Tissue engineering, *Science* 260 920–926 (1993)
9. L Huang et al, Synthesis of biodegradable and electroactive multiblock polylactide and aniline pentamer copolymer for tissue engineering applications, *Biomacromolecules ASAP*, published on the Internet (Feb 9, 2008)
10. CH Lee, A Singla and Y Lee, Biomedical applications of collagen, Int J Pharmaceutics 221 (2001)
11. W Friess, H Uludag, S Foskett, R Biron and C Sargeant, Characterization of absorbable collagen sponges as rh BMP.2 carriers, *Int J Pharmaceutics* 187 91 (1999)
12. S Yunoki, N Nagai, S Suzuki and M Munekata, Novel biomaterial from reinforced salmon collagen gel prepared by fibril formation and cross-linking, *J Biosci Bioeng* 98 40 (2004)
13. S Yunoki and T Matsuda, Simultaneous processing of fibril formation and cross-linking improves mechanical properties of collagen, *Biomacromolecules ASAP*, published on the Internet (Feb 9, 2008)
14. KY Lee and DJ Mooney, Hydrogels for tissue engineering, *Chem Rev* 101 1869 (2001)
15. AS Hoffman, Hydrogels for biomedical applications, *Advanced Drug Delivery Reviews* 54 3 (2002)
16. LG Griffith and MA Swartz, Capturing complex 3D tissue physiology in vitro, Nature Reviews Molecular Cell Biology 7, 211 (2006)
17. D-Q Wu, Y-X Sun, X-D Xu, SX Cheng, Xi-Z Zhang and R-X Zhuo, Biodegradable and pH-sensitive hydrogels for cell encapsulation and controlled drug release, *Biomacromolecules ASAP*, published on the Internet (Feb 29, 2008)
18. TP Richardson, MC Peters, AB Ennett and DJ Mooney, Polymeric system for dual growth factor delivery, *Nature Biotechnology* 19 1029 (2001)
19. KC Wood, HF Chuang, RD Batten, DM Lynn and PT Hammond, Controlling interlayer diffusion to achieve sustained, multiagent delivery from layer-by-layer thin films, *Proc Nat Acad Sci* 103 10207 (2006)
20. C Picart et al, Molecular basis for the explanation of the exponential growth of polyelectrolyte multilayers, *Proc Natl Acad Sci* 99 12531–12535 (2002)
21. K Kamburova, V Milkova, I Petkanchin and T Radeva, Effect of Pectin Charge Density on Formation of Multilayer Films with Chitosan, *Biomacromolecules*, published on Internet (Feb 22, 2008)
22. NA Peppas and SL Wright; Drug diffusion and binding in ionizable interpenetrating networks from poly(vinyl alcohol) and poly(acrylic acid); *European J Pharm Biopharm* 46 15 (1998)

23. C-C Lin and AT Metters, Bifunctional monolithic affinity hydrogels for dual-protein delivery, *Biomacromolecules ASAP*, published on the Internet (Feb 8, 2008)

24. YM Chen, N Shiraishi, H Satokawa, A Kakugo, T Narita and JP Gong, Cultivation of endothelial cells on adhesive protein-free synthetic polymer gels, *Biomaterials* 26 4588 (2005)

25. SE Kirkland, RM Hensarling, SD McConaughy, Y Guo, WJ Jarrett and CL McCormick, Thermoreversible hydrogels from RAFT-synthesized BAB triblock copolymers: steps toward biomimetic matrices for tissue regeneration, *Biomacromolecules* 9 681 (2008)

26. DS Jones, BCO Muldoon, AD Woolfson, GP Andrews and FD Sanderson, Physiochemical characterization of bioactive polyacrylic acid organogels as potential antimicrobial implants for the buccal cavity, *Biomacromolecules* 9 624 (2008)

27. D Paolino, D Cosco, M Licciardi, G Giammona, M Fresta and G Cavallaro, Polyapastylhydrazide copolymer based supramolecular vesicular aggregates as delving devices for anticancer drugs, *Biomacromolecules ASAP*, published on Internet (Feb 29, 2008)

28. J Ouimet and M Lafleur, Hydrophobic match between cholesterol and saturated fatty acid is required for the formation of lamellar liquid ordered phases, *Langmuir* 20 7474 (2004)

29. J Zhang, H Cao and SL Regen, Cholesterol-phospholipid complexation in fluid bilayers as evidenced by nearest-neighbor recognition measurements, *Langmuir* 23 405 (2007)

30. K Chandrasekar, R Vijay and G Baskar, Ionic polymeric amphiphiles with cholesterol mesogen: Adsorption and organization characteristics at the air/water interface, from *Langmuir Film Balance Studies*, *Biomacromolecules ASAP*, published on the Internet (Feb 29, 2008)

31. W Yinsong, L Lingrong, W Jian and Q Zhang, Preparation and characterization of self-aggregated nanoparticles of cholesterol-modified O-carboxymethyl chitosan conjugates, *Carbohydrate Polymers* 69 597 (2007)

32. J Kisiday et al, Self-assembling peptide hydrogel fosters chondrocyte extracellular matrix production and cell division: Implications for cartilage tissue repair, *Proc Natl Acad Sci* 99 9996 (2002)

33. RG Ellis-Behnke et al, Nano neuro knitting: Peptide nanofiber scaffold for brain repair and axon regeneration with functional return of vision, *Proc Natl Acad Sci* 103 5054 (2006)

34. DA Salick, JK Kretsinger, DJ Pochan and JP Schneider, Inherent antibacterial activity of a peptide-based β-hairpin hydrogel, *J Am Chem Soc* 129 14793 (2007)

35. C Valéry et al, Biomimetic organization: Octapeptide self-assembly into nanotubes of viral capsid-like dimension, *Proc Natl Acad Sci* 100 10258 (2003)

36. MG Ryadnov and DN Woolfson, MaP peptides: Programming the self-assembly of peptide-based mesoscopic matrices, *J Am Chem Soc* 127 12407 (2005)

37. M Zhou, D Bentley and I Ghosh; Helical supramolecules and fibers utilizing leucine zipper-displaying dendrimers, *J Am Chem Soc* 126 734 (2004)

38. K Murasato, K Matsuura and N Kimizuka, Self-assembly of nanofiber with uniform width from wheel-type trigonal-sheet-forming peptide, *Biomacromolecules ASAP*, published on the Internet (Feb 21, 2008)

39. S Ahola, J Salmi, L-S Johansson, J Laine and M. Österberg, Model films from native cellulose nanofibrils. Preparation, swelling and surface interactions, *Biomacromolecules ASAP*, published on the Internet (Feb 29, 2008)

40. A Gandini and MN Belgacem, *Cellulose Fibre Reinforced Polymer Composites*, Old City Publishing: Philadelphia, PA, ch 3 (2007)

41. H Angellier, S Molina-Boisseau, MN Belgacem and A Dufresne, *Langmuir* 21 2425 (2005)

42. MN Belgacem, A Blayo and AJ Gandini, *J Colloid Interface Sci* 182 431 (1996)

43. A Cunha, S Fernandes, C Freire, A Silvestre, C Neto and A Gandini, What is the real value of chitosan's surface energy?, *Biomacromolecules* 9 610 (2008)

CHAPTER 42

A Green, Solvent-free Biocatalytic Method to Produce Cosmetic Esters

Neil W. Boaz, PhD, and Stephanie K. Clendennen, PhD

Eastman Chemical Company, Kingsport, TN, USA

KEY WORDS: *biocatalytic, enzymatic, green, ester, 4-HBA*

ABSTRACT: *Cosmetic esters can be produced effectively via a solvent-free, biocatalytic method. This green process, described by the authors, involves combining two reactants and an enzyme, and is driven to high conversion by the removal of by-products through a nitrogen purge—in turn producing high purity materials directly from the reactor.*

Natural ingredients have always been important in the cosmetics market, and the demand for the use of greener processes is becoming more important to both formulators and consumers. In the present article—and to emphasize the distinction—*natural* refers to the source of raw materials, an example set by the Natural Products Association, while *green* refers to the process used to convert starting materials to a finished ingredient.

The US Environmental Protection Agency (EPA) has adopted a series of principles to guide the development of environmentally responsible and sustainable manufacturing, called "The 12 Principles of 'Green' Chemistry."[1] These principles have guided the development of the current biocatalytic process.

The green nature of biocatalysis— along with its mild reaction conditions, high and sometimes unique reaction selectivities, and the potential to work solvent-free—suggest that biocatalysis is a natural fit for the green preparation of cosmetic ingredients. Since petroleum-based organic solvents are undesirable for green processes, biocatalytic processes (enzymatic or microbial transformations) can instead be used since they generally are considered green.

Green Production of Esters

Green processing is especially relevant in the manufacture of naturally derived cosmetic ingredients. Natural starting materials typically are derived from plants or microbes via fermentation with minimal processing. Cold-pressed seed oils are examples of plant-derived starting materials with broad cosmetic utility. Oils (triglycerides) can be converted to the humectant glycerol or to fatty acids—both of which are starting materials for esters.

Esters are an important class of cosmetic ingredients, encompassing actives, emollients, emulsifiers and surfactants. They are employed in antiaging ingredients such as retinyl palmitate, in emollients such as fatty alcohol/fatty acid esters, and in emulsifiers such as mono- and diglycerides. Traditionally, esters are made by condensation of an alcohol and an acid in the presence of a strong acid catalyst and elevated to temperatures to both drive the reaction and remove the water by-product.[2]

Acid-catalyzed, high-temperature esterification reactions are energy-intensive and the reaction conditions are harmful to many starting materials, such as unsaturated fatty acids. Under harsh conditions, these starting materials produce undesirable color, odor and by-products that impact yield. In addition, further process steps must be included to remove the acid catalyst.[2]

In contrast, biocatalytic processes involve mild reaction conditions that do not degrade sensitive reactants or products, resulting in a reduced number of by-products as well as improved color and odor production.[2] Numerous reports of biocatalytically prepared cosmetic esters exist. A few examples include plant monoterpenes as fragrance molecules (geranyl acetate),[3] sugar fatty acid ester surfactants[4] and fatty acid esters of plant phenolic antioxidants such as rutin and naringin.[5] However, these examples are not green since they require the use of organic solvents for both the reaction and post-reaction processing to purify the final product.

A breakthrough in the deeper "greening" of biocatalytic processes, described here, is the elimination of organic solvents. Reactions similar to those described above have been performed in the absence of organic solvents and address the same classes of cosmetic ingredients: plant monoterpenes as fragrance molecules (citronellyl acetate),[6] sugar fatty acid ester surfactants[7] and fatty acid esters of plant phenolic antioxidants (ferulic acid).[8]

Eliminating the solvent from a biocatalytic reaction can have a significant environmental impact. In the authors' experience, when solvent and solvent-free biocatalytic processes for manufacturing fatty acid esters are compared, the solvent-free biocatalytic process saves more than 10 L organic solvent/kg of product in reaction and post-processing waste. Solvent-free systems also offer better volumetric production than solvent-borne reactions and in many cases, the products are sufficiently pure so that no post-reaction processing is required.[2, 9, 10]

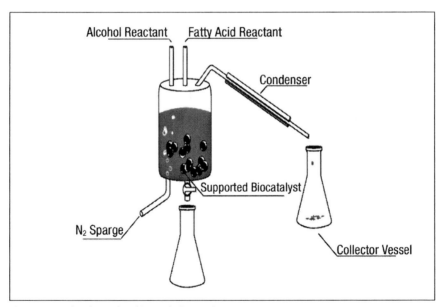

Figure 1. Batch solvent-free biocatalytic reaction

Solvent-free biocatalytic reactions can be carried out continuously[2] or as batch reactions.[11] A typical stirred tank batch reaction scenario is depicted in **Figure 1**. The two reactants are loaded along with the biocatalyst, and the mixture is heated to the desired temperature.

The reaction is then driven to high conversion by removal of the volatile by-products such as water or a lower alcohol by one of several methods including evaporation, pervaporation or by purging the reaction mixture with inert gas (shown in **Figure 1**). Removal of these by-products perturbs the equilibrium of the enzymatic reaction and affords high conversion without the need for large excess of either reactant. A semi-batch or continuous process, along with an evaporative method to remove the water by-product of the reaction, has been described for the economical production of higher-volume cosmetic ingredients.[2, 10]

Case Studies: Esters for Skin Illuminating and Emulsifying

Skin-illuminating ingredients: Inhibitors of tyrosinase—a key enzyme in melanin biosynthesis from tyrosine in mammalian skin—are useful for reducing undesirable pigmentation of the skin, resulting in a more even skin tone. The ability of a compound to address skin pigmentation can be effectively predicted in vitro by measuring the tyrosinase-inhibiting activity.[12]

Different tyrosinase inhibitors exist on the market, including hydroquinone, kojic acid, ascorbic acid and arbutin. Kojic acid is a natural product formed by fermentation with a history of use as a cosmetic ingredient for achieving even skin tone. Structurally related to kojic acid, 4-hydroxybenzyl alcohol (4-HBA) is a generally regarded as safe (GRAS) flavoring substance (Flavor and Extract Manufacturers Association substance No. 3987) that has also shown potential as a ingredient for evening skin tone. The EC_{50} or concentration of these ingredients at which the tyrosinase exhibits only 50% of its normal activity is shown in **Table 1**. A low EC_{50} value indicates the material is an effective inhibitor. The activity of 4-HBA was found to be higher than ascorbic acid, hydroquinone and arbutin in the tyrosinase inhibition assay.

Table 1. Tyrosinase inhibition values of skin illuminating ingredients

EC_{50} (mM)	Compound
0.016	Kojic acid
0.19	4-Hydroxybenzyl alcohol (4-HBA)
0.39	Ascorbic acid
0.62	Hydroquinone
1.0	Arbutin

Two distinct monoesters can be prepared from 4-HBA since the parent molecule has both a phenol and a primary alcohol. Esterification using standard chemical means such as acid chlorides or anhydrides selectively occurs at the phenol because this is the most acidic hydroxyl. However, enzymatic esterification of 4-HBA is selective for the benzyl alcohol, often resulting in > 98% selectivity for the primary ester.

Using the protocol shown in **Figure 1**, 4-HBA can be esterified enzymatically with an acid or ester reactant under solvent-free conditions and with a high conversion to ester, which is achieved by purging the mixture with nitrogen to remove the water or alcohol by-product. After removal of the enzyme, 4-HBA esters of high purity are obtained. These enzymatically prepared esters function as highly effective tyrosinase inhibitors (see **Table 2**), demonstrating enhanced tyrosinase inhibiting activity as compared to the parent diol and the chemically prepared ester (4-hydroxymethylphenyl ester) and diester.

The esters are also significantly more lipophilic than the parent molecule, as demonstrated by their increased solubility in non-polar media. Fatty acid esters of skin-illuminating ingredients improve permeability, activity, pH and heat stability of an ingredient in a formulation. These performance benefits have been demonstrated for kojic acid[13,] and can be inferred for structurally related 4-HBA.

Emulsifiers: Plant oil-derived esters can form the basis for emulsifier and emollient esters, and are also targets for a green biocatalytic production process. The naturally occurring mixture of fatty acids in the starting plant oil is reflected in the composition of the final product. As fatty acid chain length and degree of unsaturation alter the properties of the final product, the specific needs of the formulator can be addressed and tailored by judicious choice of plant oil. In addition, mono- and poly-unsaturated fatty acids, such as conjugated linoleic acid and gamma linolenic acid, can be processed via biocatalysis without compromising the structural integrity of the fatty acid or producing undesired color in the reaction product. [11]

Emulsifiers are an important class of cosmetic ingredients used to stabilize creams and lotions. Lecithin is the only green and natural emulsifier used in cosmetic formulations today. More familiar in food applications, lecithin is a naturally derived mixture of compounds including phospholipids, which impart the emulsifying properties. Lecithin is typically separated from soybean oil by steam precipitation, qualifying the product as a green and natural ingredient. However, more versatility in the portfolio of natural and green emulsifiers for cosmetics is needed.

One class of emulsifiers commonly used in food and cosmetic products is glycerides. These fatty acid esters of glycerol currently are available as synthetically produced ingredients, but solvent-free enzymatic synthesis of fatty acid mono- and diglycerides as emulsifiers has also been reported.[9-11, 14]

Table 2. Tyrosinase inhibition values of selected esters of 4-HBA

Compound	EC$_{50}$ (mM)	Structure
4-HBA	0.19	
Enzymatic 4-HBA acetate	0.038	
Chemical 4-HBA acetate	0.92	
Enzymatic 4-HBA propionate	0.017	
Chemical 4-HBA propionate	1.0	
Chemical 4-HBA dipropionate	> 10.0	
Enzymatic 4-HBA hexonoate	0.049	

Mixtures of glyceride esters can be prepared from glycerine and fatty acid ethyl esters derived from plant oils by biocatalytic, solvent-free transesterification. These reactions are pushed to high conversion by removal of the ethanol liberated in the transesterification using a nitrogen purge, resulting in glycerides with > 95% purity (based on gas chromatographic analysis for residual fatty acid ethyl ester).

To evaluate the glycerides, the rheological properties of a simple 1:1 mixture of golden jojoba oil and water emulsified with 5% w/w of each glyceride were investigated. Glycerides have a unique property among emulsifiers in their ability to interact with polysaccharides and polypeptides to dramatically change the rheological properties of the emulsion. This interaction is well-known in the food industry and can be leveraged in the formulation of cosmetic emulsions as well. To demonstrate the interaction of glycerides with polysaccharides, samples were also prepared where the water phase contained 1% w/w soluble potato starch (dissolved by heating). The mixtures were each homogenized and held at RT. The viscosities of the resulting emulsions were measured at 23°C using a viscometer[a].

In **Figure 2**, viscosity is plotted as a function of shear rate. The solid lines depict the broad range of emulsion viscosities—a function of the natural fatty acid composition of the oil (related to chain length and degree of unsaturation) and any natural minor components present in the oil. Glyceryl oleate resulted in the thickest emulsion, while glyceryl pomegranate had a thinner, cream-like consistency. When 1% w/w soluble potato starch was added to the water phase, the viscosity of the emulsions increased (dotted lines). An interaction between the glyceride and an additive was also apparent in the presence of other biological polymers such as agar and lactalbumin. The interaction between glycerides and polysaccharides/proteins varies with the additive and suggests that a wide and interesting variety of textures could be achieved.

---

[a]Model AR2000 Viscometer is a product of TA Instruments.

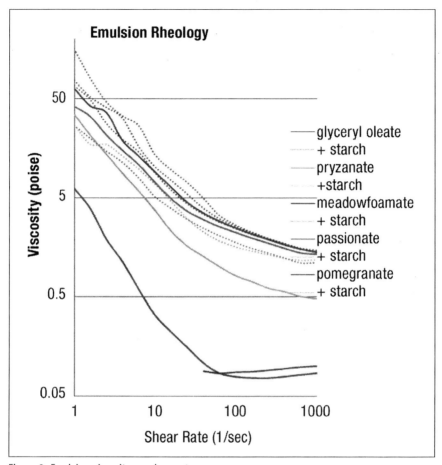

Figure 2. Emulsion viscosity vs. shear rate.

Conclusion

Consumers are becoming much more educated about the efficient use of resources, particularly as expressed by natural ingredients prepared using green chemistry. In addition, many consumer product companies are developing and communicating a sustainability strategy that includes more environmentally responsible manufacturing practices. Good communication between suppliers and customers is crucial to developing greener ingredients, and suppliers will be challenged to come up with creative ways of communicating a green story to their customers.

A comprehensive picture will compare the overall ecological impact of green ingredients with more traditional synthetic counterparts. This picture will include such diverse considerations as the geographical source of raw materials, annual renewability, competition with the food supply, processes used in manufacture, solvents used in manufacture, manufacturing energy used and its source, processes used to clean and maintain the manufacturing equipment, choice of ingredient packaging, mode of shipping, and shelf-life and biodegradability of the ingredient, among others.

The biocatalytic production of cosmetic ingredients has advantages. Communicating the green story will require an in-depth analysis of the biocatalytic process and a comparison with the corresponding synthetic processes in terms of energy saved and solvent/other waste eliminated. The widespread use of biocatalysis for the production of green and natural ingredients has yet to occur, although a combination of biocatalyst technology and process engineering developments will lead to more uses for these green processes in cosmetics, and eventually, across all markets.

Published July 2009 *Cosmetics and Toiletries* magazine

References

1. P Anastas and J Warner, *Green Chemistry: Theory and Practice*, Oxford University Press: New York (1998)
2. T Veit, Biocatalysis for the production of cosmetic ingredients, *Eng Life Sci* 4(6) 508–511 (2004)
3. A Trusek-Holownia, A Noworyta, An integrated process: Ester synthesis in an enzymatic membrane reactor and water sorption, *J Biotechnol* 130, 47–56 (2007)
4. US Pat 5,505,938, Straight chain saturated or unsaturated C8-C18 alkyl aldonolactone esters and an enzymatic process for their preparation, DJ Pocalyko, AJ Carchi, B Harichian and R Vermeer, assigned to Lever Brothers Company (Apr 9, 1996)
5. E Passicos, X Santarelli, D Coulon, Regioselective acylation of flavonoids catalyzed by immobilized Candida Antarctica lipase under reduced pressure, *Biotechnol Lett* 26(13) 1073–1076 (2004)
6. F Fonteyn, C Blecker, G Lognay, M Marlier and M Severin, Optimization of lipase-catalyzed synthesis of citronellyl acetate in solvent-free medium, *Biotechnology Letters* 16(7) 693–696 (1994)
7. M-P Bousquet, R-M Willemot, P Monsan, and E Boures, Enzymatic synthesis of unsaturated fatty acid glucoside esters for dermo-cosmetic applications, *Biotechnol Bioeng* 63(6) 730–736 (1999)
8. JA Laszlo, DL Compton, FJ Eller, SL Taylor, TA Isbell, Packed bed reactor synthesis of feruloyl monoacyl- and diacylglycerols: clean production of a green sunscreen, *Green Chemistry* 5, 382–386 (2003)
9. P Tufvesson, A Annerling, R Hatti-Kaul, D Adlercreutz, Solvent-free enzymatic synthesis of fatty alkanolamides, *Biotechnol Bioeng* 97(3), 447–453 (2006)
10. J Aracil, M Martinez, and R Soriano, Valorisation of glycerol. Enzymatic synthesis of fatty acid monoglycerides, *Proceedings of 1st World Conference on Biomass for Energy and Industry*, London, James & James, Ltd. (2001) pp 1047–1050

11. Z Guo and Y Sun, Solvent-free production of 1,3-diglyceride of CLA: Strategy consideration and protocol design, *Food Chemistry* 100(3) 1076–1084 (2007)

12. SJ Um, MS Park, SH Park, HS Han, KJ Kwan, HS Sin, Synthesis of new glycerrhetinic acid (GA) derivatives and their effects on tyrosinase activity, *Bioorganic & Medicinal Chemistry* 11(24) 5345–5352 (2003)

13. US Pat 4,369,174, Cosmetic composition containing kojic acid ester, S Nagai and T Isumi, assigned to Sansho Pharmaceutical Co, Ltd (Jan 18, 1983)

14. AM Fureby, P Adlercreutz and B Mattiasson, Glyceride synthesis in a solvent-free system *Journal of the American Oil Chemists Society* 73(11) 1489–1495 (1996)

Index